Aromatherapy for Massage Practitioners

Aromatherapy for Massage Practitioners

Ingrid Martin

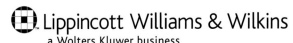

Lippincott Williams & Wilkins
a Wolters Kluwer business
Philadelphia · Baltimore · New York · London
Buenos Aires · Hong Kong · Sydney · Tokyo

Acquisitions Editor: John Goucher
Managing Editor: Karen Ruppert
Marketing Manager: Hilary Henderson
Signing Publisher Representative: Susan Schlosstein
Production Editor: Sirkka E.H. Bertling
Designer: Doug Smock
Development Editor: Betsy Dilernia
Illustrator: Joyce Lavery
Compositor: Nesbitt Graphics, Inc.
Printer: Courier Corporation—Westford

Printed in the United States of America

Library of Congress Cataloging-in-Publication Data

Martin, Ingrid.
  Aromatherapy for massage practitioners/Ingrid Martin.
    p. ; cm.—(LWW massage therapy & bodywork educational series)
  Includes bibliographical references and index.
  ISBN 0-7817-5345-7
  1. Aromatherapy.   2. Massage therapy.   I. Title.   II. Series.
  [DNLM: 1. Aromatherapy.   2. Massage—methods.   3. Oils, Volatile—adverse effects.   4. Oils, Volatile—isolation & purification.   5. Oils, Volatile—therapeutic use.   WB 925
M381a 2006]
RM666.A68M36 2006
615'. 3219—dc22

                                                                2005032888

About the Author

Ingrid Martin has more than 15 years of experience working in the fields of therapeutic massage and aromatherapy. She is a licensed massage practitioner, with specialized training in deep tissue massage and acupressure. She first studied aromatherapy in 1992 at the Institute of Traditional Herbal Medicine and Aromatherapy in London, England, with Gabriel Mojay, a well-known authority and author in the aromatherapy world. Over the years, she has done intensive training with some of the leading educators in the field, including Bob and Rhiannon Harris, Lora Jansson, and John Steele.

Ingrid has created and run successful private practices in both Britain and the United States and has taught aromatherapy professionally for the past 10 years, primarily to massage students. She also designs and teaches advanced courses for established aromatherapists and advises professional massage therapists in aromatherapy. She currently lives and works in Seattle, Washington.

Preface

As a professional massage therapist and aromatherapist, as well as a teacher of aromatherapy to established massage practitioners and to students in massage schools, I have been searching for the ideal textbook for a long time. Although there are dozens of aromatherapy books on the market, I have come to realize that none of them deals adequately with the practical issues that my students raise in class every day. These questions usually relate directly to their massage practice. For example: How do I price my sessions to account for the cost of the oils? What dilution of essential oils should I use? Can I send my products home with clients? How do I decide on a formulation for an ailment such as fibromyalgia? The only reliable, useful answers to such questions come from years of experience in using aromatherapy with massage clients.

The use of alternative healthcare modalities is exploding in the United States, and massage and aromatherapy are among the most popular. According to the American Massage Therapy Association, 18% of the adult population had a massage during the past 12 months. Although no reliable data are available, the clear consensus among professional massage practitioners is that aromatherapy is increasingly popular with their clients. It is no coincidence that most aromatherapy practitioners in the United States and in other English-speaking countries, such as Great Britain and Australia, began as licensed massage practitioners. Yet, surprisingly, to date there are no practice-based books on aromatherapy and massage, written especially for professional massage practitioners or students and addressing their specific concerns and needs.

Massage therapists who become interested in using aromatherapy tend to get their information from popular books on the subject. These books often have content that is not particularly relevant to the professional needs of the massage practitioner. They also fail to cover many subjects that are vital to an aromatherapy massage session, such as pricing, dilution and blending, how to label products for clients, safety, client assessment, and how to deal with the more serious ailments commonly seen in massage practices. This book fills that gap. It integrates the two realms of aromatherapy and massage in a practical manner that will be immediately useful to busy professionals and students alike. The material in the book has been developed and tested over my many years of experience as a classroom and workshop teacher. It is designed as a textbook for use by aromatherapy teachers in class, as well as by massage practitioners, or by students for self-study. Because the book is written for practicing or prospective massage professionals, it is assumed that the reader will already have a thorough training in massage techniques and related subjects, such as kinesiology and anatomy and physiology; therefore, I do not attempt to cover these subjects in depth. The emphasis is on aromatherapy and its application to the massage practice.

Aromatherapy is a useful remedy for many problems that a massage therapist encounters in his or her practice. However, it is important to remember that it is a complementary health modality. For the more serious conditions described in various chapters in the book, aromatherapy is never considered a primary treatment. It is helpful for the relief of symptoms but is not intended to replace conventional treatment.

Organizing Principles

The book's introductory chapter presents a definition of aromatherapy and explores its different forms of use in various parts of the world. It also provides some historical background and context and discusses the scope of practice of an aromatherapist.

The book is then divided into five main parts. Part I: The Essential Oils (Chapters 2–6) constitutes the important foundation material of aromatherapy. It covers growing and extraction methods, buying and storing essential oils, how aromatherapy affects the mind and the body, and the chemistry of essential oils. Chapter 6 presents 50 profiles of individual essential oils, giving information on their traditional uses, safety considerations, and most effective uses within massage therapy. The profiles are listed in alphabetical order for ease of reference.

Part II: Practical Matters (Chapters 7–11) addresses the safe and effective use of essential oils. Chapters discuss aromatherapy applications that are appropriate in a professional massage setting, measurements and dilutions, carriers, safety considerations, and how to blend therapeutically and aesthetically.

Part III: The Aromatherapy Massage (Chapters 12–14) goes step by step through a typical aromatherapy massage session, with chapters on necessary equipment and supplies, how to conduct an aromatherapy consultation, how to select essential oils, what to charge for aromatherapy sessions, and suitable products to send home with clients.

Part IV: Client Issues (Chapters 15–24) begins with a chapter on stress, how it affects the mind and body, and how to use aromatherapy to relieve stress. Subsequent chapters cover the systems of the body, providing information on how to use aromatherapy to relieve the symptoms of various problems.

Part V: Special Considerations (Chapters 25 and 26) addresses the particular issues of elderly care and end-of-life care, which often require specialized use and knowledge of essential oils.

How to Use This Book

Aromatherapy for Massage Practitioners is designed as a textbook to be worked through systematically by the reader. Each section builds on the previous one, from the more theoretical foundation knowledge of aromatherapy, in Part I, to the more practical aspects of safe use in Part II, an actual aromatherapy session in Part III, and ending with how to deal with specific problems and issues in Parts IV and V.

Parts II and III are meant to be practiced either in a classroom setting or with friends and colleagues, before being applied to professional massage sessions. Activities provide guided exercises to strengthen understanding and proficiency with the different techniques. If used as teaching material, Part III can be worked through several times as in-class case studies, with the supervision of the teacher.

Part IV has the same basic structure in each chapter, with the following components:

- A brief review of the body system and its functions
- How aromatherapy affects the body system

- Specific problems and ailments massage therapists are likely to encounter within their practice, and the most appropriate essential oils and methods of application for relieving symptoms
- Case studies as examples of how aromatherapy is used in real-life scenarios

Parts IV and V may also serve as reference material for the practitioner who has completed the book, as the need arises in his or her practice.

Other Pedagogical Features

A chapter outline, summary, and review questions are provided for each chapter. These elements help clarify and reinforce material new to the reader. Illustrations further explain the concepts presented. Key terms are boldfaced and explained as they are introduced, and are also included in a glossary in the back of the book.

The book includes the following appendices:

- A therapeutic guide for ailments and the most suitable essential oils for relieving symptoms, for use as a reference
- A list of recommended suppliers
- Information on training courses in aromatherapy
- A list of suggested resources, such as aromatherapy journals and websites

A Note on Language

The phrase "essential oils" (and occasionally "volatile oils") is used throughout the book to describe various different types of aromatic extracts. Strictly speaking, essential oils are the product of one specific extraction method, and other aromatic extracts have different names. However, for ease of use, it is a convention to use the term "essential oils" to denote most types of extracts commonly used in aromatherapy.

Ingrid Martin

Reviewers

Laura Allen, BA, MS, LMBT
Administrator and Nationally Certified CEU Provider
Shaw University, Walden University, The Whole You School
of Massage & Bodywork
Rutherfordton, North Carolina

Stella Gesner, NCT, MB
Deptford, New Jersey

Kelly Holland-Azarro, CCAP, RA, LMT
LMT, Reg. Aromatherapy, Cert. Clin.
Ashi Therapy Ashi Aromatics, Inc
Banner Elk, North Carolina

Jane Langone
Bodyworker, Aromatherapist
Addiston, Illinois

Gabriel Mojay, LicAc, MBAcC, MIFPA
Institute of Traditional Herbal Medicine and Aromatherapy
Chelmsford, Essex, United Kingdom

Amelia Morgan, BS
Editor
Naha
Coeur d'Alene, Idaho

Lisa Roth, RN, BS
Ohio Academy of Holistic Health
Milford, Ohio

Craig Sauer
Program Administrator
Provo College
Sandy, Utah

Sylla Sheppard-Hanger, LHCP/LMT
Director
Atlantic Institute of Aromatherapy
Tampa, Florida

Tomi Lynn Wilson, LMT
Portland, Oregon

Fairin Woods, BS
President
PT Townsend School of Massage
PT Townsend, Washington

Cheryl Young, BA, RN, LMP
Instructor
Ashmead College
Gig Harbor, Washington

Acknowledgments

I am greatly indebted to the following people who generously provided input, encouragement, and advice during the writing of this book. I am especially grateful to those who gave their time to review selected chapters: Daniel Bromberger, Kate Bromley, William Chambers, Catherine Cohen, Aaron Glaser, Lora Jansson, Janis Lynne, Steve McKinney, Jeff Owens, Keith Shawe, Jane Shofer, Anne Williams, Cynthia Wold, and Cheryl Young.

I also wish to acknowledge the reviewers chosen by Lippincott Williams & Wilkins, who read the text and gave useful feedback. I am very thankful to the team at Lippincott Williams & Wilkins, especially Pete Darcy, Karen Ruppert, and, above all, Betsy Dilernia, without whom this book would have made much less sense.

Last, but certainly not least, I would like to thank all the aromatherapy and massage students and clients over the years, who have been my most important teachers, and all my friends in Europe and the United States for their love and support.

Contents

Expanded Contents

1 An Introduction to Aromatherapy

Over the course of the past decade, there has been an amazing amount of growth in the popularity, awareness, and practice of aromatherapy. Now accepted as a legitimate complementary modality, it is being used increasingly in hospitals and clinics in both Europe and the United States. Many massage clinics and spas offer aromatherapy treatments, and the word "aromatherapy" is used on the labels of many products in pharmacies and health food stores. Yet aromatherapy is often misunderstood. Many people have an uninformed but distinct impression of what they think it is, and that impression may be very different from how it is practiced by trained aromatherapists. Some people assume that aromatherapy consists of using scented candles and potpourri or sniffing a pretty smell to help them relax.

Aromatherapists often spend more time re-educating people than simply informing them, and the somewhat frivolous image that aromatherapy has gained, mostly through marketing campaigns by cosmetic and toiletry companies, disturbs most professionals. In the words of Bob Harris, editor of the *International Journal of Aromatherapy*: "The popularization, trivialization and sometimes sensationalism created by the need to promote the therapy as a commercial product have masked and harmed the true therapeutic potential of aromatherapy."[1]

Defining Aromatherapy

Aromatherapy is the use of extracts from aromatic plants for healing purposes. But what exactly is an aromatic plant? What kinds of extracts are used? And what constitutes healing?

Aromatic plants are plants that have a distinct smell in at least one part of the plant. For thousands of years they have been used for cooking, for medicine, and for sacred ceremonies. Not all plants, of course, are aromatic—a dandelion or a tulip, for instance. These flowers may have a faint smell common to all plant material but there is no distinctive fragrance by which we could recognize a tulip or dandelion if we smelled it with our eyes closed. Other plant material, like ripe apples or pears, have a strong, individual aroma, but they possess no volatile oils that can be extracted by the methods normally used to obtain aromatic oils. For the purposes of aromatherapy, therefore, when we talk about aromatic plants we are discussing only a tiny proportion of the plant kingdom—plants that have unique fragrances that can be extracted.

Herbalism and Aromatherapy

Many practitioners regard aromatherapy as one branch of herbal medicine. There is a lot of merit to this view, as many aromatic plants, such as rosemary or juniper, are used both in standard herbal practice in many cultures and in aromatherapy. However, many plants commonly used in aromatherapy, such as cedarwood and geranium, are not found in standard herbal usage, and information about their herbal properties is not available.

In **herbalism,** extracts are obtained by steeping plants in either water (decoctions or infusions) or alcohol (tinctures). Aromatherapists, on the other hand, use extracts produced by distillation (essential oils), by solvent extraction (absolutes), by CO_2 extraction (CO_2 extracts), or by cold expression (expressed oils or essences). Different extraction methods result in products with different chemical constituents. Comparing herbal extracts and aromatic oils from the point of view of their uses or safety can be both misleading and harmful. A lot of information about the properties of essential oils is taken directly from herbal books, and as a result, some of it may be inaccurate.

Methods of using herbal extracts and aromatic oils are also very different. Although herbal preparations are sometimes applied externally, by and large these are local remedies, intended, for example, to treat skin problems or to relieve muscle or joint pain. Standard herbal remedies are internal, taken by mouth. Aromatherapists, on the other hand, usually apply preparations externally, even when treating internal ailments, such as digestive discomfort or menstrual cramping. This variation in mode of application makes a substantial difference in how the substance affects the body and what dosages and safety precautions should be used.

Healing Effects

What exactly is healing? Many books have been written on this subject. Perhaps we can say that healing often includes an improvement in a person's quality of life—physical, mental, or emotional. Aromatherapy has been shown to produce beneficial results in all of these areas, and it can therefore be considered a truly holistic healing art. Extensive studies demonstrate the effectiveness of essential oils in physical healing. Examples are their use in medical aromatherapy to combat chronic bacterial infections,[2] the obvious sedative effects of certain aromatic extracts, and the anti-inflammatory properties of others.[3] Enough evidence has been collected, both clinically and in individual practice, to substantiate the fact that essential oils have effects on the body. Anyone who has put undiluted peppermint essential oil directly onto the skin has experienced the intense cooling effect, and those who have tried clove oil for a toothache are instant believers in its pain-killing quality.

The mental and emotional effects of essential oils have also been studied and recorded since the early twentieth century. As early as the 1920s, two Italian physicians, Gatti and Cayola, published their observations of how aromatics can be beneficial for both anxiety and depression. Aromatherapy has been shown to improve mood, heighten alertness, and increase a person's ability to perform math problems faster and more accurately.[4] Perhaps most conclusively, several studies of the effects of using essential oils with people who have Alzheimer's disease cite "significant benefits" in calming agitation.[5] This is particularly interesting because these patients often lose their sense of smell, so the benefits of aromatherapy in this case are more than a simple placebo effect from a pleasant aroma.

Different Forms of Aromatherapy

Aromatic healing is used in many different cultures in a wide variety of ways. In South America, for example, many traditional healers work shamanistically, traveling in spirit to other dimensions to bring back information for healing their clients. Among these traditional practitioners are the perfumeros, who use aromatic oils in their healing rituals, spraying them from their mouths over the person asking for help.[6] Another example is the extensive use of aromatic smoke from sage, cedar, and other North American plants in smudging, or cleansing rituals, in Native American healing. Figure 1.1 shows a Native American ceremony, in which a smudge stick made of aromatic herbs is burned.

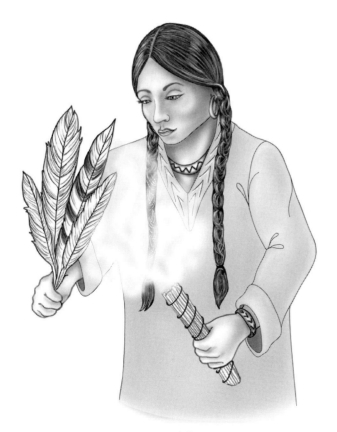

Figure 1.1 A Native American smudging ceremony.

Holistic Aromatherapy

This book concentrates on not all the uses of aromatic healing around the world but on Western aromatherapy. The form that is practiced in most English-speaking countries—Britain, the United States, Canada, and Australia—is often referred to as **holistic aromatherapy.** This form usually is combined with massage and practiced by qualified massage therapists, as well as by other complementary health practitioners such as reflexologists, acupressure practitioners, and hypnotherapists.

The holistic aspect is shown in the importance placed not just on helping clients to improve their physical situation but also on working with mental or emotional difficulties. For example, a holistic aromatherapist will ask his client about the levels of stress in her life while he explores the possible physical causes of her low-back pain. Holistic aromatherapists regard health not as an absence of illness but as the establishment of ease and enjoyment in all areas of the client's life, with a strong emphasis on restoring balance and happiness. The comforting, soothing effects of touch obviously play a large role in this form of aromatherapy, and the relationship between therapist and client can also be an important part of the healing process.

The amounts of essential oils used in holistic aromatherapy are fairly low, and the degree of risk attached to the modality is correspondingly slight. The most common adverse side-effect is occasional mild skin irritation, which generally clears up with no treatment in a short time—often after only an hour or two. The selection of essential oils is usually made by consultation with the client, taking into account any physical ailments, emotional difficulties, and the preferences of the client for a particular scent. The application methods are almost always external, usually by skin absorption via massage, compress, or hydrotherapy; or by inhalation, usually from a bottle or tissue, or via diffusion into the air.

Holistic aromatherapy is particularly suited to chronic ailments, such as arthritis, asthma, or low-back pain; to stress-related problems, such as irritable bowel syndrome, insomnia, or borderline high blood pressure; and to emotional difficulties, such as depression or anxiety. (These conditions are discussed in later chapters.) It is less well suited to acute or severe physical or psychological problems, which most massage therapists, and other complementary therapists, would be less likely to encounter regularly in any case.

Medical Aromatherapy

Medical aromatherapy, sometimes called aromatic medicine, is the form most often practiced in France. Modern French aromatherapy originated with medical doctors, and the trend in France has always been to regard the use of essential oils as a specialized part of medical practice. Medical aromatherapy is practiced today almost exclusively by physicians, who often use other therapies, such as osteopathy or homeopathy, in conjunction with their allopathic treatments.

In medical aromatherapy, the approach is primarily scientific, with the emphasis on treating physical illnesses and diseases. The selection of essential oils is made after consultation with the patient and often after various laboratory tests have been completed. The oils are usually chosen for their effectiveness in treating viral, bacterial, or fungal infections, or for their effect on internal organs such as the large intestine or the liver.

Doses are often much higher than in holistic aromatherapy. Application methods may be external or internal, including the oral ingestion of capsules and the use of suppositories and pessaries. In medical aromatherapy there is a higher risk of irritation of skin or mucous membranes, possible allergic reaction, or toxic overdose. This methodology seems to be most suited to severe and acute forms of physical illness, such as a serious bacterial infection. It is probably less effective for more chronic types of ailments, stress relief, and emotional problems.

Clinical Aromatherapy

It is interesting that two such divergent forms of aromatherapy developed in France and England, countries that are not far apart geographically. But until recently, the differences between the two countries have been extreme. In France, only medical doctors can legally practice aromatherapy, and any nonmedical person who uses a therapeutic modality is regarded as illegally practicing medicine without a license. In England, conversely, most aromatherapists condemn the French-style internal use of essential oils as dangerous and unnecessary. During the last few years, however, there has been some meeting of the ways and attempts to marry the best aspects of both systems. In England, Shirley Price has encouraged health professionals, such as nurses, to use essential oils in hospital settings, as has Jane Buckle in the United States.[7] This style, often called **clinical aromatherapy,** uses mostly external applications, as in traditional holistic aromatherapy, and concentrates on both the physical and emotional well-being of the client, but with a lot more emphasis on using aromatherapy as a support modality (or even as a primary care tool) during serious illnesses.

Merging Traditions

In France, Dr. Daniel Pénoël, a respected general practitioner and naturopathic doctor who has worked extensively with essential oils, has done much to promote a more in-depth use of aromatherapy for an increasing number of serious health problems, by both complementary practitioners and the general public. He has lectured in England on the French style of aromatherapy, including internal applications, and his book *Natural Home Health Care Using Essential Oils* advises the use of essential oils applied both in "the English way" and in very small amounts internally.[8] This seems to the author to be a good adaptation of the more intensive French style, applied in a sensible, safe way for the English-speaking complementary practitioner who has less medical training. A few other people are working in this area, including Bob and Rhiannon Harris, two English aromatherapy consultants living and working in France. They run workshops and courses for aromatherapists from other countries who want to learn something about the French methods of using essential oils.[9]

We can hope this merging of the two traditions will continue, with French doctors absorbing the lesson that using smaller amounts of essential oils externally can be extremely beneficial for the relief of stress and chronic ailments, and with holistic aromatherapists overcoming their fear of using stronger dilutions of essential oils for treatment work and acute situations. The internal use of essential oils, even in very small amounts, is regarded in most countries as practicing medicine, and it certainly requires more medical training than most massage therapists receive. For this reason, only the external use of essential oils is covered in this book, with techniques including essential oil use in massage and hydrotherapy.

Historical Perspectives

Massage and aromatherapy have been regarded as a natural pairing for thousands of years. Vegetable oils, such as olive, sesame, and linseed, were extracted from plants as early as Neolithic times, and steeping herbs to produce an aromatic oil was also done. The two obvious ways to use a scented oil were to cook with it or rub it on the body. The first written accounts of herbal medicine from ancient Egypt indicate that this is exactly what people did with them. "Some of the scents suspended in fat were used in treatment as well as for pleasure. In the days of the New Kingdom the greasy substance was applied either by massaging it into the skin, or by fixing it to the area in question as a bandage or poultice."[10] Figure 1.2 shows an inlaid panel found in Tutankhamun's tomb, showing him being anointed with scented oils by his queen.

In many ancient civilizations people used oil or fat infused with aromatic plants to rub on the skin. In Central and South America, the Aztecs, Olmecs, Incas, and Mayans all used steam baths and massage. "Pinewood ointments were rubbed on the chest for lung ailments and elsewhere for muscular aches and pains. Other ointments made from herbs, animal fats, or oils and a variety of special leaves were used in the application of massage during the steam."[11] The Aboriginal peoples of Australia have used the *Melaleuca*

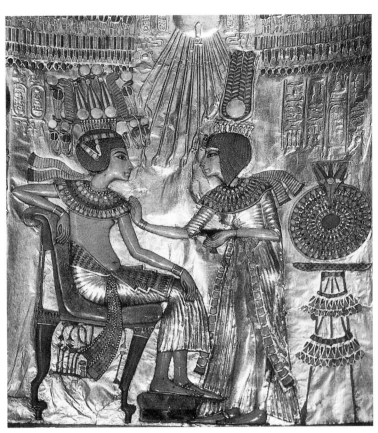

Figure 1.2 Tutankhamun being anointed with scented oils. (Reprinted with permission from Manniche, L. Sacred Luxuries: Fragrance, Aromatherapy, and Cosmetics in Ancient Egypt. Ithaca, NY: Cornell University Press. Text © 1999 by Lise Manniche, Photographs © 1999 Werner Forman, © 1999 Opus Publishing Limited. Used by permission of the publisher, Cornell University Press.)

species medicinally for possibly thousands of years, and massage with scented oils has always been an important part of Ayurvedic medicine.

In Europe, the ancient Greeks learned much about aromatic oils from the Egyptians. Hippocrates recommended daily scented baths and massage to maintain proper health, and the use of aromatic oils as an external treatment was continued for centuries. Hildegard of Bingen, the famous twelfth-century mystic and healer, wrote about many aromatic herbs that were rubbed into the skin to treat internal problems. The juice of violets, for example, in olive oil and goat's fat was used to treat cancer: "Salve the body parts all around, and also right there where the cancer and other viruses are devouring the person."[12] Gradually, however, the use of pharmaceutical medications in Europe replaced the older tradition of herbal medicine, and the herbal/aromatic form of treatment fell out of favor.

Aromatherapy in its modern form began in the 1920s, when the French chemist René-Maurice Gattefossé became interested in the therapeutic properties of essential oils. He named this new field "aromathérapie" and published his findings in 1928.[13] These writings influenced various medical doctors in France, among them Jean Valnet, an army physician who started to use essential oils in his practice. Valnet published a now classic book, The Practice of Aromatherapy, and taught others about the new discipline of aromatherapy.[14]

Up to this point, aromatherapy was regarded mostly as an interesting medical specialty, but Marguerite Maury, an Austrian nurse working in France, helped popularize the subject. She was particularly interested in the effects of essential oils on the entire body, through more dilute applications on the skin. Maury was also the first practitioner of aromatherapy to place a strong emphasis on the individuality of each client, stating in her book, Le Capital "Jeunesse," that one had to make an "individual prescription" for the person, rather than for the ailment.[15] These principles shaped the philosophy of holistic aromatherapy, in which practitioners almost always apply essential oils topically.

Combining Massage and Aromatherapy

Essential oils work on the body and the mind in two main ways:

1. They are **volatile,** or evaporate easily into the air, and are inhaled and smelled; thus, they directly affect the brain, and therefore mood and emotion.

2. Essential oil components are readily absorbed through the skin; they enter the bloodstream and have an effect on the internal organs (including the brain).

Aromatherapy and massage thus make an ideal marriage.

Because essential oils have a therapeutic effect when components permeate the skin, they combine well with massage, a therapy that includes touching and applying substances to the skin. Also, the warmth of the client's body, the therapist's hands, and the air in the massage room will cause the essential oils to evaporate and be inhaled—the other way of introducing essential oils into the body. In fact, most aromatherapists outside of France tend to be massage therapists, so much so that the official Website of the International Federation of Professional Aromatherapists in Britain states: "Your aromatherapist will then select and blend the essential oils appropriate to your individual needs, and will *in most cases apply them through massage* [my italics]."

Essential oils dissolve easily in oils and fats. Most aromatherapists agree that diluting essential oils in oil or lotion before applying them to the skin is a safer form of application than applying them **neat,** or undiluted. Massage oils and lotions are mostly oil-based or fat-based and therefore are ideal vehicles for diluting essential oils.

Essential oils also combine well with hydrotherapy. They do not dissolve in water, but studies have shown that skin that is hydrated by soaking or bathing in water will absorb essential oils much more easily, and the beneficial effects will be greater.[16] If the hydrotherapy technique includes warmth, the oils will tend to permeate even more easily, as warmth opens the pores of the skin, making for higher absorption rates.

Many massage techniques can be enhanced and expanded on by using aromatherapy. For example, essential oils with pain-relieving properties may be helpful for injuries, the use of sedative oils will deepen relaxation massage, and aromatic oils that increase lymphatic flow will benefit lymphatic drainage work. Essential oils have been proven to help relieve stress, relax muscles, ease muscular and arthritic pain, deepen breathing, reduce muscle spasm, and so on. Many massage therapists become excited during their first weeks of aromatherapy training, when they begin to see dramatic improvements in their clients. Injuries heal faster, muscle knots melt away under their fingers, headaches clear up within minutes, and clients leave looking and feeling more relaxed and rested than they have in weeks.

Aromatherapy may benefit clients for whom massage is difficult or contraindicated. Aromatherapy lotions can be gently smoothed over varicose veins or areas of severe bruising with good results. Clients with flare-ups in arthritic joints can gain relief from analgesic and anti-inflammatory essential oils. Hospital or hospice patients, who can tolerate only very short and limited massage, can receive aromatherapy diffusers to lift their mood or help with insomnia.

Another benefit of aromatherapy to the massage therapist is the aromatherapy "homework." Sending a client home with aromatic blends can extend the practitioner's treatment time and maximize results, as the soothing, energizing, or pain-relieving effects from the oils can continue whenever the client uses the blend. Many ailments, such as dermatitis, frequent headaches, chest or sinus congestion, and joint pain, respond much better to a daily routine of essential oil application combined with weekly or monthly massage treatments. Massage therapists can also help clients with problems that may be difficult to address within the massage session. A client who has problems sleeping but typically schedules his massage sessions in the mornings or afternoons may be helped by a sedative aromatherapy blend at bedtime. Someone who is terrified of flying might be calmed by taking on the plane the aromatherapy blend her massage therapist uses in their regular relaxation sessions. Massage therapists who use aromatherapy can help clients even when they are not present, thereby enhancing their health and satisfaction.

The Scope of Practice

Unlike massage therapy, there are no licensing laws for holistic aromatherapy in the United States, Britain, and most other countries. Medical aromatherapy has strict licensing laws in France. Some aromatherapy organizations have their own codes of professional conduct for members, but the use of aromatherapy as an external application is not regulated by law in any country. If a school or an individual advertises certification courses in aromatherapy, it is important to remember that a graduate is certified only by the school or the individual teaching the course. Some of these programs may follow guidelines set up by various aromatherapy organizations, such as the National Association of Holistic Aromatherapists (NAHA). However, these are guidelines only, and organizations such as NAHA have no legal authority to license aromatherapists.

Holistic aromatherapy is almost always practiced in combination with another modality that requires a license, such as massage therapy, hypnotherapy, or nursing. Aromatherapists should examine local licensing laws governing massage therapy to determine their scope of practice. However, local licensing laws tend to be general and often make no mention of secondary modalities such as aromatherapy.

The official Website of the British organization International Federation of Professional Aromatherapists states: "It is the responsibility of a practicing aromatherapist to bear in mind her/his own standard of training and level of knowledge, as well as any insurance limitations when deciding how the essential oils are to be used for each individual client."[17] In a profession that has no licensing, training standards and course content vary widely, and self-accountability is extremely important. In the words of Diane Polseno, former chair of the National Ethics Subcommittee of the American Massage Therapy Association (AMTA): "Educational training individualizes SOP [scope of practice] and it becomes a personal issue rather than a collective one."[18]

The most important consideration in self-regulation is to be realistic, with yourself and your clients, about your skills and experience. A practitioner who has just completed 50 hours of training in aromatherapy will not have the same depth of knowledge as someone with 200 hours of training and several years of experience using essential oils in a massage practice. Do not be tempted to go beyond the level in which you are competent and comfortable, and do not attempt to treat issues for which you have no knowledge or training.

Massage therapists who practice aromatherapy should be careful to avoid any appearance of practicing medicine without a license. Here are three essential guidelines:

- Diagnosing is outside the scope of practice of massage therapists and aromatherapists. Massage therapists can assess clients in terms of their own modality—for example, they can decide which muscles are tight and which areas of the body to work on to relieve pain and improve posture. However, they cannot diagnose illness or disease.

- Prescribing is outside the scope of practice of aromatherapists. They should not advise a client to start or stop taking medications, nor recommend using essential oils instead of medication prescribed by a physician.

- Aromatherapists should never advise clients to use essential oils internally. External use only is within the scope of practice. This includes using essential oils on the skin, in hydrotherapy treatments, or as inhalation.

SUMMARY

- Aromatherapy is the use of extracts from aromatic plants for healing purposes.
- Aromatherapy and herbalism differ in the type of plants used, the methods of extraction, and the modes of application.
- Aromatherapy has proven effects on physical, mental, and emotional states.
- Holistic aromatherapy uses low amounts of essential oils and external applications. It is mostly practiced by massage therapists and other complementary health practitioners.
- Medical aromatherapy uses larger amounts of essential oils, and applications may be internal or external. It is mostly practiced by naturopathic and medical doctors.
- Clinical aromatherapy uses essential oils in external applications, with an emphasis on aromatherapy as a support modality for serious illnesses. It is mostly practiced by nurses and other health professionals.

- Aromatic oils have been used together with massage for thousands of years, but modern aromatherapy with essential oils was developed in the early twentieth century.
- Essential oils affect the body and the mind via inhalation and via absorption through the skin into the bloodstream.
- Aromatherapy can enhance the effects of massage therapy, and it can also sometimes be used with clients who are contraindicated for massage.
- Aromatherapists should consult local licensing laws for massage therapy for guidance about scope of practice.
- Essential oils should never be recommended for internal use by massage therapists.

Review Questions

1. Herbal extracts and aromatherapy extracts have the same chemistry, properties, and uses. (T/F)
2. In what ways does holistic aromatherapy use essential oils? (a) orally, (b) topically, (c) in various internal applications.
3. Medical aromatherapy uses essential oils in quite _____ doses, whereas holistic aromatherapy uses them in _____ amounts.
4. Medical aromatherapy is more suited to chronic problems and stress relief. (T/F)
5. Clinical aromatherapy uses mostly external applications, as in holistic aromatherapy. (T/F)
6. In aromatherapy massage, the client is affected by essential oils in two main ways: _____ and _____.
7. Essential oils dissolve in _____ but do not dissolve in _____.
8. A "neat" essential oil means: (a) diluted with carrier oil, (b) blended with other essential oils, (c) undiluted, (d) stronger than other essential oils.

Notes

1. Harris B. Editorial comment. Int J Aromather 2002;12(1):1.
2. Von Frohlich E. A review of clinical, pharmacological, and bacteriological research into *Oleum spicae*. Wiener Medizinische Wochenschrift 1968;15:345–350.
3. Rossi T, Melegari M, Bianchi A, et al. Sedative, anti-inflammatory and anti-diuretic effects induced in rats by essential oils of varieties of *Anthemis nobilis:* a comparative study. Pharmacol Res Comm 1988; 20:71–74.
4. Diego MA, Jones NA, Field T, et al. Aromatherapy positively affects mood, EEG patterns of alertness and math computations. Int J Neurosci 1998;96:217–224.
5. Ballard CG, O'Brien JT, Reichelt K, et al. Aromatherapy as a safe and effective treatment for the management of agitation in severe dementia: the results of a double-blind, placebo-controlled trial with Melissa. J Clin Psychiatry 2003;64(6):732.
6. Notes from a workshop with John Steele, Seattle, WA, 1999.
7. Price S, Price L. Aromatherapy for Health Professionals. Edinburgh, UK: Churchill Livingstone, 2001; and Buckle J. Clinical Aromatherapy: Essential Oils in Practice. Edinburgh, UK: Churchill Livingstone, 2003.
8. Pénoël D, Pénoël R. Natural Home Health Care Using Essential Oils. La Drôme, France: Éditions Osmobiose, 1998.
9. Harris B, Harris R. Essential oil resource consultants. Available at: www.essentialorc.com. Accessed April 15, 2005.
10. Manniche L. Sacred Luxuries: Fragrances, Aromatherapy and Cosmetics in Ancient Egypt. Ithaca, NY: Cornell University Press, 1999:114.
11. Calvert RN. The History of Massage. Rochester, VT: Healing Arts Press, 2002:17.
12. Strehlow W, Hertzka G. Hildegard of Bingen's Medicine. Santa Fe, NM: Bear & Co., 1988:129.
13. Gattefossé RM. Aromathérapie. Paris, France: Girardot éditeur, 1928.
14. Valnet J. The Practice of Aromatherapy. Saffron Walden, UK: CW Daniel, 1992.
15. Maury M. Marguerite Maury's Guide to Aromatherapy. Saffron Walden, UK: CW Daniel, 1995.
16. Buckle J. Clinical Aromatherapy: Essential Oils in Practice. Edinburgh, UK: Churchill Livingstone, 2003:25.
17. Website of the International Federation of Professional Aromatherapists. Available at: www.ifparoma.org/html/practicecodes.html. Accessed November 22, 2004.
18. Polseno D. The Scope of Your Practice: Part II. Massage Ther J 2000;38(1):27.

2

Extracting Essential Oils From Plants

The Function of Essential Oils in Aromatic Plants
Growing and Harvesting
Methods of Extraction
    Distillation
    Solvent Extraction
    Carbon Dioxide Extraction
    Cold Expression
    Enfleurage
    Maceration
Hydrosols

Before an aromatherapist can use an essential oil, a large amount of work has to be done to get the volatile oils from the plant into the bottle. Many people are involved in the various stages of this process, which include growing and harvesting the plants and extracting the essential oils. The techniques involved in cultivating aromatic plants and extracting the oils vary widely, depending on the climate, the size of the farm, the poverty or wealth of the country where the plants grow, and other factors. It is useful to understand something of this complex process, as it affects the availability of certain essential oils, their prices, and even possibly their properties.

The Function of Essential Oils in Aromatic Plants

As mentioned in Chapter 1, aromatic plants are plants with a distinct, individual smell. But what exactly makes a plant aromatic, and what is the function of the plant's scent? Aromatic plants contain essential oils (or volatile oils), composed of particular chemical compounds (discussed in Chapter 5). Out of an estimated 250,000 to 1 million plant species, only about 3000 are known to produce essential oils. Of these, only about 300 are used for the commercial production of essential oils.[1]

The word "oil" is somewhat misleading; it is a fluid, but a nongreasy one, and so volatile that it evaporates easily at room temperature. This is not how we would normally think about an oil. This quick evaporation of essential oils is what makes aromatic plants appealing to the senses—think of walking through a garden of roses on a warm day, or grating a lemon, or chopping ginger for cooking.

Most essential oils are antibacterial, some are antiviral, and some are antifungal. The oils protect the plants against pathogens, which are disease-causing microorganisms. For example, resins such as frankincense and myrrh, which are very high in antibacterial essential oils, are released by the tree to seal off cuts in the outer bark, which would be susceptible to infection. Other components of the volatile oils may mimic the sex pheromones of a particular insect: the wasp, moth, or bee that the plant needs to attract to be pollinated.[2] Still others, like the sagebrush that grows in the North American deserts, produce large amounts of volatile oils that are toxic when they fall onto other plants, ensuring the producers enough space around them so that they can receive the sunlight, water, and nutrients needed for growth. Volatile oils may also help discourage insects and animals from eating the leaves of the plant because of their bitter taste. Producing these toxic chemicals gives a plant some advantages when it comes to survival.

Essential oils occur in these plants in different parts, depending on what function the plant has for them. They can be extracted from flowers and buds, leaves, the wood and the resin of trees, fruit and the peel of fruit, roots, grasses, and even mosses. To follow are examples of essential oils from different plant parts:

- *Flowers*: rose, neroli, jasmine, chamomile
- *Buds*: clove
- *Leaves of trees*: eucalyptus, tea tree, myrtle, bay laurel, pine, spruce, fir
- *Flowering tops of herbs*: lavender, sage, rosemary, basil, thyme, mint, lemon balm
- *Wood*: sandalwood, cedarwood, rosewood
- *Bark*: cinnamon, sweet birch
- *Resins*: frankincense, myrrh, benzoin, elemi
- *Fruit*: juniper berry, cardamon, may chang (litsea), black pepper
- *Peel of fruit*: orange, lemon, lime, bergamot, mandarin, grapefruit
- *Roots*: ginger, sandalwood, vetiver, spikenard
- *Grasses*: lemongrass, citronella, palmarosa, ginger grass
- *Mosses*: Greenland moss, oak moss

Figure 2.1 shows some plant parts from several aromatic plants.

Growing and Harvesting

Many aromatic plants are harvested from the wild; in fact, 90% of all medicinal and aromatic plants are "wild-crafted."[3] Aromatherapists have to be particularly careful when choosing essential oils because some of the plants from which the oils are made have been overharvested, to the extent that they are in danger of becoming extinct. Plants that are endangered in this way are often those in which the volatile oils are concentrated in the wood or the roots, and the whole plant must be destroyed to obtain the oil.

According to the United Nations Convention on International Trade in Endangered Species (CITES), plants that have been subjected to this destructive harvesting, and that may be endangered, include spikenard (*Nardostachys jatamansi*), distilled from the roots of a shrub growing in the Himalayas; sandalwood (*Santalum album*), whose export is restricted by the Indian government as its situation is so dire; and rosewood (*Aniba roseadora*). It would be a responsible move for aromatherapists to promote alternatives to these oils. Australian sandalwood (*Santalum spicatum*), for example, although arguably not such a beautiful fragrance as the Indian species, possesses many of the same therapeutic qualities,[4] and rosalina (*Melaleuca ericifolia*) has been suggested as a possible substitute for rosewood oil.[5]

Other plants are not wild-crafted but are deliberately cultivated for their aromatic oils. Vast fields of lavender are grown in the south of France, roses are tenderly cared for in Bulgaria, and jasmine is part of the traditional crop of India. Many of these aromatic plants are grown in developing

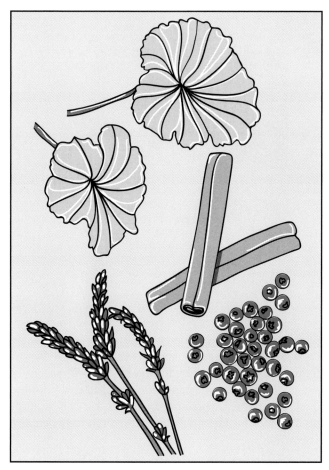

Figure 2.1 Different plant parts of aromatic plants. The plant parts shown are geranium leaves, cinnamon bark, juniper berries, and lavender flowers.

countries, where lower labor costs minimize the expense of cultivation and harvesting. For example, jasmine and tuberose flowers have to be carefully handpicked to avoid bruising the delicate flowers.

Growing and harvesting are complex processes, and farmers often specialize in plants that have been cultivated by the same family for generations. We can begin to appreciate why rose oil is so expensive, for example, when we learn that the soil around the roses has to be shifted several times during a growing season, to balance moisture and discourage diseases, and that roses must be picked by hand the first day that they open and taken to the distillation plant before midday, to get the finest quality and quantity of essential oil.[6]

Many aromatherapists prefer organic essential oils because of a desire for greater purity of product and also for ethical and environmental reasons. These oils are likely to be more expensive than those grown by conventional methods because of the greater amount of labor involved. A good example is a small French organic farmer and distiller I visited in Provence, who told me that she was having great problems eliminating a bug that was eating one of her crops. Because she is a certified organic producer, she cannot use

any pesticides, so her solution was to patrol the crops at night, when the bugs would crawl up to the top of the plants, and use a vacuum cleaner to suck them up—not only labor-intensive, but also sleep-depriving!

Some essential oils are available only from conventionally cultivated plants, but most can be obtained, with a little effort and searching, from ethically wild-crafted or organic sources.

Methods of Extraction

Aromatic oils are extracted from the plants in various ways, including distillation, solvent extraction, and cold expression. The extraction method used will depend on various factors, including the **yield,** which is the amount of essential oil it is possible to extract from the plant, and the plant's tolerance for high temperatures.

Distillation

The most common method of extraction is **distillation,** a very old technique whose product is **essential oils.** Distillation equipment dating back to around 3000 B.C. has been found by archaeologists in Pakistan, and traditional stills for producing essential oils or alcohol can be found in many areas of the world, from Britain to Siberia to South America.[7] They can range widely in size and in complexity, from small homemade stills, cobbled together from tin cans and other scraps of metal, found on farms that carry out "backyard" distillation in poorer countries, to huge stainless steel, commercial distillation equipment that can hold tons of plant material. Even small tabletop distilling equipment can be bought by the aromatherapist who wants to experiment with extracting his or her own essential oils. Whatever the sophistication or size of the still, the basic principles are the same for steam distillation, water distillation, and hydrodiffusion.

Steam Distillation. In **steam distillation,** steam is passed through the plant material in the still (Figure 2.2). The heat and pressure cause the plant structures that hold the essential oil to burst open and release the oil, which is vaporized with the steam. This aromatic steam is then channeled into another container, where it is exposed to a cool surface, causing it to condense into a liquid containing both essential oil and water. Essential oil and water have different densities, which allows a natural settling out of the essential oil and makes the final stage of separating the water from the oil much easier. Usually the essential oil floats on top of the water, but in some cases the denser oils, like vetiver, may sink to the bottom.[8] At this stage the essential oil may not smell particularly appealing, as it contains what are called "**still notes,**" which are extremely volatile components; they smell rather like boiled vegetables. Distillers will let the oil settle, or "age," for quite some time to let the still notes evaporate before selling the oil.

Although it may seem like a fairly simple procedure, each plant requires different treatment, and the heat and

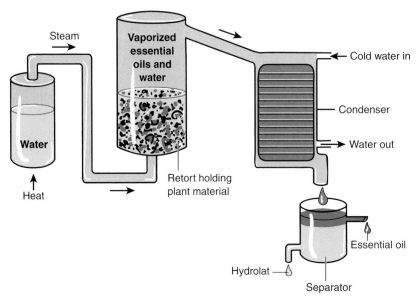

Figure 2.2 The steam distillation process.

distillation time needed can vary widely depending on the plant material and on the type of still being used. Lavender, for example, requires a short, quite hot distillation and may be finished in 2 or 3 hours, while vetiver typically requires a distillation time of 24 hours or longer. Some plants may need to be distilled immediately after picking, like rose, while lavender is often dried for a day or two to allow the harsher chemicals to evaporate, making the resulting essential oil sweeter. The dampness of the steam has to be controlled, and again may need to vary for different plant material. All of this requires specialized knowledge for each plant, often handed down from generation to generation of distillers.[9]

As with any extraction method, steam distillation has its advantages and disadvantages. It is a fairly inexpensive production method, at its simplest requiring only basic equipment, and therefore can be carried out by both small and large producers. Sometimes the smaller distillers are the ones who produce the most exquisite essential oils, designed primarily for the aromatherapy trade. It is a traditional method, so we know a lot about the products of distillation, their chemistry, their properties, and their safety aspects. On the other hand, there is a lot of heat involved in this process, and the essential oils are inevitably changed by the high temperatures. German chamomile (*Matricaria recutita*) is a good example. The flower from which it is extracted looks like a large daisy, with yellow and white flowers, yet the essential oil is a deep blue color. There is nothing chemically in the plant itself that would account for this color; it is due to the presence in the essential oil of chamazulene, a chemical created by the heat of the distillation process. This is not necessarily bad; chamazulene, for example, is a good anti-inflammatory agent. For other plants, however, the heat can

be disastrous. Jasmine cannot be easily extracted by any form of distillation because the intense heat will distort the aroma; for this reason, jasmine is not available as a distilled essential oil. It is important to remember that only aromatic oils obtained by any distillation method can truly be called essential oils.

Water Distillation. In **water distillation,** another method of extracting essential oils, plant material is placed directly into water in the distilling vessel (the retort). It is generally used for flower petals, or for powdered plant material such as sandalwood, as both these types of material have a tendency to clump together when steam is applied, making steam distillation more difficult. Water distillation needs very close attention, as there is a chance of scorching the plant material when the water level drops, which would negatively affect the fragrance and the therapeutic components.[10] It is ideal for plants that are heat-sensitive, as it tends to be gentler than steam distillation. However, because the plants are immersed in hot water for long periods of time, it is not the best choice for producing essential oils such as clary sage and lavender, which are high in chemicals that tend to break down in such conditions.

Hydrodiffusion. **Hydrodiffusion,** another type of distillation, is not as common as steam or water distillation. In the hydrodiffusion process, steam is forced through the plant material from above, rather than from below, resulting in an essential oil that, according to one supplier, "can be richer, often denser and of a superior aromatic bounty."[11]

Solvent Extraction

How is jasmine extracted if not by distillation? A lot of the essential oils from flowers are produced by **solvent** extraction, which uses solvents, such as hexane or butane, to "wash" the aromatic oils out of the plant material. The first result is a waxy, semisolid substance known as a **concrete,** which has many other plant constituents, such as fatty acids and waxes, contained in it. The concrete then undergoes various processes, such as washing with alcohol, vacuum separation, evaporation by distillation, and freezing, to eliminate the original solvents, plant waxes, and so on. The end product is a highly aromatic liquid called an **absolute,** which is often colored and frequently quite thick. An absolute tends to smell more like the original plant than an essential oil does, probably because it has not been subjected to the same heat and because the solvent process extracts a wider range of aromatic molecules than does the distillation process. If we compare a rose essential oil with a rose absolute (both are commonly produced), we can smell that the absolute has a deeper, richer fragrance. If we compare the colors and viscosity, we will see that the essential oil is a clear, thin liquid, while the absolute is reddish-colored and thick.

Solvent extraction has three important advantages over distillation:

1. The absolute generally has a stronger, richer aroma.

2. Solvent extraction gives a greater yield than distillation. This is important when working with plants that contain extremely small amounts of essential oil, such as hyacinth (*Hyacinthus orientalis*).

3. Some oils, such as jasmine, that would be damaged by the heat of distillation can be extracted.

Some aromatherapists, however, are dismayed by the toxic chemicals used and by the fact that the absolutes may still contain tiny trace amounts of these chemicals. They maintain that absolutes, while wonderful to diffuse in the air, should not be used on the skin because it is possible to absorb the chemical residues into the body. Also, traces of solvent may increase the risk of allergic skin reactions. However, other aromatherapists insist that you would probably absorb many more toxic chemicals in a cup of decaffeinated coffee or on a short walk near a highway, and that the beauty of using absolutes on the body outweighs the potential risks. Absolutes have become safer in the last few decades as the use of the harsher solvents has declined, and the industry has limited the solvent residue to 10 parts per million—generally regarded as extremely safe. Their use within aromatherapy remains a highly debated topic, and every aromatherapist must make his or her own choice whether or not to use them.

Carbon Dioxide Extraction

Carbon dioxide extraction (also called CO_2 extraction or hypercritical CO_2 extraction) is a fairly new process that is essentially a type of solvent extraction because no heat is used and the plant material is dissolved in a solvent. The big difference is in the type of solvent used. Carbon dioxide, of course, is a natural substance we breathe in and out all the time and unlike other solvents is completely environmentally friendly. To convert it from a gas into a usable solvent, the CO_2 is put under enormous amounts of pressure (about 200 times normal atmospheric pressure). The pressure changes it into a liquid, which acts as a solvent. The release of pressure converts the CO_2 back into a gas, avoiding the need for other processes that are usually required to separate the solvent from the aromatic oils.

The products of CO_2 extraction have many advantages and few disadvantages. **CO_2 extracts** have the full aroma and the wide range of molecules found in absolutes, but without the solvent traces. Also, the lower temperatures at which this process is performed result in an extract with chemical components closer to the natural chemicals in the plant. An example is the CO_2 extract of German chamomile (*Matricaria recutita*). Unlike the blue color of the steam-distilled oil, it is clear because it contains matricin. This chemical is usually converted to chamazulene by the heat of the distillation process, giving the essential oil its blue color. Laboratory testing on CO_2 extracts yields significant differences in chemical composition between them and essential oils from the same plant.[12] The safety aspects of CO_2 extracts have not yet been thoroughly tested.

Cold Expression

Another common method of extracting essential oils is **cold expression,** or the cold pressing of a plant. This process is used only with citrus fruits because they contain large amounts of volatile oils in high quantities near to the plant surface. The products are called **expressed oils** or **essences.**

The rind of the fruit, where the aromatic oils are concentrated in tiny pockets, is pierced or pressed to give a mixture of juice and volatile oils, which have different densities and therefore separate out easily. There are several traditional methods of expression, including using a sponge to press out and collect the oil and piercing the citrus skins on a vessel with spikes at the top and a collecting tube at the bottom.[13] More modern methods include machines with large steel rollers, or expeller presses, which crush the entire fruit; the expressed oil is separated later by high-speed centrifuges.

As in solvent extraction, this process uses no heat, so the resulting oil has a strong, natural quality. Unlike in solvent extraction, there are no chemicals added, so the oil is completely free of any trace amounts of toxins. However, it is important when buying citrus oils to make sure the plants have been organically grown, as the pesticides and herbicides that are often used in citrus cultivation remain on the rind and are easily included with the essential oil in this relatively simple process.

Enfleurage

Enfleurage is a traditional extraction method, not used often today, except occasionally for more expensive flowers such as tuberose and jasmine. The entire process is extremely labor-intensive and time-consuming, resulting in a product with an extraordinary fragrance but one that is also expensive.

The essential oil is extracted with a fatty substance, rather than a solvent. Glass sheets are coated with a fat, traditionally tallow and lard, and flowers are then placed on the fat. The sheets are carefully stacked in piles and left for the essential oils to disperse into the oily solvent. After 24 hours, the depleted flowers are removed by hand and a fresh layer of flowers is laid onto the sheet. This process is repeated many times (for jasmine, the process lasts about 70 days) until the fat is completely saturated with the volatile oils, at which point the infusion, known as a pomade, is collected and washed with alcohol to remove the essential oils from the fat. The alcohol is then evaporated off, leaving a pure **enfleurage,** often called an absolute (this term is used for the products of both solvent extraction and enfleurage). The absolute is usually darkly colored and semisolid.[14]

Maceration

Also known as **infusion, maceration** is the oldest method of extracting essential oils, probably going as far back as Neolithic times when humans first learned how to press vegetable oils, such as olive and linseed. This process enabled them to use the oils to soak plant material, to extract the aromatic oils. These fatty infusions were frequently used by the ancient Egyptians as perfumes or medicines, recorded by them as ointments or salves. Figure 2.3 is a limestone relief from ancient Egypt showing the maceration of lilies in oil. In the words of Lise Manniche, a professor of Egyptology, "oil was the most obvious medium for capturing and administering a fragrance medicinally."[15]

The process consists of placing the herbs or flowers in some kind of fat and leaving the fat in the sun or another warm place to let the aromatic molecules saturate the fat. The advantages of this extraction method are the ease and low cost of the process and the fact that various herbs that are difficult to distill can easily be infused. St. John's wort is a good example. This plant yields a rich red infusion with strong healing properties, but the essential oil has an ex-

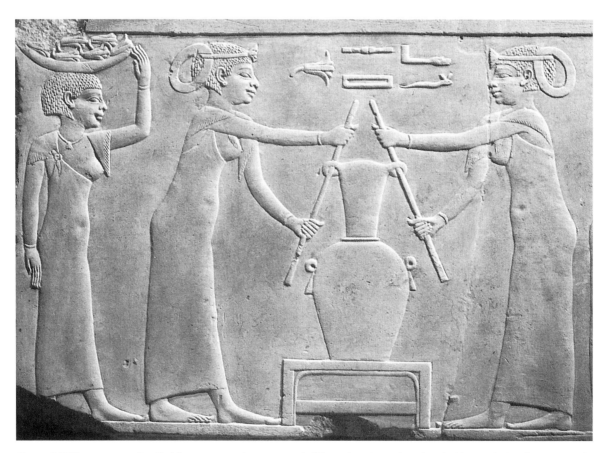

Figure 2.3 Women squeezing lily blossoms to make macerated oil in ancient Egypt. (Reprinted with permission from Manniche L. Sacred Luxuries: Fragrance, Aromatherapy, and Cosmetics in Ancient Egypt. Ithaca, NY: Cornell University Press. Text © 1999 by Lise Manniche, Photographs © 1999 Werner Forman, © 1999 Opus Publishing Limited. Used by permission of the publisher, Cornell University Press.)

tremely low yield, making it prohibitively expensive to extract by distillation.

Macerated oils are a valuable resource for massage therapists. We use oils or lotions when we work with clients, and the infusion can either be used as an aromatic massage oil itself or act as a healing carrier oil for a blend of essential oils. The other advantage of this extraction method is that you can do it yourself quite easily at home in a spare hour or two. For the massage therapist who has a garden with a few aromatic herbs in it, maceration is an ideal way to obtain scented, therapeutic massage oils. You can be absolutely certain of the purity of both the plant and the extraction method.

To make your own infused oils, pack a jar tightly with plant material, cover it completely with vegetable oil, put on the lid, and leave it in a sunny or mildly warm place for a week or two (Figure 2.4). Or you can put the plant material and oil into a bowl over a pan of simmering water for 2 or 3 hours. After either method, strain the oil and pour it into clean, airtight bottles for storage. Some plants, such as rosemary, seem to respond better to the hot method, while others, such as St. John's wort, require the cold one.[16] You may have to experiment a few times to find the right method, length of time, plant material-to-oil ratio, and so on. The first few times I tried to infuse lavender, I ended up with a slimy mess, until I discovered that lavender is one of the plants that should be dried for a day or two before being infused. These oils can then be used for massage or to make lotions, creams, or ointments.

Hydrosols

Hydrosols are the by-products of the distillation process, the aromatic water that condenses from the water vapor used to distill the essential oil. They are water-based substances, rather than substances that dissolve in oil or lotion. Many aromatic molecules in plants are water-soluble, and they readily dissolve in the distillation water to make the hydrosol. Hydrosols from citrus fruits generally do not exist, as these oils are expressed and only very occasionally are distilled.

Hydrosols were traditionally called "floral waters." Rosewater is a well-known example, especially in the Middle East and India, where it is used in sweet drinks, candies, and desserts. In aromatherapy circles the term "floral water" is still used, but less so than before, as many new and unusual aromatic waters are being sold, and calling a hydrosol "seaweed floral water" might sound somewhat strange. These substances are now commonly called hydrosols, solutions in water, or

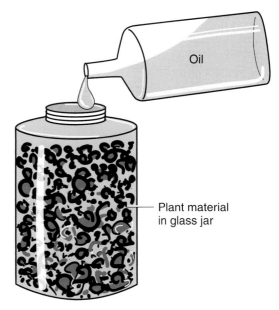

Figure 2.4 The maceration of plant material in oil.

hydrolats, from the Italian *latte* for milk, because they often are cloudy or milky immediately after distillation.[17]

Hydrosols have different chemical constituents than their corresponding essential oils, being higher in water-soluble chemicals and lower in lipophilic (fat-soluble) chemicals. In spite of the chemical differences, they often smell very similar to the essential oil with which they are distilled and often are considered to have some similar therapeutic properties. However, because they dissolve in water and not in fats, they have very different application methods from essential oils because they do not mix well with the oils or lotions normally used with massage. Hydrosols are often used instead to spray the body after a session, especially on a hot day, or to spray the face to wake and refresh a client. They can be given to clients to take home to use as a spritz or in the bath.

Hydrosols have become increasingly popular in aromatherapy in recent years. When I started my practice in the late 1980s, it was difficult to find more than the traditionally used rose, neroli, and lavender waters. Now it is possible to find 30 different hydrosols from one supplier, and many more than that if you shop around. Hundreds of liters of hydrosol are produced during the distillation of only 1 L of essential oil, so it would seem as if there should be a lot of hydrosol available! However, because it is bulky and sells for much less than the essential oil, distillers are often reluctant to ship it for price reasons, and in the past it has often simply been dumped.

SUMMARY

- Essential oils help protect aromatic plants against bacteria, viruses, fungi, and predators. They also attract insects to pollinate the plant.

- Essential oils may occur in any plant part.

- Aromatic plants may be wild-crafted or cultivated. The cultivation may be organic or conventional. Most aromatherapists prefer wild-crafted or organically produced essential oils because of the lower risk of chemical traces.

- Some aromatic plants are endangered because of overharvesting.

- Extraction methods include distillation, solvent extraction, carbon dioxide extraction, cold expression, enfleurage, and maceration.

- Distillation produces essential oils. Steam distillation is the most common method used today, but water distillation and hydrodiffusion are also used. In all types of distillation, heat is used to release the essential oil from the plant.

- Solvent extraction produces absolutes. Absolutes often have stronger, fuller aromas than essential oils, but may contain chemical traces from the solvent. This method is used for plants with oils that are distorted by heat or that have low amounts of essential oils.

- Carbon dioxide extraction produces CO_2 extracts. Liquid CO_2 is used as a solvent. The products have strong, full aromas, similar to absolutes, but with no chemical traces.

- Cold expression produces expressed oils or essences. It involves crushing or piercing the plant material. This method is used only with citrus rinds.

- Enfleurage produces enfleurages or absolutes. Fat is used to extract the essential oils. An extremely time-consuming and expensive process, it is used today only for expensive flowers, such as tuberose and jasmine.

- Maceration produces infused oils. Plant material is left to soak in oil. The aromatic oil can be used for massage or in cooking.

- Hydrosols are by-products of the distillation process. They are very mild. They dilute in water, not in fats.

Review Questions

1. Essential oils are anti-_____, anti-_____, and anti-_____.
2. Plants use essential oils to protect themselves from _____, _____, and other _____.
3. Most aromatic plants are: (a) organically grown, (b) harvested from the wild, (c) conventionally grown.
4. Plants that are particularly endangered are those in which the essential oils are mainly found in the _____ and _____.
5. Aromatic plants are often grown in developing countries because _____ are lower.
6. Essential oils are extracted by _____.
7. Absolutes are extracted by _____.
8. Citrus oils are extracted by _____.
9. One of the disadvantages of distillation is that the heat may change the chemicals or the aroma of an essential oil. (T/F)
10. Some aromatherapists dislike using absolutes on the skin because of the risk of _____ traces.
11. To use CO_2 as a solvent, it has to be: (a) heated, (b) cooled, (c) put under pressure, (d) frozen.
12. Expressed oils tend to be much more expensive than other types of aromatic oils. (T/F)
13. Hydrosols are by-products of the _____ process.
14. Hydrosols are completely soluble in _____.
15. Infused oils can easily be made at home. (T/F)

Notes

1. Shawe K. Course notes from Botany for Aromatherapists workshop, Seattle, WA, August 2000.
2. Shawe K. Course notes from Botany for Aromatherapists workshop, Seattle, WA, August 2000.
3. Baker S. Environmental issues and aromatherapy. Int J Aromather 2003;13(2/3):63.
4. Webb M. Bush Sense—Australian Essential Oils and Aromatic Compounds. Adelaide, Australia: Griffin Press, 2000:91.
5. Burfield T. Unethical use of rare and threatened plant and animal products in the aroma industry. Endangered Species Update 2003; 20(3):97–106.
6. Grace K. Aromatherapy Journeys. Video distributed by Terra Entertainment, 1998.
7. Firth G. Secrets of the Still. McLean, VA: EPM Publications, 1983: 23–50.
8. Guenther E. The Essential Oils, Vol. 4. New York: Van Nostrand Co., 1948:161.
9. Guenther E. The Essential Oils, Vol. 4. New York: Van Nostrand Co., 1948:168.
10. McMahon C. Attars: Traditional Perfumes of India. The World of Aromatherapy III Conference Proceedings, Seattle, WA, 2000.
11. Essential Aura Aromatics. Available at: www.essentialaura.com. Accessed November 28, 2004.
12. Ehlers D, Färber J, Martin A, et al. Investigating fennel oils—CO_2 extraction and steam-distillation. Deutsche Lebensmittel-Rundschau, 2000;96(9):330–335.
13. Guenther E. The Essential Oils, Vol. 3. New York: Van Nostrand Co., 1948:6–14.
14. Guenther E. The Essential Oils, Vol. 1. New York: Van Nostrand Co., 1948:189–195.
15. Manniche L. Sacred Luxuries: Fragrance, Aromatherapy and Cosmetics in Ancient Egypt. Ithaca, NY: Cornell University Press, 1999.
16. Ody P. The Complete Medicinal Herbal. New York: Dorling Kindersley, 1993:122.
17. Catty S. Hydrosols: The Next Aromatherapy. Rochester, VT: Healing Arts Press, 2001:9.

3 Buying and Storing Essential Oils

Guidelines for Smart Purchasing
  Finding a Reputable Supplier
  Checking the Basic Information
  Learning the Vocabulary
  Questioning Your Supplier
  Using Your Senses
Guidelines for Storage
  Why Essential Oils Deteriorate
  Keeping Your Essential Oils Fresh

When using essential oils for therapeutic purposes, it is extremely important that they are of the highest quality, very pure, and as fresh as possible. If essential oils are not pure and fresh, aromatherapists will not achieve the expected results when using them, as the chemical makeup becomes unpredictable. Essential oils that have been carelessly distilled, mixed with other substances, or allowed to deteriorate can cause problems. There is an increased risk of skin irritation or allergic reaction, and the fragrance of the essential oils will definitely be affected negatively. It is extremely important that aromatherapists use essential oils of the highest quality possible, to ensure safe and effective outcomes for their clients.

Guidelines for Smart Purchasing

Buying essential oils may seem like the easiest part of incorporating aromatherapy into a massage practice, much easier than remembering what each oil is good for or the safety indications. However, purchasing is perhaps the most difficult part of practicing aromatherapy because the commercial side of aromatherapy is complex. Aromatherapy is the smallest market segment for consumers of essential oils—constituting about 5% of the total. The other 95% of the market consists of products for the perfume industry, food flavorings, and pharmaceuticals.[1] The food and pharmaceutical industries are concerned primarily with the main chemical components of essential oils. Certain minimum compliance standards exist, and as long as an essential oil falls within these guidelines, these industries are not concerned with how the plant was grown, if it was extracted without damaging the aroma, or even if other essential oils or isolated chemical components have been added later, a process known as **adulteration.**

Likewise, the main focus of the perfume industry is the fragrance of the essential oil and its consistency from season to season. It would be impossible for a fragrance house to effectively market a perfume that smells different from year to year, which is what would happen if these companies relied solely on pure essential oils. It is taken for granted within the perfume world that a large part of the perfume will consist of chemical components made within a laboratory, and that any essential oils in the mixture will have been adulterated (or "standardized") to yield a consistent aroma. Many of the most expensive perfumes from the more famous houses still use large amounts of the finest essential oils, such as rose and jasmine, to create their aromas, but consumers have become accustomed to synthetic fragrances, especially in the cheaper perfumes and in shampoos, soaps, deodorants, and so on. In the words of Barillé and Laroze, authors of *The Book of Perfume,* "the evolution of the perfume industry is such that a return to entirely natural compositions is out of the question, since consumers are now used to the power and impact, the tenacity and trail of the synthetic products."[2]

Adulteration is also carried out by manufacturers of essential oils simply to increase their profits. Franklin and Chopra, writing on essential oil integrity, remark:

"It is a known fact that the volume of essential oils such as rose, lavender and rose geranium traded in the market is far in excess of the world-wide production of these oils. Adding synthetic chemical components, or in some cases low-value oils, makes up the volumes traded. The price that these essential oils fetch in the marketplace makes it a worthwhile exercise to adulterators of these oils."[3]

If we consider that rose (*Rosa damascena*) essential oil costs more than 10 times that of geranium (*Pelargonium graveolens*) essential oil, it is not difficult to see how major profits can be made by adding large amounts of geranium to rose (or in some cases substituting it for rose) and labeling it as rose essential oil. Laboratory tests can be performed to determine the specific chemicals in the essential oil. However, synthetic chemicals can be added to make the adulterated oil fit the usual chemical profile of rose so that even laboratory analysis cannot always detect adulteration. In an address to the International Federation of Aromatherapists, Tony Burfield remarked: "It is particularly economically attractive to extend high value floral absolutes such as rose (*Rosa* spp.), jasmine (*Jasminum grandiflora* other spp.) and osmanthus (*Osmanthus fragrans* var. *auranticus*), and the more valuable oils such as neroli oil and rose otto, and this practice occurs extensively within the trade."[4]

Unfortunately, it is difficult to guarantee that you are buying an essential oil that has not been tampered with in some way. However, you can do certain things to minimize that possibility.

Finding a Reputable Supplier

One of the most vital things for an aromatherapist to have is one or more suppliers who sell only to the aromatherapy market and who supplies **therapeutic-grade essential oils**—oils that have been carefully and knowledgeably extracted from a single, good-quality botanical source, unadulterated, bottled and transported carefully, and sold in a timely manner to the therapist. Many suppliers meet these standards, and they sell essential oils ranging from good to absolutely superb. However, a large number of companies and individuals sell essential oils that are not top quality, but they market themselves aggressively as the leaders in the field. How can practitioners who are new to aromatherapy begin to tell the difference, and where should they start looking for oils?

Just as with any other product—whether it's kayaking gear or cooking implements—the best people to ask are those who have been in the field for some time. Get in touch with aromatherapists in your area who have good training and experience, and find out who they buy their oils from. Consult Appendix B in this book for reputable suppliers. If you take a workshop or go to a lecture on aromatherapy, ask the teacher to talk about his or her favorite suppliers. Go to aromatherapy conferences and trade shows and sniff your way around the exhibits, and don't be afraid to ask questions. Look for suppliers who have been selling essential oils for at least a few years and are well known within the aromatherapy community. And be aware that, as with most other products, you generally get what you pay for. Therapeutic-grade oils are not inexpensive because they require a lot of time, energy, and knowledge to produce.

Checking the Basic Information

You should look for certain things when buying essential oils, and your supplier should be able to give you particular information. Some of this information should be clearly written on the bottle, or at least on the supplier's price list. They include the following:

Botanical Name. In botanical and therapeutic circles, plants are identified by their **botanical names,** which are in Latin. The first part of the name, the **genus** (capitalized), refers to a small group of closely related plants, while the second part, the **species** (lower case), identifies the particular plant in the group. Both names often give some information about the plant or the person who named it. For example, *Lavandula angustifolia* refers to the small group of plants commonly called lavender (from the Latin word *lavare*, meaning "to wash," as this was a commonly used laundry herb); the specific plant is the *angustifolia*, or the one with "narrow leaves." It is also useful to know what **family** (a larger group of related plants) a particular genus belongs to (lavender belongs to the Lamiaceae family); it can provide more information about the uses and properties of the essential oil.[5]

This method of naming plants is used worldwide. Common names are unreliable, varying among different countries and even from region to region. Also, a common name may be used for several different species within one genus, such as eucalyptus, which has more than 700 different species, or it may even be used for completely unrelated plants, like cedarwood, which is the common name both for the European *Cedrus atlantica*, a member of the Pinaceae family, and

for various species of the Juniperus family in America. To illustrate, Table 3.1 lists some of the common and botanical names for various plants commonly called lavender.

Because lavandin (*Lavandula x intermedia*) is about half the price of "true" lavender (*Lavandula angustifolia*) and can legitimately be sold as lavender because it is from the *Lavandula* genus, it is definitely worthwhile to check on the botanical name! Many of the lavender-scented toiletries in stores are made with the cheaper lavandin.

Plant Part. Many plants store essential oils in several different plant parts. Sometimes the entire plant is distilled, a good example being thyme, which is highly aromatic in all its parts and which is too small a plant to pick only one part. Other plants may produce very different oils from the different parts, so it is vital to know exactly what you are getting because properties or safety indications may differ. For example, cinnamon is distilled from either the bark or the leaves; the leaf oil is less irritating to the skin. The bitter orange tree (*Citrus aurantium* var. *amara*) produces three different essential oils: neroli from the flowers, bitter orange from the peel of the fruit, and petitgrain from the leaves and twigs. It is very important here to know which plant part has been used, especially since neroli oil often is up to 10 times more expensive than bitter orange oil.

Cultivation Method. Many good suppliers list whether the plant has been wild-crafted or cultivated organically or conventionally. Some may list other cultivation methods, such as "ethical," which in most cases means that the crop has been grown without pesticides or herbicides but has not been certified organic. Particularly in the case of citrus oils, absolutes, and CO_2 extracts, it is important to know whether the plant has been grown organically, as pesticides are more likely to come across in cold expression and solvent extraction.

Country of Origin. The country of origin is the country where the plant was grown, which may be a different country from where it underwent extraction. The specific soils, climates, and altitudes in various regions of the world will

Table 3.1	**Common and Botanical Names for Different Lavenders**		
Common Name	**Alternate Name**	**Botanical Name(s)**	**Family Name**
Lavender	True lavender	*Lavandula angustifolia (Lavandula vera, Lavandula officinale)*	Lamiaceae
Lavender	Spike lavender	*Lavandula latifolia (Lavandula spica)*	Lamiaceae
Lavender	Lavandin	*Lavandula x intermedia*	Lamiaceae
Lavender	Spanish lavender	*Lavandula stoechas*	Lamiaceae

produce a very individual chemical composition, even from the same species of essential oil. It is amazing to smell the differences in several oils of *Lavandula angustifolia* from England, France, the United States, Madagascar, and even Kashmir. Some countries are regarded as the finest producers of a particular essential oil, such as ginger from Jamaica, geranium from the Reunion islands, or vanilla from Madagascar, and these oils often command a higher price than the same species from another country.

Chemotypes. Some plants adapt so much to a particular area that over time, many decades or even centuries, they become distinct in their chemical composition from the original plant. Called **chemotypes,** they are the same species but have consistently different chemistry from each other, season after season. Thyme (*Thymus vulgaris*) is an excellent example, having several different chemotypes that occur in various countries in Europe, all with different properties and safety indications.[6] An essential oil supplier should be able to tell you the main chemical constituents in any essential oil that you buy, thereby establishing which chemotype it is. A particular chemotype is indicated by the letters "CT" followed by the chemical group that distinguishes the chemotype, for example, *Thymus vulgaris* CT thymol or *Thymus vulgaris* CT linalool.

Extraction Method. As we discussed in Chapter 2, essential oils may be extracted from the plant in a variety of ways. The extraction method affects the plant's chemical makeup and therefore its aroma, its color and viscosity, and its properties. For example, citrus oils usually are expressed from the rind but occasionally are steam-distilled, the most common example being lime. The expressed oil of lime is sharp and crisp, very like the smell of the peel itself, while the steam-distilled essential oil is sweeter and smoother, almost like a lime candy. Rose absolute and **rose otto** (a common name for rose essential oil) are both common, but the absolute has a different color, aroma, and chemical composition from the essential oil. In the last few decades, CO_2 extracts have become increasingly available, and suppliers will often sell them as well as essential oils. I recently saw a price list with eight distinct types of *Lavandula angustifolia*, including the CO_2 extract, the essential oil, and the absolute.

Even if the properties of the various extracts are not significantly different, their fragrances certainly are, and the extraction method must be clearly stated by the supplier. Occasionally the type of extract available will make a dramatic difference to the therapeutic properties of a particular oil. Ylang ylang, for example, undergoes an unusual form of extraction, called **fractional distillation,** in which the distillation is interrupted every few hours and the essential oil from those few hours is removed. The distillation then continues with the same plant material. The result is several different grades of ylang ylang. The essential oil from the first few hours of dis-

tillation, called ylang ylang **extra,** is the most highly prized and the most expensive. The next most desirable is ylang ylang first grade, then second, and then third.

Perfumers and aromatherapists alike prefer the extra, because it has both a superior fragrance and much more pronounced therapeutic effects because of the higher ester content in the essential oil. (Esters are chemicals that tend to have antispasmodic, calming, and sedative effects, as well as a pleasant floral aroma.) The ester content decreases in the first grade, though it is still significant, and it almost disappears completely in the second and third grades, with the result that their aroma and therapeutic effects usually are disappointing.[7]

Yet another form of ylang ylang is created by some distillers who combine the extra and first grade (and sometimes also the second grade) to make what is called a ylang ylang **complete.** The confusion is compounded by the fact that there is no consensus among distillers about how long each stage of distillation should take, with the result that every ylang ylang is different, depending on the distiller. However, the grade of this essential oil should be clearly marked so consumers have some idea of what they are buying.

Packaging. Essential oils should be bottled in colored glass. They will react with plastic, causing the bottles to deteriorate and possibly leak, and creating changes in the essential oil. Colored glass should be used because light can cause the oils to deteriorate. The bottles should have tamper-proof seals, as reactions with oxygen will cause them to degrade more quickly.[8] Some suppliers record on the label the month and year the essential oil was bottled. This is a welcome innovation because otherwise it is extremely difficult to determine the age of the essential oil.

Learning the Vocabulary

Specific terminology is used in the production of essential oils. It is useful to know certain terms when deciding whether an oil is of high quality.

- **Pure oils** and **natural oils** are names that have little legal meaning in the United States.

- **Rectified oils** or **redistilled oils** have been distilled at least twice to remove certain chemical components. Bergamot, for example, can be found in a "bergapten-free" form, in which the furocoumarins have been removed for safety reasons because of their phototoxic effects.

- **Folded oils** are usually citruses that have been redistilled several times, making them more concentrated and therefore more desirable for the food industry.[9]

- **Reconstituted oils** or **extended oils** have had natural or synthetic ingredients added to them. Sometimes this is entirely legitimate, as in the case of the pharmaceutical industry, which often requires that an essential oil have a minimum percentage of a particular chemical constituent.

Less innocent is the practice of adding chemicals to an oil simply to increase its value. Some suppliers have even been known to extend their essential oils with vegetable oil or alcohol, without informing their clients. (It is, however, completely acceptable to sell expensive essential oils, such as rose or neroli, diluted in a high-grade carrier as long as the labeling is clear—for example, "10% rose essential oil in jojoba.")

- **Nature identical oils** are either compounded completely from naturally extracted or synthetic chemicals or have had synthetic chemicals added that are ostensibly "identical" to those found in the naturally extracted essential oil. This term is becoming increasingly common, and it is alarming to those aromatherapists who do not want their oils tampered with in any way.

- **Aromatherapy oils** are not essential oils and usually contain a blend of essential oils, carrier oils, and possibly absolutes.

Questioning Your Supplier

Even for a well-trained, experienced aromatherapist, it is impossible to know, just by smelling an essential oil, if it is pure or not. Aromatherapists must rely on various laboratory tests to ensure that what they are getting is authentic and unadulterated. Unfortunately, most of these tests are extremely expensive and require at least one fluid ounce of essential oil, so they are beyond the means of those who simply want to buy small amounts of good-quality aromatics. Suppliers will put essential

oils through these tests, but it is generally the larger suppliers, with more resources, who will do so.

The main techniques used for analysis are gas-liquid chromatography and mass spectroscopy. Gas-liquid chromatography (GC) is used extensively to separate and identify the different chemical components of a substance. (The abbreviation GLC is also used.) Figure 3.1 shows a typical GC analysis, with several high peaks and many low ones. Basically, the higher the peak in the chart is, the higher the percentage of this component is in the essential oil. The components can be identified by where the peaks appear on the chart. The pattern can be compared with that of a chart from a known sample, to see if they match up.

Mass spectroscopy (MS) can determine the atomic and molecular masses of components within an oil, thus identifying the separate components. This test is very useful if done together with a GC test. A reputable supplier should be able to provide you with a GC or GC-MS analysis chart, though these can be difficult to read for those without training in this type of analysis. Other lab tests include infrared spectroscopy (IR), optical rotation, specific gravity (SG), and refractive index.

You can ask suppliers if these lab tests have been performed on their oils. You can ask to see the results, or ask for a summary of the results. Even if suppliers are too small to have these kinds of tests done, it is still worthwhile to ask about testing because their response can be very revealing. If they appear not to know what you are

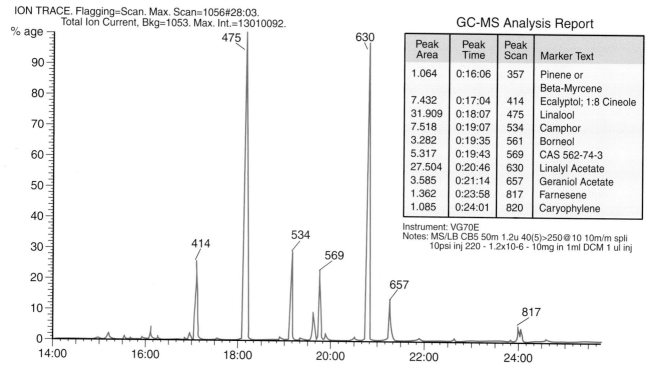

Figure 3.1 Gas–liquid chromatography (GC) analysis of lavender essential oil. MS, mass spectroscopy. (Available at: www.dreamingearth. com. Accessed June 1, 2005.)

talking about, that will give you some indication of their experience and/or training. For the same reason, it is worthwhile to ask about extraction methods, cultivation methods, and so on. You can ask your supplier for Safety Data Sheets on any essential oil you buy for information on chemical constituents; known contraindications for use; safety information in case the oil is spilled in large quantities, swallowed, or ignited; and data on handling, storing, transporting, and labeling. However, Safety Data Sheets are generally written for the use of essential oils in industry and they are less informative about small-scale use of essential oils by an aromatherapist.

A recent survey of essential oil suppliers indicated that many of them were not particularly helpful when asked for information, with fewer than half the companies willing to reply: "Generally the responding companies were more willing to forward price lists and publicity information than respond directly to requests for specific details. However, the few companies who did respond appropriately appeared genuinely keen and enthusiastic in terms of offering their support and providing information."[10]

Using Your Senses

Even an experienced aromatherapist may find it difficult to assess the quality of an essential oil by smelling it, and it is almost impossible to tell if it is adulterated. However, the nose is extremely sophisticated, capable of assessing quality in subtle ways that even laboratory tests and instruments cannot: "In spite of great technological advancements in analysis techniques the trained nose can still be the single most important arbiter of quality."[11]

You can read descriptions of the smell, color, and viscosity of an aromatic oil and check to see if the oil you have bought corresponds, even approximately. For example, sandalwood (*Santalum album*) oil is generally pale yellow in color, has an oily, almost sticky feel to it, and is quite thick, often taking a long time to pour from a bottle with a dropper top. If your sandalwood oil is darkly colored, feels watery, and pours very quickly, you can tell that you need to ask your supplier a few questions about it. *The Illustrated Encyclopedia of Essential Oils* by Julia Lawless is a good resource; it has photographs of the oils in clear bottles, so the colors are visible.[12]

Guidelines for Storage

The correct way to store oils to maximize their life span and how long that life span actually is are areas of debate among aromatherapists. Some aromatherapists keep their essential oils for many years, while others maintain that they will not last longer than a few years and should be discarded at the end of this time. The truth is that no one actually knows for sure how long these products last and to what extent they change over time. Certainly aromatic oils can keep their smell and character for an extremely long time. When the tomb of Tutankhamun was opened, archaeologists found clay pots containing aromatic extracts; when the extracts melted in the heat of the hand they still emitted a faint odor, more than 3000 years after they were made.[13] Aromatic oils were considered to have a long life in ancient times: "Ten years or more would be the life of myrrh unguent, with cinnamon and cassia a close second. An exception among the ephemeral floral scents, iris perfume would last for six years and, properly stored, even as long as twenty years."[14] And this was in the hot climate of Egypt with no refrigeration.

Why Essential Oils Deteriorate

All aromatic oils are not equal—their chemical compositions and volatilities vary dramatically. It would seem logical that the essential oils that contain the most reactive and most volatile chemicals would be the ones to change in aroma, or fade, most quickly. In fact, most aromatherapists agree that the citrus oils, which follow this description, are notorious for not lasting long, especially the lighter ones such as grapefruit. The citrus oils and the needle oils (pine, spruce, and fir) are very high in chemical constituents that **oxidize,** or react readily with oxygen, making these essential oils the shortest-lasting in aromatherapy. Essential oils that smell like lemon but are not citruses are also high in chemicals that react with oxygen and deteriorate quickly. Examples in this category are lemongrass, melissa, eucalyptus citriodora, and citronella. Studies have shown that oils that are oxidized tend to be more irritating to the skin. Therefore, it is wise to buy these oils in smaller quantities and use them up quickly—perhaps within 1 year or 18 months.

Most essential oils will last for at least two years if stored in good conditions, and some will last for much longer. As a rule of thumb, I calculate roughly how long an essential oil will stay good by looking at its volatility. If an oil is extremely volatile—for example, certain peppermints—then I try not to keep it longer than about 18 months. For oils with mid-range volatility—herbs like rosemary and clary sage—I calculate around 2 or 3 years. For those that are extremely stable—sandalwood, patchouli, or some of the heavy flower absolutes—the sky is the limit. I have owned a patchouli essential oil for over 12 years, and it seems to get better and better! According to Guenther, "some oils (e.g., vetiver, sandalwood, and patchouly) show very good keeping qualities and may actually improve upon aging."[15] One of my suppliers informed me recently that geranium oil is not considered therapeutic quality in India until it is more than 5 years old.

Generally speaking, essential oils made from woods, roots, and resins are the most stable; many herbs and flowers have medium stability; and citruses, needle oils, and some herbs such as mint are quite unstable and unlikely to last for a long time. Many absolutes seem to last longer, and possibly also CO_2 extracts, as they are a type of solvent extract, although documented studies are not available at this time.

Keeping Your Essential Oils Fresh

Although much debate exists about how long essential oils can be kept, most aromatherapists agree on the methods of storage. Here are some guidelines:

- Keep your essential oils somewhere cool and dark. They do not keep well in sunlight or in very warm conditions, as these factors accelerate chemical reactions, which may cause deterioration.
- Store essential oils in a dry place. Moisture also seems to speed up chemical reactions, which cause oils to degrade more quickly.[16]

- Keep essential oils at a constant temperature. Refrigeration is a good idea, but it is probably more important to keep them at a constant cool temperature. According to Sue Clarke, author of *Essential Chemistry for Safe Aromatherapy*, "the rate of deterioration *doubles* for every 10°C rise in temperature."[17]
- Limit the exposure of essential oils to air to minimize oxidation. If you buy in bulk, pour your essential oil into several smaller colored glass bottles and use one at a time, leaving the others sealed against oxidation.
- Store essential oils in colored glass because they may react with plastic, changing the chemical composition of the oil. The bottle may also be weakened by this reaction, eventually bulging or leaking. Suppliers store larger amounts of essential oil in aluminum or steel containers that have been lacquered inside.

SUMMARY

- The aromatherapy market consumes only about 5% of the total amount of essential oils produced. The biggest consumers of essential oils are the perfume, food, and pharmaceutical industries.
- Adulteration of essential oils to increase profits is common. Essential oils can be adulterated by adding cheaper essential oils, natural or synthetic chemicals, vegetable oil, or alcohol.
- Laboratory tests, such as gas-liquid chromatography and mass spectrometry, are used to test for impurities in essential oils, but they cannot always detect adulteration.
- Information on essential oils provided by suppliers should include the botanical name, plant part, cultivation method, country of origin, specific chemotype (if appropriate), and extraction method.

- Essential oils should be bottled and stored in colored glass with tamper-proof seals.
- The color, consistency, and usual aroma of an essential oil can help determine its authenticity and quality.
- Some essential oils deteriorate faster than others. Essential oils from citrus fruits, the needles of evergreen trees, and oils that smell lemony react more easily with oxygen and degrade faster. Degraded oils may be more irritating to the skin, and they should be used within 12 to 18 months.
- Most other essential oils can be kept for up to two years. Some heavier, less volatile oils, such as patchouli and vetiver, may keep well for many years.
- Store essential oils in a cool, dry place with a constant temperature. Avoid exposure to oxygen and sunlight.

Review Questions

1. Which industries are the major consumers of essential oils?
2. What is adulteration?
3. Why do we use the botanical name (Latin name) of the essential oil?
4. What three essential oils are extracted from the bitter orange (*Citrus aurantium* var. *amara*)?
5. It is important to know whether the plant was grown with pesticides, especially for which extraction methods?
6. The climate, soil, and altitude of an area can significantly affect both the aroma and the chemistry of an essential oil. (T/F)
7. A chemotype is the same species of plant, but with a different _____ makeup.
8. Ylang ylang (*Cananga odorata*) comes in different grades, of which the _____ is considered the finest.
9. Essential oils should not be stored in _____ bottles, as they may react with this material.
10. Rectified means that some constituents have been added to an essential oil. (T/F)
11. An aromatherapy oil is the same thing as an essential oil. (T/F)

12. The main techniques used for essential oil analysis are _____ chromatography and _____ spectrometry.

13. Essential oils can only be kept for 6 months to 1 year. (T/F)

14. Essential oils should be kept somewhere: (a) warm and dark, (b) sunny and warm, (c) cool and dark.

Notes

1. Clarke S. Essential Chemistry for Safe Aromatherapy. Edinburgh, UK: Churchill Livingstone, 2002:91.
2. Barillé E, Laroze C. The Book of Perfume. Paris, France: Flammarion, 1995:40.
3. Chopra A, Franklin J. Integrity of Essential Oils. Available at: www.positivehealth.com. Accessed February 16, 2004.
4. Burfield T. The Adulteration of Essential Oils—and the Consequences to Aromatherapy & Natural Perfumery Practice. Presented at the International Federation of Aromatherapists Annual AGM, London, UK, 2003.
5. Mabberley DJ. The Plant-Book. Cambridge, UK: Cambridge University Press, 1993.
6. Guenther E. The Essential Oils, Vol. 3. New York: Van Nostrand Co., 1948:745.
7. Guenther E. The Essential Oils, Vol. 5. New York: Van Nostrand Co., 1948:295.
8. Guenther E. The Essential Oils, Vol. 1. New York: Van Nostrand Co., 1948:377.
9. Clarke S. Essential Chemistry for Safe Aromatherapy. Edinburgh, UK: Churchill Livingstone, 2002.
10. Godfrey H, Duerden T. Essential oils: how do commercial suppliers respond to requests for information? Int J Aromather 2003; 12(2/3):68.
11. Burfield T. The Adulteration of Essential Oils—and the Consequences to Aromatherapy & Natural Perfumery Practice. Presented at the International Federation of Aromatherapists Annual AGM, London, UK, 2003.
12. Lawless J. The Illustrated Encyclopedia of Essential Oils. Rockport, MA: Element Books, 1995.
13. Manniche L. Sacred Luxuries: Fragrance, Aromatherapy and Cosmetics in Ancient Egypt. Ithaca, NY: Cornell University Press, 1999:86.
14. Manniche L. Sacred Luxuries: Fragrance, Aromatherapy and Cosmetics in Ancient Egypt. Ithaca, NY: Cornell University Press, 1999:63 quoting Theophrastus "On Odors" 34.38
15. Guenther E. The Essential Oils, Vol. 1. New York: Van Nostrand Co., 1948:236.
16. Guenther E. The Essential Oils, Vol. 1. New York: Van Nostrand Co., 1948:377.
17. Clarke S. Essential Chemistry for Safe Aromatherapy. Edinburgh, UK: Churchill Livingstone, 2002:167.

4

The Effects of
Essential Oils
on the Body

Inhalation: Smell and the Olfactory System
Olfactory Pathways
The Effects of Smell on the Brain
The Effects of Smell on Hormones
Olfaction and Emotion
The Absorption of Essential Oils Through the Skin
Factors That Affect Absorption

The word "aromatherapy" suggests that essential oils work only through the sense of smell, and people may imagine that aromatherapy is merely a technique for relaxation, using pleasant smells to soothe the spirit. In fact, essential oils enter the body and affect it, on a chemical level as well as a psychological one. Aromatic molecules are very small compared with a lot of other substances that we take into our bodies: most essential oils have molecules with only 10 or 15 carbon atoms, while a cholesterol molecule has 27 carbon atoms and a typical vegetable oil molecule may have about 56. This means that essential oil molecules may have a much easier time getting into the body than many other compounds because of their extremely small size.

There are many ways by which essential oils can enter the body and affect it. In France, where medical aromatherapy is practiced, essential oils may be administered orally in capsules, sublingually in drop form, anally via suppositories, or vaginally via pessaries. These methods of application let essential oils reach the bloodstream in high concentrations, and this form of aromatherapy is closest to the prescribing of drugs in conventional Western medicine. However, this internal use of essential oils is outside the scope of practice for massage therapists, who practice holistic aromatherapy, used in topical applications. In these methods, essential oils affect the body via inhalation and by absorption through the skin, or the lungs, into the bloodstream. For those who find it difficult to imagine that inhaling an essential oil may have an effect on brain chemistry, they only have to be reminded of the powerful effects caused by glue sniffing. For those who insist that essential oils could not strongly influence body chemistry via skin absorption, hormone replacement therapy and antinausea patches are a reminder that medicinal substances are often applied topically, yet they enter the bloodstream quickly and easily.

Inhalation: Smell and the Olfactory System

The sense of smell is somewhat mysterious; in fact, smells affect us in ways we often don't even notice. Faint odors, even at a subliminal level, have a noticeable impact on our behavior, and we develop a keen and discriminating sense of smell when we are very young. For example, small babies can identify their mothers by smell alone, just as mothers can identify their babies. This is an indication of the importance of smell as a survival mechanism, a concept that is reinforced by a brief look at how **olfaction,** the sense of smell, works.

Olfactory Pathways
With every breath we take, volatile, aromatic molecules enter our nostrils and are trapped in a thin layer of sticky mucus at the top of the nose. The molecules dissolve in this layer and are picked up by specialized receptor cells on the end of microscopic hairlike cilia protruding from olfactory neurons (nerve cells). About 5 million neurons grow out from the olfactory bulb through tiny holes in the cribriform plate of the ethmoid bone. The **olfactory bulb,** the primary organ of smell, is made up of nervous tissue. It is a direct outgrowth of the brain and contains the only neurons in the body to replace themselves regularly (about once every 60 days).[1]

When aromatic molecules and receptors link up, a nerve signal in the form of an electrical impulse is generated and sent back to the olfactory bulb, which initially processes the impulse, before sending it along the **olfactory tract,** a bundle of nerve fibers, to the **olfactory cortex** (part of the cerebral cortex) and from there to the limbic system. The **limbic system** is a collection of structures that include the thalamus, the hypothalamus, and the amygdala. Figure 4.1 shows the olfactory pathways and their connection to the limbic system.

The Effects of Smell on the Brain
Smell and taste are known as the chemical senses because both of them derive sensory information from chemicals entering the body. This mechanism often gives smell and taste an immediacy and intimacy the other senses lack, through direct interaction with molecules from the outside world. As Diane Ackerman writes in *A Natural History of the Senses* about olfactory neurons, "unlike any other neurons in the body, they stick right out and wave in the air current like anemones on a coral reef."[2] Also, the part of the brain that interprets olfactory signals from aromatic molecules is significant. Smell is processed primarily by the limbic system, a portion of the brain that is involved with memory and emotions. In fact, according to leading neurologists, when we smell something, neural signals go first to the **amygdala,** "that part of the limbic system specialized in recognizing the emotional significance of events in the external world."[3] In other words, smells can result in feelings of joy, anger, or fear—emotions that in different situations help the individual (and therefore the species) survive by prompting appropriate behavior. A strong smell of smoke, for example, produces feelings of fear, which in turn trigger the fight-or-flight response of the sympathetic nervous system, thereby flooding the tissues with adrenaline to help cope with the emergency.

If odors can activate the sympathetic nervous system, there is also evidence demonstrating that they can calm the body and mind, putting us into the healing parasympathetic mode. One study showed that the odor of orange oil diffused in a dental waiting room reduced anxiety and produced a greater feeling of calm in patients.[4] Another study showed changes in EEG readings, suggesting increased relaxation and drowsiness in human subjects after sniffing lavender essential oil.[5]

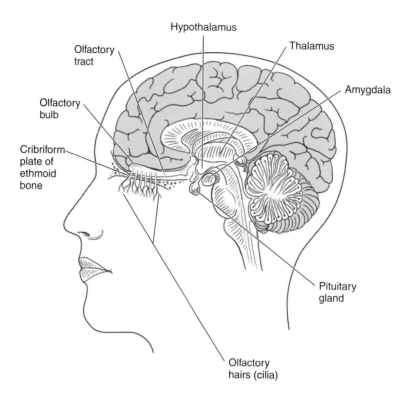

Figure 4.1 The olfactory pathways and the limbic system.

This is important and useful information for massage therapists because many clients have high levels of stress, whether generated by mental, emotional, or physical situations in their lives. Massage therapists can use aromatherapy in various ways to soothe and calm clients, thereby decreasing the symptoms of disorders that are often triggered or exacerbated by stress. These disorders include asthma, irritable bowel syndrome, and fibromyalgia. Reducing anxiety levels through massage and aromatherapy can lower pain perception, help decrease high blood pressure, and improve the quality of life.

The Effects of Smell on Hormones

One important structure in the limbic brain is the **hypothalamus,** which is often referred to as the "master gland" of the endocrine system. It releases many chemical messengers that trigger other parts of the endocrine system to start or stop producing hormones. It also has nerve fibers specialized for both the reception of nerve signals and the secretion of hormones,[6] making it the vital part of the brain where the nervous system and the endocrine system overlap and exchange information.

As part of the limbic brain, the hypothalamus is also sensitive to signals from aromatic molecules, and it is well established that the endocrine system is particularly strongly influenced by the chemicals that we inhale. Every woman who has shared a living space with another woman has experienced the phenomenon wherein their menstrual cycles will coincide after living together for some time. In 1998,

experiments by two research physiologists, McClintock and Stern, showed that applying female underarm secretions under the nose of another female could significantly delay or hasten her menstrual cycle, demonstrating clearly that it is the inhalation of chemicals from another female's body that produces this effect.[7]

The endocrine system has a significant effect on all the systems of the body, particularly the reproductive system. Understanding this is useful for massage therapists working with clients who have severe PMS, menstrual cramping, and menopausal symptoms because aromatherapy has the potential to help with all of these issues, through its effect on mood, and more directly on the endocrine system itself. A 1996 study by Yamada et al. showed that inhaling chamomile essential oil (*Matricaria recutita*) may reduce anxiety and depression in menopausal women by acting on the hypothalamus.[8]

Olfaction and Emotion

In addition to the chemical effects of aromatic molecules on various brain structures, aromas can be incredibly evocative and personal. Just for a moment, imagine the most memorable aromas of your childhood. I frequently ask students in my classes to do this and the responses are surprisingly varied. Many people mention food smells—frying bacon, hot chocolate, pumpkin pie—but many also talk nostalgically about diesel fumes, melting tar, and chemicals from swimming pools. The interesting thing is that, no matter what they mention, the effects are the same: For an instant they are back in childhood, feeling the emotions of that time, whether pleasant or not. Smells have the ability to resurrect emotions and memory, to delight and to disturb. As Ackerman puts it, "smells detonate softly in our memory like poignant land mines, hidden under the weedy mass of many years and experiences. Hit a tripwire of smell, and memories explode all at once."[9]

This personal "smellscape" that we all possess can be both immensely problematic and very useful for aromatherapists. It is impossible to accurately predict any one person's subjective response to an essential oil, no matter how much research we have done on its usual effects on the brain and the body. For this reason, it is sensible and advisable to check out the oils we would like to use with our clients, to determine if they have any strong emotional reaction to them, before we start using them in a session. We can also deliberately evoke pleasant memories. An aromatherapist friend of mine was working with a woman from the Caribbean, who was very homesick in our grey Seattle winter. He blended all the exotic, tropical fragrances that he had available, which reminded her of home, thus lifting her spirits.

Another way to use the association of smell and emotion is to create new sensory connections for clients. For example, if we use a particular blend for which a client has no existing emotional associations, we can create a smell-mood memory, perhaps by using the blend in a soothing relaxation massage. A link starts between this particular aroma and the calming mood of the massage. When repeated several times with the same blend of oils, a strong connection can be made in the brain between the smell and the relaxation. The blend can then be used by the client in more stressful situations, where the same feeling of calm is desired. Because the brain gets the same aromatic signals from the essential oils through the olfactory system, it sends messages to the body to respond in much the same way as it did the last time this smell was encountered, and the body relaxes, as it did in the massage session. This kind of reaction is sometimes called a **learned odor response,** and it can be very powerful. It is useful, for instance, for clients who are afraid of flying or who have exam phobia.

The impact of smell can be extremely strong and multilayered, with a cascade of effects on memory, mood, and emotion, mediated by brain chemistry. Some of these effects are predictable and can be charted, and many others are purely personal and subjective and very difficult to predict, even from one occasion to another with the same client.

The Absorption of Essential Oils Through the Skin

Essential oils seem to penetrate the skin and enter the bloodstream without much difficulty. One study used lavender oil (*Lavandula angustifolia*) in a 2% dilution, massaged over the stomach area for 10 minutes. Traces of the essential oil's main components were found in the test subject's blood 5 minutes after the massage ended, and the concentration reached peak levels after about 20 minutes.[10] Thus, if we give a client even a 30-minute massage, she may already have absorbed a certain amount of the essential oil into her bloodstream by the time we have finished the massage. This can be very useful for the quick relief of unpleasant sensations, such as nausea or headaches.

Essential oils are ideal for skin absorption, as they have a small molecular size, are **lipophilic** (fat-soluble), and thus can penetrate the barrier of the outer layer of skin, the **stratum corneum** (Figure 4.2). Essential oil constituents also use hair follicles and sebaceous glands as shortcuts to bypass the stratum corneum, with the result that absorption in areas rich in hair and sweat glands tends to be good, even where the outer skin is thick, such as on the soles of the feet. Not all constituents are absorbed, and some may penetrate faster than others.

It is almost impossible to give an aromatherapy massage without the client inhaling the aroma of the oils being used. As a result, there has been some debate in aromatherapy circles about whether skin absorption is actually effective or if the good results during and after the session are due primarily to the effects of inhalation on the brain.[11] Research shows that essential oils do, in fact, get absorbed into the blood; oils have been investigated by pharmaceutical researchers as "skin penetration enhancers," to help topically applied medical drugs enter the bloodstream more easily.[12] However, it would seem to make sense that if only very mild dilutions of aromatic oils are applied to the skin, they may not have much of an impact on the body, and that many of the effects, especially on the nervous system, may well be due to the effect of the aromatic molecules on the brain via inhalation. But it is also clear that applying essential oils in stronger dilutions may have a significant effect on body systems.

Figure 4.3 illustrates the routes of absorption for essential oils, which parts of the body they may travel to, and their eventual excretion.

Factors That Affect Absorption

The means by which essential oils are applied to the skin also makes a significant difference in the amount that is absorbed and the effects they will have. Essential oils are by nature volatile, so they may easily evaporate from the skin, rather than be absorbed by it. An aromatherapist may choose to **occlude,** or cover, an area that has been treated with essential oils to slow the rate of evaporation, thereby increasing the skin's absorption rate.[13] The less permeable the covering is, the less oil will evaporate. This technique is fairly straightforward on a small area; it is not a problem to apply a strong dilution of essential oils to an arthritic knee and then cover it with an occlusive dressing,

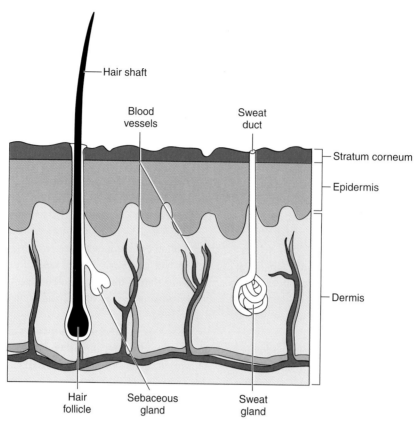

— Hair shaft

Blood
vessels

Sweat
duct

— Stratum corneum

— Epidermis

— Dermis

Hair
follicle

Sebaceous
gland

Sweat
gland

Figure 4.2 The absorption of essential oils through the skin. Essential oils are absorbed through the stratum corneum, sweat ducts, and hair follicles.

or even with plastic wrap. But it is not as easy or convenient to occlude the entire body after giving a full body massage, unless some kind of spa treatment is being used, such as a body wrap, which enfolds most of the body in some combination of sheets, plastic wrap, space blankets, and wool blankets.

Heat may also affect the rate and amount of absorption, as blood vessels dilate with warmth and can absorb essential oils more readily. Even the heat generated by massage is sufficient to speed up rates of absorption through the skin. Hot water will increase skin penetration even more dramatically, warmth and hydration of the epidermis seeming to be an ideal combination. Many massage therapists use foot baths to relax clients before a massage, or work in a spa setting where clients receive their treatment after being in a bath, sauna, or steam room.

Another factor affecting the rate and amount of essential oil absorption is the nature of the carrier used. A **carrier** is any substance used to dilute an essential oil. Essential oils diluted in an oil or lotion will take longer to permeate the skin than essential oils that are applied undiluted, or neat. Various types of carriers may slow down skin penetration more than others. Lotions made of an emulsion of oil and water seem to absorb most quickly, with plain vegetable oils

or gels being somewhat slower.[14] The slowest to absorb are heavy ointments and pastes, which are often made with waxes or saturated fats, such as cocoa butter or Shea butter. The choice of carrier depends on its function, whether to provide fast skin permeation or to nourish the skin itself, or even to give a slow release of essential oils to a localized area.

Two other variables in the rate and amount of absorption are the quality and integrity of the client's skin and the size of the area being treated. The skin of older people and young children tends to be much thinner and therefore absorbs well in a short period of time. Broken or abraded skin has a very high and unpredictable level of permeation, and the use of essential oils should generally be avoided here. As a general rule, the larger the area of skin is to which essential oils are applied, the higher the levels of absorption are overall.

Topical application has many advantages for massage therapists. It is extremely easy to incorporate aromatherapy into a hands-on treatment session, and done responsibly it has a low risk of adverse reactions and is generally well tolerated by most clients. The disadvantages are the difficulty in achieving very high levels of absorption if this is desired, the risk of skin irritation or allergic reaction, and the unpredictability of absorption rates.

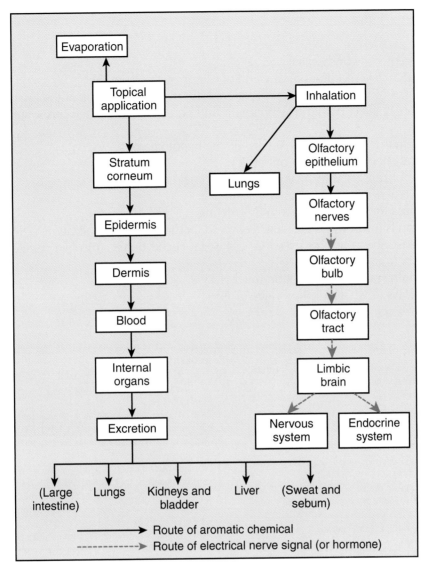

Figure 4.3 Routes of absorption of essential oils.

SUMMARY

- In holistic aromatherapy, essential oils affect the body via inhalation and skin absorption.

- In the olfactory system, aromatic molecules are picked up by specialized receptors on the ends of cilia growing out from the olfactory bulb, the organ of smell, which is an outgrowth of the brain.

- Aromatic molecules stimulate the olfactory bulb to send nerve signals to the limbic brain.

- The limbic brain can affect emotions, the sympathetic and parasympathetic branches of the nervous system, and the endocrine system.

- Due to their small molecular size, essential oils absorb easily through the skin into the bloodstream, where they may affect various body systems.

- The rate and levels of absorption are affected by temperature, the type of carrier used, skin type and quality, and whether the skin is covered after application.

Review Questions

1. Why do essential oils enter the body easily?
2. Aromatic molecules stimulate receptors on the end of cilia, growing from the _____.
3. Nerve signals stimulated by aromatic molecules are sent directly to which area of the brain?
4. Essential oils can strongly affect both the sympathetic and parasympathetic nervous systems, via the limbic brain. (T/F)
5. The _____ system is also affected by smells, via the hypothalamus.
6. Smells have a chemical effect on the brain only. (T/F)
7. The learned odor response is used by aromatherapists to help the skin. (T/F)
8. Essential oils take several hours to penetrate the skin. (T/F)
9. Essential oils can bypass the stratum corneum by entering _____ and _____.
10. Essential oil absorption is lower when the skin is covered (occluded) after application. (T/F)
11. The best carrier for fast absorption of essential oils is: (a) cocoa butter, (b) plain vegetable oil, (c) lotion made of oil and water.
12. Heat and hydration both speed up absorption rates. (T/F)
13. Broken or thin skin slows down absorption rates. (T/F)

Notes

1. The Memory of Smells, The Howard Hughes Medical Institute. Available at: www.hhmi.org. Accessed July 23, 2004.
2. Ackerman D. A Natural History of the Senses. New York: Vintage Books, 1995:10.
3. Ramachandran VS, Blakeslee S. Phantoms in the Brain. New York: William Morrow & Co., 1998.
4. Lehrner J, Eckersberger C, Walla P, et al. Ambient odor of orange in a dental office reduces anxiety and improves mood in female patients. Physiol Behav 2000;71(1-2):83–86.
5. Diego MA, Jones NA, Field T, et al. Aromatherapy positively affects mood, EEG patterns of alertness and math computations. Int J Neurosci 1998;96:217–224.
6. Campbell N, Reece J. Biology, 6th Ed. San Francisco, CA: Benjamin Cummings, 2002:962.
7. Stern R, McClintock M. Regulation of ovulation by human pheromones. Nature 1998;392:177–179.
8. Yamada K, Miura T, Mimake Y, et al. Effect of inhalation of chamomile oil vapour on plasma ACTH level in ovariectomized rats under restriction stress. Biol Pharm Bull 1996;9:1244–1246.
9. Ackerman D. A Natural History of the Senses. New York: Vintage Books, 1995:9.
10. Jager W, Buchbauer G, Jirovetz L, et al. Percutaneous absorption of Lavender oil from a massage oil. J Society Cosmet Chem 1992; 43(1):49–54.
11. Watt M. Essential oils: their lack of skin absorption, but effectiveness via inhalation. Aromatherapy Global Online Research Archive. Available at: www.nature-helps.com/agora/skinabso.htm. Accessed March 15, 2005.
12. Williams AC, Barry BW. Essential oils as novel human skin penetration enhancers. Int J Pharm 1989;57:R7–R9.
13. Fuchs N, Jager W, Lenhardt A, et al. Systemic absorption of topically applied carvone: influence of massage technique. J Society Cosmet Chem 1997;48(6):277–282.
14. Harris B, Harris R. Course notes from Advanced Clinical Aromatherapy, September 2002, Essential Oil Resource Consultants, La Martre, France.

5

Essential Oil Chemistry

This chapter discusses the main groups of chemicals that make up most essential oil components. The chemical properties of essential oils apply to later discussions on effects and safety precautions. More information on the basics of organic chemistry can be found in textbooks and aromatherapy books.[1]

Understanding Chemical Compounds

Like all matter, essential oils are collections of chemical compounds. A few oils are simple in their makeup, but most of them contain a large and diverse range of chemicals. We study the chemistry of essential oils for various reasons:

- To understand generally how and why aromatherapy works
- To understand safety and essential oil purity issues more clearly
- To be able to communicate with medical doctors and other trained scientists and explain in their own language the benefits of aromatherapy
- To explain the actions of specific essential oils that we notice in practice
- To give us insight about the possible uses and hazards of unfamiliar essential oils that have familiar chemical components

Understanding the chemistry of essential oils provides a scientific basis for aromatherapy that helps us to establish it as a serious discipline with potential applications in the medical field as well as alternative health care. However, by focusing on their main components and ignoring their complexity and versatility, one can oversimplify the properties of essential oils. In the words of Simon Mills, a leading herbalist, "any assumption about the action of a plant that relies solely on the basis of the action of a constituent should be resisted. It should always be recalled that the action of the whole plant is more than the action of its parts."[2] In other words, the effect of any essential oil is due to the collective interactions of its chemical components.

When we examine the chemistry of an essential oil, we tend to focus on the largest two or three compounds. However, trace amounts of 0.001% may have a larger influence on the smell of an oil. Often there is no correlation between the percentage concentration of a chemical and its impact on the odor of an essential oil. If these trace amounts can have such a huge influence on smell, it is possible that they may have an equally large effect on the oil's therapeutic properties.

The Production and Composition of Chemical Compounds in Plants

Plants absorb water (H_2O) from the ground and carbon dioxide (CO_2) from the air, and use the energy of sunlight in the process of **photosynthesis** to split up these molecules and recombine them to form **glucose,** a simple sugar (Figure 5.1). The plant uses glucose to make products of metabolism called **primary metabolites,** such as carbohydrates, proteins, and lipids. All plants produce these primary metabolites, which are needed by most living organisms to survive and grow. Many plants also make **secondary metabolites,** which include color pigments and essential oils. Secondary metabolites vary from plant to plant and are not essential for the plant's survival, though they may increase its strength and competitiveness. According to Dewick, author of *Medicinal Natural Products—A Biosynthetic Approach,* "in the vast majority of cases the function of these compounds and their benefit to the organism is not yet known . . . but it is logical to assume that all do play some vital role for the well-being of the producer. It is this area of secondary metabolism that provides most of the pharmacologically active natural products."[3]

As Figure 5.1 shows, the main building blocks of primary and secondary metabolites are the atoms in water and carbon dioxide, in other words, carbon (C), oxygen (O), and hydrogen (H). Most molecules in essential oils are made from these three elements, though small amounts of sulphur and nitrogen are also sometimes found.

Plants make secondary metabolites through a long series of steps, modifying the molecules slightly in each step. A series of steps with a distinct sequence is called a pathway. The two most common pathways that produce essential oil components are the **mevalonate pathway,** which starts off in the plant with mevalonic acid, and the **shikimate pathway,** which starts with shikimic acid. (The acetate pathway also yields some essential oil components, but it is primarily involved in making vegetable oil constituents.) Because the compounds in essential oils have evolved along these various pathways, sometimes two compounds have molecules that are structurally similar to each other but differ in their properties because of their different origins.

Carbon Compounds

Organic chemistry is the branch of chemistry concerned with substances that have carbon in their structures. All living things—including people, animals, and plants—are composed of carbon compounds. Essential oils, being plant extracts, are also organic substances with carbon forming the backbone of all their molecules. Carbon atoms have an affinity for bonding together, creating chains or rings, and bonding with hydrogen atoms, making **hydrocarbons**—molecules consisting only of hydrogen and carbon atoms. Short chains, with few carbon atoms, tend to be gases, like methane or butane; medium chains, with up to 20 carbon atoms, are liquids, like essential oils; and long chains create solids, like rubber. Molecules found in essential oils are generally 20 carbon atoms or less because the bigger and heavier a molecule is, the less likely it is to be volatile—a necessary characteristic for an aromatic substance.

A **functional group** is a different atom or group of atoms added to the hydrocarbon structure, and one that is

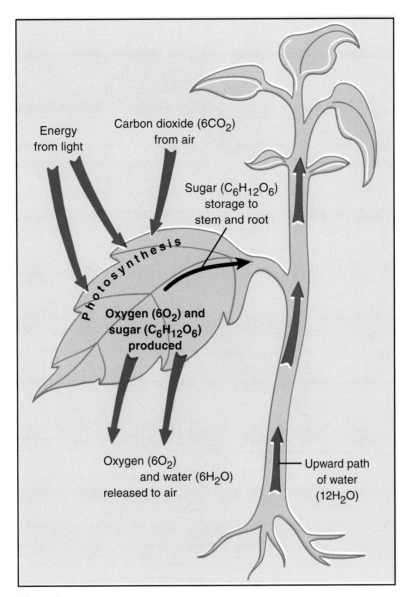

Figure 5.1 The process of photosynthesis.

more likely to create or undergo chemical reactions. In essential oils, functional groups usually contain oxygen. The molecules in an essential oil that contain oxygen affect the aroma, the volatility, and the properties of the oil. Essential oils that contain oxygenated compounds tend to be less volatile and more viscous, or thick, than oils with unoxygenated hydrocarbons. Also, oxygenated molecules tend to be more **hydrophilic,** or soluble in water, than those without oxygen, which are more **lipophilic,** or soluble in fats.[4]

Chemical Groups in Essential Oils

Two main groups of compounds are found in essential oils. **Terpenoids** are formed along the mevalonate pathway in the plant; this pathway is the most common way for essential oil components to be made. All of them have molecules based on the **isoprene unit,** a branched chain of five carbon atoms. These building blocks join together to form molecules with 10, 15, or 20 carbon atoms—all multiples of the five-carbon isoprene unit. They may have functional groups attached to the molecule. Terpenoids are also called **aliphatic compounds.**

Phenylpropanoids are a much smaller group of compounds formed along the shikimate pathway. All of them have molecules based on the **phenyl ring,** a ring of six carbon atoms with stable bonds between them.

Although the pathways of development for terpenoids and phenylpropanoids are quite distinct, the chemicals formed along these different pathways may have similar structures, due to the functional groups. As a result, they can be grouped together in chemical groups. For example, in the group of chemicals called aldehydes, there are terpenoid aldehydes and phenylpropanoid aldehydes. Some chemical groups contain only terpenoids, some only phenylpropanoids, while some groups have components formed along both pathways.

Hydrocarbons

As already mentioned, hydrocarbons are compounds consisting of only hydrogen and carbon. Their individual names end in "-ene," as in limonene. They are all terpenoids.

Monoterpene Hydrocarbons. **Monoterpenes** are the smallest (two isoprene units, so 10 carbon atoms) and therefore the lightest molecules in essential oil chemistry. Because essential oils are extracted by distillation, which favors small, very volatile molecules, monoterpenes are the most common chemical group among essential oils. They are found in high quantities in the citrus oils, such as lemon (*Citrus limon*) and the oils from the needles of conifer trees, such as pine (*Pinus sylvestris*). Figure 5.2 shows two diagrams of the δ-limonene molecule, an example of a monoterpene found in citrus expressed oils and pine essential oil.

Monoterpenes have the following effects and characteristics:

- *Skin penetration.* Because hydrocarbons are fat-soluble, monoterpenes can penetrate the skin very easily; they have a fluidizing effect on the lipid structure of the stratum corneum.[5] Therefore, essential oils high in monoterpenes could have a faster physiological effect than other oils when applied to the skin because they may absorb more quickly into the bloodstream.

- *Immune stimulation.* Animal tests show that applying monoterpenes significantly increased white blood cell production, indicating the potential of these compounds to boost the immune system.[6] It is common in many countries to make drinks or syrups of citrus fruits like lemon, or of needles, especially pine, to help the body fight off infections.

- *Antiseptic action.* Citrus and pine oils have been used for a long time as effective cleansers and antiseptics. The monoterpenes in these oils provide a natural antibacterial action.[7]

- *Volatility.* Because of their small size, monoterpenes are extremely volatile, making them useful for respiratory problems and for deodorizing air.

- *Oxygenation leading to skin irritation.* Citrus, needle, and juniper berry oils, all very high in monoterpenes, are prone to spoiling because monoterpenes react very easily with oxygen.[8] It is important to keep these oils in full bottles, tightly closed, to avoid reaction with oxygen because old oils with oxygenated monoterpenes are more likely to irritate skin than fresh ones.

Some individual monoterpenes have specific actions. Limonene, for example, has been studied for its ability to dissolve gallstones when taken internally,[9] as well as its tendency to improve hepatic, or liver, function.[10] Citruses have long been used in herbalism and cooking as **cholagogues,** substances that have the ability to stimulate the release of bile to help digestion. Studies show myrcene to have **analgesic,** or pain-killing, qualities.[11]

Sesquiterpene Hydrocarbons. **Sesquiterpenes** have 15 carbon atoms, or three isoprene units. Slightly less volatile than monoterpenes because of their larger size, they are still quite common among essential oil constituents. Figure 5.3 shows a diagram of farnesene, an example of a sesquiterpene, in its abbreviated form. Farnesene is found in rose essential oil (*Rosa damascena*).

Sesquiterpenes have the following effects and characteristics:

- *Anti-inflammatory effects.* Many studies have shown the anti-inflammatory and anti-allergenic properties of German chamomile (*Matricaria recutita*), which contains high levels of the sesquiterpenes chamazulene and bisabolene. A member of the same family, *Helichrysum italicum*, or everlasting, is also high in sesquiterpenes and shares these properties.[12]

- *Calming effects.* Sesquiterpenes may have a calming, hypotensive action. Essential oils high in sesquiterpenes traditionally have been used to help relieve stress and tension.

Diterpene Hydrocarbons. **Diterpenes** rarely occur in essential oils because they are rarely volatile, due to their larger

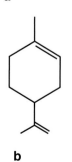

a

b

Figure 5.2 A monoterpene hydrocarbon. δ-Limonene is a constituent of citrus (*Citrus* ssp.) expressed oils and pine (*Pinus* ssp.) essential oils. (**a**) Carbon and hydrogen atoms. (**b**) Carbon skeleton.

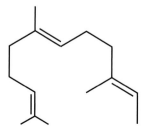

Figure 5.3 A sesquiterpene hydrocarbon. Farnesene is a constituent of German chamomile (*Matricaria recutita*) essential oil.

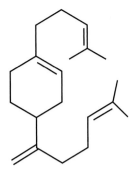

Figure 5.4 A diterpene hydrocarbon. Camphorene is a constituent of camphor (*Cinnamomum camphora*) essential oil.

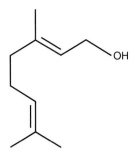

Figure 5.5 A monoterpene alcohol. Geraniol is a constituent of geranium (*Pelargonium graveolens*) essential oil.

size (20 carbon atoms, or four isoprene units). Hydrocarbons with molecules larger than this are not found in essential oils, although they are important starting materials for steroids, cholesterols, and various vitamins. Figure 5.4 shows camphorene, a diterpene.

Alcohols

Alcohols are terpenoids with a functional group of oxygen and hydrogen (OH), which is known as a **hydroxyl group.** Because terpenes can be monoterpenes, sesquiterpenes, or diterpenes, depending on their size, alcohols that are based on these hydrocarbons can also be monoterpene alcohols (10 carbon atoms), sesquiterpene alcohols (15 carbon atoms), or diterpene alcohols (20 carbon atoms). Because they are oxygenated compounds, they are more soluble in water than the hydrocarbons. Their names end in "-ol," for example, geraniol. They are generally regarded in aromatherapy as the safest essential oil components, and oils rich in alcohols are often used with young children and with the very old or frail.[13]

Monoterpene Alcohols. **Monoterpene alcohols** are common essential oil constituents. The more popular essential oils among aromatherapists often have high levels of monoterpene alcohols, perhaps because of their usefulness combined with their reputation for mildness and safety. Figure 5.5 shows geraniol, a monoterpene alcohol, with its –OH functional group. Geraniol is found in geranium (*Pelargonium graveolens*), palmarosa (*Cymbopogon martinii*), and many other essential oils.

Monoterpene alcohols have the following effects and characteristics:

* *Antimicrobial action.* Monoterpene alcohols are found to be effective against a variety of microorganisms, especially bacteria.[14] **Primary alcohols** (those with the hydroxyl group bonded to a carbon at the end of a chain) such as nerol, citronellol, and geraniol have also been found to be antifungal, an important discovery for skin fungi, such as athlete's foot, in which essential oil remedies need to be mild enough to be easily tolerated by the skin.[15]

* *Immune support.* Many alcohols are considered to be immunostimulant, especially on a long-term basis, because of their mildness and lack of toxicity.

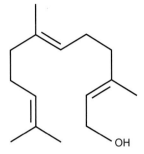

Figure 5.6 A sesquiterpene alcohol. Farnesol is a constituent of rose (*Rosa damascena* or *centifolia*) essential oil.

Individual monoterpene alcohols have been found to be sedative and hypotensive, for example, linalool,[16] while others are antispasmodic, for example, menthol and borneol.[17]

Sesquiterpene Alcohols. **Sesquiterpene alcohols** are sesquiterpenes with a hydroxyl group attached. Figure 5.6 shows farnesol, a sesquiterpene alcohol found in rose (*Rosa damascena*) essential oil.

Sesquiterpene alcohols have the following effects and characteristics:

* *Anti-inflammatory action.* Essential oils high in sesquiterpene alcohols, such as German chamomile (*Matricaria recutita*) and sandalwood (*Santalum album*), have been used in various cultures for many years to ease inflammation of both the skin and internal tissue.[18]

* *Antispasmodic effect.* Extensive studies have been done on the antispasmodic qualities of German chamomile, with the conclusion that the antispasmodic effect is due to the sesquiterpene alcohol a-bisabolol.[19]

* *Sedative action.* Many essential oils rich in sesquiterpene alcohols are used in aromatherapy for calming and sedative effects. Investigations show that these are definite chemical effects.[20]

Diterpene Alcohols. **Diterpene alcohols** are rarely found in essential oils because of their larger size. Some diterpene alcohols, such as sclareol, may have an influence on the endocrine system, perhaps having some effects similar to estrogen; however, these effects are not firmly documented.

Phenols

Phenols are hydrocarbons with a hydroxyl group attached, making them structurally similar to the alcohols. But instead of having a skeleton made of isoprene units (the branched chains with five carbons), the phenols have their hydroxyl group attached to a phenyl ring. Phenols evolve along the mevalonate pathway for terpenoids; these are called **aromatic phenols.** They are also formed along the more unusual shikimate pathway; these are called **phenylpropanoid phenols.** Essential oils high in phenols tend to have aggressive, penetrating smells, especially the phenylpropanoids. Like alcohols, their names end in "–ol." Figure 5.7 shows thymol, a phenol, with its functional group –OH. Thymol is found in a chemotype of thyme essential oil (*Thymus vulgaris* CT thymol).

Phenols have the following effects and characteristics:

- *Strong antiseptic action.* Oils high in phenols are among the strongest antiseptics in aromatherapeutic use. It is no accident that aromatic plants high in phenols, such as thyme (*Thymus vulgaris*) and oregano (*Origanum vulgare*), were traditionally burnt in hospitals as fumigants and disinfectants. Modern studies reinforce this view.[21]

- *Antifungal action.* A lot of research shows the significant topical antifungal properties of phenols.[22]

- *Anti-inflammatory effect.* Essential oils high in phenols, as well as the pure phenolic compounds themselves, have been shown in both laboratory tests and personal observation to be strongly anti-inflammatory, especially in the treatment of rheumatic inflammation or insect bites. Their action appears to inhibit the synthesis of **prostaglandins,** chemicals the body produces during the inflammatory response.[23]

- *Skin irritation.* One of the major risks with phenol-rich essential oils is that of irritation to skin and mucous membranes. These oils usually are not applied undiluted to the skin, and they generally are used in diffusion only in small amounts after being blended with other milder oils.

- *Hepatotoxic effect.* Research shows that phenol-containing essential oils may cause **hepatotoxicity,** or liver damage, when used in large amounts or for long periods of time.[24] However, other tests suggest that they may actually protect the liver against damage when used in small amounts.[25] It is probably best to use these oils in low dosages for short time periods and to substitute essential oils that have a high content of alcohols when longer-term use is required.

Aldehydes

Aldehydes have a **carbonyl group** (a carbon atom and an oxygen atom double-bonded and attached to a carbon atom on the hydrocarbon skeleton). Aldehydes may evolve as terpenoids, with both 10-carbon and 15-carbon foundations (monoterpene aldehydes and sesquiterpene aldehydes), or they may be phenylpropanoid aldehydes. **Terpenoid aldehydes** and **phenylpropanoid aldehydes** share some characteristics, but they also have significant differences, especially in fragrance and safety. All aldehydes have a powerful fragrance, even in small amounts, but the aliphatic aldehydes, such as citral, neral, and geranial, have a lemony odor, while the phenylpropanoid aldehydes, such as cinnamic aldehyde, tend to be more pungent and spicy. Their names end in "–al," as in citral, or in "aldehyde," as in cinnamic aldehyde. Figure 5.8a shows citronellal, a terpenoid aldehyde found in melissa (*Melissa officinalis*) and citronella (*Cymbopogon citratus*) essential oils. Figure 5.8b shows cinnamic aldehyde, a phenylpropanoid aldehyde found in cinnamon (*Cinnamomum verum*) essential oil.

Aldehydes have the following effects and characteristics:

- *Antimicrobial action.* Both types of aldehyde seem to have a powerful fungicidal effect, though typically the phenylpropanoid aldehydes have a stronger effect.[26] Many essential oils high in aldehydes, such as lemongrass (*Cymbopogon citratus*), have a recognized antibacterial action in aromatherapy, which is borne out by laboratory studies.[27] Aldehydes react very easily with oxygen, and studies show that oxidized aldehydes lose much of their antibacterial effect, so essential oils used for this purpose should be as fresh as possible.[28] Aldehydes may also have an antiviral effect. This is suggested by the research done on melissa (*Melissa officinalis*) as an effective remedy for herpes simplex, as well as by research on other plant extracts high in aldehydes.[29]

- *Sedative effect.* The sedative effect is strongest in the terpenoid, lemony smelling aldehydes.[30]

- *Skin irritation.* Most of the case histories citing skin irritation from aldehydes involve cinnamic aldehyde or cinnamon essential oil.[31] However, anecdotal evidence from other aromatherapists suggests that many aldehydes of both types can cause skin irritation if used in high doses.

- *Possible hormonal effects.* Some research seems to suggest that aldehydes in general and citral in particular may have an effect on the endocrine system. Female rats treated with citral showed a marked decrease in ovarian follicles, and this study states that "the observations raised serious

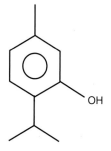

Figure 5.7 A phenol. Thymol is a constituent of thyme (*Thymus vulgaris* CT thymol) essential oil.

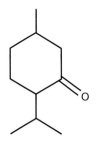

Figure 5.9 A ketone. Menthone is a constituent of peppermint (*Mentha piperita*) essential oil.

a

b

Figure 5.8 Aldehydes. (**a**) Citronellal is a terpenoid aldehyde, a constituent of melissa (*Melissa officinalis*) essential oil. (**b**) Cinnamic aldehyde is a phenylpropanoid aldehyde, a constituent of cinnamon essential oil.

questions regarding the effects of citral on human reproduction."[32] Another study showed that the topical application of citral had an effect on sebum production due to an increase in testosterone levels,[33] while a third study showed that citral had "estrogenic activity."[34] All of these studies used citral in extremely high doses, and as it is not restricted in any way, in foods, perfumes, and so on, it is obviously not regarded as a particular hazard.

Ketones

Ketones are structurally similar to aldehydes in that they have a carbonyl group, but in ketones the carbonyl group is bonded to the hydrocarbon structure in a different way. Like most other terpenoids, ketones occur in various sizes, but by far the most common are monoterpene ketones. Their names end in "-one," like fenchone, with the exception of one of the most common ketones, camphor. Figure 5.9 shows menthone, a ketone found in peppermint (*Mentha piperita*) essential oil.

Ketones have the following effects and characteristics:

- *Mucolytic effect.* Many ketones are **mucolytic,** they break down and liquefy mucus. This effect is useful for infections that cause thick, sticky mucus in the respiratory system.

- *Antimicrobial action.* They show both antibacterial and antiviral actions.[35]

- *Skin-healing effect.* Traditionally, essential oils that contain significant amounts of ketones have been used in skin care and specifically to treat scarring. Such oils include rock rose (*Cistus ladaniferus*), helichrysum (*Helichrysum italicum*), and jasmine (*Jasminum grandiflorum*).

- *Toxicity.* Research on ketones and many case histories of accidental ingestion of ketone-rich essential oils indicate the possible negative effects of this chemical group, such as hepatotoxicity and **neurotoxicity,** or damage to the nervous system. Various cases have been reported of intoxication and convulsions from the ingestion of commercial preparations of sage (*Salvia officinalis*), hyssop (*Hyssopus officinalis*), thuja (*Arbor vitae*), a type of cedar (*Chamaecyparis thyoides*), Spanish sage (*Salvia lavandulaefolia*), and camphorated cottonseed oil. These negative responses were shown to be caused by extreme stimulation of the central nervous system.[36] Other studies suggest that some ketones may be damaging to the liver.[37] However, there are several ketones—such as jasmone, fenchone, verbenone, and carvone—that are nontoxic. Care should be taken with any essential oils that are high in the more toxic ketones—thujone, pulegone, and camphor—because some evidence indicates they may accumulate in body tissues because of their slow metabolism, thus leading to chronic toxicity.[38]

Esters

Esters are formed by reactions between alcohols (or phenols) and carboxylic acid. This reaction can go both ways; in other words, an alcohol plus an acid will yield an ester plus water, and an ester will also react with water to yield an alcohol and an acid. For this reason, esters always occur in essential oils together with their related alcohol. For example, linalyl acetate is found with linalool and geranyl acetate with geraniol. Because of this reversible reaction, essential oils high in esters can degrade with time, especially if there is water in the oil.

Esters are the most diverse group of chemical compounds in essential oils, though there are relatively few oils in which they are present in large quantities. Esters are prized in perfumery because they give essential oils a pleasant floral or fruity scent. Both terpenoid and phenylpropanoid esters exist. They have double names, the first from their derivative

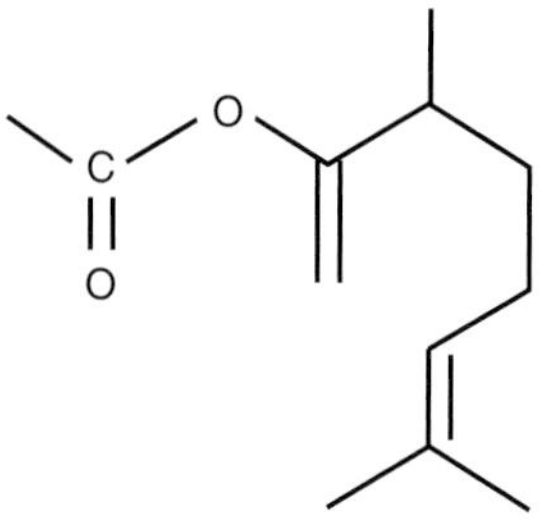

Figure 5.10 An ester. Linalyl acetate is a constituent of lavender (*Lavandula angustifolia*) essential oil.

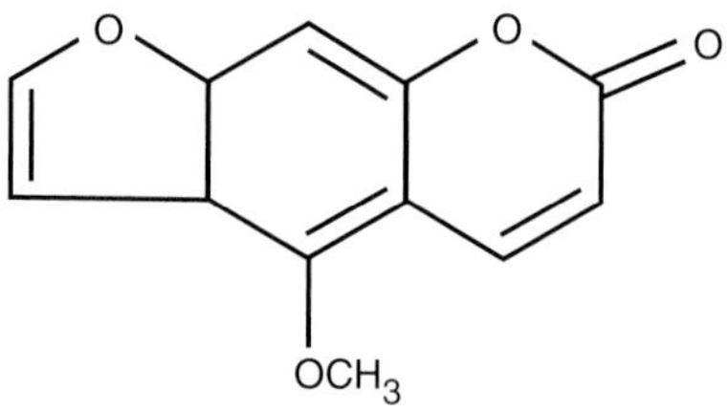

Figure 5.11 A lactone. The furocoumarin bergapten is a constituent of bergamot (*Citrus x bergamia*) expressed oil.

alcohol, the second from the acid. These names always end in "-yl" and "-ate," as in bornyl acetate. Figure 5.10 shows linalyl acetate, an ester found in lavender (*Lavandula angustifolia*), clary sage (*Salvia sclarea*), petitgrain (*Citrus aurantium* var. *amara*), and many other essential oils.

Esters have the following effects and characteristics:

- *Antispasmodic effect.* Essential oils that are high in esters, such as lavender (*Lavandula angustifolia*) or petitgrain (*Citrus aurantium var. amara*), often are used in aromatherapy treatments to help with muscular spasm.

- *Sedative effect.* Many studies show the calming, sedative qualities of both essential oils high in esters and the ester components themselves.[39]

- *Adaptogenic action.* Components and oils are considered to be **adaptogenic** when they help the body return to homeostasis and to respond to stress. This may mean that they can produce seemingly contradictory results at different times: warming or cooling, sedative or stimulant. Oils high in esters appear to have this ability quite markedly.

- *Anti-inflammatory effect.* Studies done on linalyl acetate clearly show it to have anti-inflammatory properties,[40] and those essential oils having a high percentage of esters are often used as anti-inflammatories in aromatherapy.

Most esters are extremely safe and mild, with little risk of skin irritation or toxicity. However, methyl salicylate, the major constituent of wintergreen (*Gaultheria procumbens*) and sweet birch (*Betula lenta*) essential oils, does seem to pose some risks. It is extremely analgesic and antispasmodic,[41] but even with topical application care should be taken because it can increase the effects of any anticoagulant medication being taken, thereby heightening the risk of hemorrhage. There are also some concerns about possible long-term toxicity.[42]

Lactones

Lactones are esters in which the functional group has been incorporated into a carbon ring. Lactones are common in plants, but the large, heavy molecules rarely come through the distillation process. They are most commonly found in expressed citrus oils or in some solvent extracted oils. There have been cases reported of contact dermatitis with lactones.[43] Their name endings are variable. Certain

sesquiterpene lactones have been found to have antibacterial and antifungal actions.[44]

Coumarins and furocoumarins are types of lactones. They are important to identify in aromatic oils because they often are **photosensitizing,** or **phototoxic,** making the skin much more sensitive to ultraviolet (UV) light.[45] This makes the user more at risk, not just for sunburn but also for skin cancers. These compounds can be phototoxic in small amounts. Bergamot (*Citrus x bergamia*) has only about 3% of the furocoumarin bergapten, but it is considered strongly photosensitizing. Figure 5.11 shows bergapten.

Ethers

Ethers have an oxygen atom linking two carbon atoms in their molecules. Most are phenylpropanoid ethers, and like most compounds that evolve along the shikimate pathway they tend to have both strong aromas and effects. Figure 5.12 shows anethole, a phenylpropanoid ether found in fennel (*Foeniculum vulgare*) and aniseed (*Pimpinella anisum*) essential oils.

Ethers have similar effects and characteristics as esters:

- *Antispasmodic and carminative effects.* Traditionally, many of the oils high in ethers, such as basil (*Ocimum basilicum*), tarragon (*Artemesia dracunculus*), and fennel (*Foeniculum vulgare*), have been used as **carminatives,** substances that treat colic and other digestive spasms.[46]

- *Hormonal effect.* Research shows that anethole, the main constituent of fennel (*Foeniculum vulgare*) and aniseed (*Pimpinella anisum*) essential oils, has estrogenic effects.[47]

- *Toxicity.* Phenylpropanoid ethers, the most common being apiole, myristicin, and safrole, may be toxic to the liver[48] and the nervous system. Terpenoid ethers, such as methyl chavicol, methyl eugenol, and anethole, are generally safe, but they are still considered very powerful in effect and are not suitable for use in high dosages for long periods of time.

Oxides

Oxides have an oxygen atom within a carbon ring structure. They usually evolve from an alcohol and are often named after it, such as bisabolol oxide. The exception in essential oils is 1,8 cineole, which is a common oxide found in eucalyptus (*Eucalyptus* ssp.), rosemary (*Rosmarinus officinalis*), and many other essential oils. Most of the research on oxides re-

OCH₃

CH ═ CH ─ CH₃

Figure 5.12 An ether. The phenylpropanoid anethole is a constituent of fennel (*Foeniculum vulgare*) essential oil.

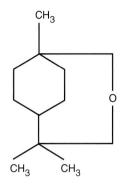

Figure 5.13 An oxide. 1,8 cineole (eucalyptol) is a constituent of eucalyptus (*Eucalyptus globulus* or *radiata*) essential oil.

lates to this component. Figure 5.13 shows 1,8 cineole (sometimes called eucalyptol).

1,8 cineole has the following effects and characteristics:

- *Expectorant action.* 1,8 cineole is extremely volatile, and the essential oils containing large amounts of it are generally recognized in aromatherapy as having a beneficial effect on the respiratory system in general, particularly in helping to clear mucus. Studies show its **expectorant,** or phlegm-loosening, properties.[49]
- *Stimulant effect.* Research shows that inhalation of 1,8 cineole increases motor activity.[50]
- *Skin penetration.* 1,8 cineole seems to be an even more potent agent for skin penetration than limonene, making oils high in this chemical ideal for fast absorption.[51]

- *Antispasmodic effect.* Some research suggests that 1,8 cineole may be useful as a relaxant for smooth muscle.[52]

Oxides are generally regarded as safe for topical use. There has been some suggestion that oils high in 1,8 cineole may be skin irritating, but the research does not support this claim.[53]

Table 5.1 summarizes the effects and characteristics of the major chemical groups and gives examples found in essential oils. It is as comprehensive as possible. Many constituents have similar name endings (e.g., the alcohols and the phenols) but very different properties and safety indications.

Table 5.1 Major Chemical Groups in Essential Oils

Name of Chemical Group	Examples in Essential Oils	Effects, Characteristics, and Safety Issues	Essential Oils High in These Compounds
Monoterpenes	α-pinene, β-pinene, camphene, carene, dipentene, fenchene, limonene, menthene, myrcene, ocimene, p-cymene, phellandrene, sabinene, terpinene, terpinolene, thujene, tricyclene	Skin penetrating, tonic and immune stimulating, antiseptic, volatile **Possibly skin irritating when old**	All expressed citrus oils, pine (*Pinus* ssp.), cypress (*Cupressus sempervirens*), fir (*Abies* ssp.), spruce (*Picea* ssp.), juniper berry (*Juniperus communis*)
Sesquiterpenes	Aromadendrene, bergamotene, bisabolene, bourbonene, bulnesene, cadinene, caryophyllene, cedrene, chamazulene, copaene, cubene, curcumene, elemene, farnesene, guaiene, gurjunene, humulene, italicene, longifolene, muurolene, patchoulene, santalene, selinene, seychellene, viridiflorene, ylangene, zingiberene	Anti-inflammatory, calming	Ginger (*Zingiber officinalis*), German chamomile (*Matricaria recutita*)
Monoterpene alcohols (monoterpenols)	Borneol, carveol, citronellol, fenchol, geraniol, lavandulol, linalol, menthol, myrtenol, nerol, pinocarveol, pulegol, terpinen-4-ol, terpineol, thuyan-4-ol	Antimicrobial, immune supportive (some are sedative, hypotensive, and antispasmodic)	Rose (*Rosa* ssp.), thyme CT linalool (*Thymus vulgaris* CT linalool), geranium (*Pelargonium graveolens*), rosewood (*Aniba roseadora*)

(Continued)

Table 5.1	(Continued)

Name of Chemical Group	Examples in Essential Oils	Effects, Characteristics, and Safety Issues	Essential Oils High in These Compounds
Sesquiterpene alcohols (sesquiterpenols)	Atlantol, bisabolol, cadinol, carotol, caryophyllene alcohol, cedrol, elemol, eudesmol, farnesol, globulol, guaiol, muurolol, nerolidol, patchoulol, pogostol, santolol, spathulenol, viridiflorol	Anti-inflammatory, antispasmodic, sedative	Sandalwood (*Santalum album*), nerolina (*Melaleuca quinquenervia* CT nerolidol)
Diterpene alcohols (diterpenols)	Manool, salviol, sclareol	Possible hormonal effects	Carrot seed (*Daucus carota*)
Phenols	Carvacrol, chavicol, cresol, eugenol, guiacol, iso-eugenol, thymol	Strongly antiseptic, antifungal, anti-inflammatory **Skin and mucous membrane irritating** **Possibly hepatotoxic**	Aniseed (*Pimpinella anisum*), star anise (*Illicium verum*), cinnamon leaf (*Cinnamomum verum*), clove (*Syzygium aromaticum*), fennel seed (*Foeniculum vulgare*), thyme CT thymol (*Thymus vulgaris CT thymol*)
Aldehydes	Acetaldehyde, anisaldehyde, benzaldehyde, caproic aldehyde, citral, citronellal, cinnamaldehyde, cuminaldehyde, decanal, farnesal, geranial, myrtenal, neral, nonanal, perillaldehyde, phellandral, piperonal, sinensal, teresantal, valeranal, vanillin	Antimicrobial terpenoids are sedative and possibly have hormonal effects **Skin irritating in large amounts**	Melissa (*Melissa officinalis*), lemongrass (*Cymbopogon citratus*), may chang (*Litsea cubeba*), *Eucalyptus citriadora*, lemon verbena (*Lippia citriadora*), cinnamon (*Cinnamomum verum*)
Ketones	Acetophenone, atlantone artemisia ketone, camphor, carvone, cryptone, dione, fenchone, ionone, irone, isopinocamphone, jasmone, menthone, methyl heptone, nootkatone, octanone, pinocamphone, pinocarvone, piperitone, pulegone, tagetone, thujone, valeranone, verbenone	Mucolytic, antimicrobial, skin healing **Hepatotoxic and neurotoxic**	Camphor (*Cinnamomum , camphora*), caraway (*Carum carvi*), dill (*Anethum graveolens*), sage (*Salvia officinalis*), spearmint (*Mentha spicata*)
Esters	There are too many to list completely. Some common examples are: benzyl benzoate, butyl angelate, cinnamyl acetate, eugenyl acetate, geranyl acetate, incensyl actetate, lavandulyl acetate, linalyl acetate, methyl anthranilate, methyl salicylate, neryl actetate, terpinyl acetate	Antispasmodic, sedative, adaptogenic, anti-inflammatory	Roman chamomile (*Chamaemelum nobile*), cardamon (*Elletaria cardamomum*), lavender (*Lavandula angustifolia*), clary sage (*Salvia sclarea*), sweet birch (*Betula lenta*), wintergreen (*Gaultheria procumbens*)
Lactones	Achilline, ambrettolide, atlantolactone, costuslactone, costunolide, isoatlantolactone, nepeta lactone	Some are antifungal and antibacterial **May be skin irritating**	Only found in essential oils in small amounts
Coumarins	Aesculatine, angelicin, aurapten, bergamottin, bergapten, bergaptol, citropten, coumarin, imperatorin, osthole, psoralen, umbelliferone, visnadin	**May be phototoxic**	Only found in essential oils in small amounts
Ethers	Anethole, apiol, asarone, chamospiroether, elemicin, isosafrole, methyl carvacrol, methyl chavicol (estragole), methyl eugenol, myristicin, phenylethyl methyl ether, safrole	Antispasmodic and carminative Anethole has an estrogenic effect **Possibly hepatotoxic**	Tarragon (*Artemesia dracunculus*), basil (*Ocimum basilicum* CT methyl chavicol), fennel (*Foeniculum vulgare*)

(Continued)

Table 5.1	(Continued)		

Name of Chemical Group	Examples in Essential Oils	Effects, Characteristics, and Safety Issues	Essential Oils High in These Compounds
Oxides	1,8 cineole, ascaridole, bisabolol oxide, bisabolone oxide, caryophyllene oxide, geranyl oxide, linalol oxide, nerol oxide, manool oxide, pinene oxide, piperitone oxide, rose oxide, sclareol oxide	Expectorant, stimulant, skin penetrating, antispasmodic	*Eucalyptus* ssp., spike lavender (*Lavandula latifolia*)
Acids	Anisic acid, atlantic acid, benzoic acid, cinnamic acid, citronellic acid, geranic acid, lauric acid, myristic acid, rosmarinic acid, valerenic acid, vetiveric acid		Only found in essential oils in small amounts

SUMMARY

* Essential oils are very complex chemically, and some oils have hundreds of different components.

* Even trace amounts of certain components may influence the aroma and effects of the essential oil.

* Essential oil chemistry is studied to help understand how aromatherapy works, safety and purity issues, and the actions and possible hazards of essential oils, and to help communicate with medical and scientific professionals.

* The plant uses sunlight, water, and carbon dioxide in photosynthesis to make glucose. The glucose is then synthesized into various useful products, including essential oils.

* Most essential oil components are made from carbon, oxygen, and hydrogen. A few may also contain sulphur or nitrogen.

* Essential oils molecules are produced along two different pathways in the plant, the mevalonate pathway and the shikimate pathway, resulting in terpenoid and phenylpropanoid components. Phenylpropanoids are generally stronger in both aroma and effects.

* The basis of an essential oil molecule is a chain or a ring of carbon atoms, with hydrogen atoms attached. Hydrocarbons are molecules made only of carbon and hydrogen; they include monoterpenes, sesquiterpenes, and diterpenes.

* The addition of another atom or group of atoms to the hydrocarbon changes the molecule; additions are called functional groups.

* When functional groups are added to hydrocarbons, they create groups of chemicals called alcohols, phenols, aldehydes, ketones, esters, lactones, ethers, and oxides. These groups have distinct properties.

Review Questions

1. The main elements in essential oil molecules are carbon, _____, and _____.
2. The most common essential oil components are called terpenoids. (T/F)
3. Essential oil molecules are all organic; in other words, they all contain carbon. (T/F)
4. Essential oil constituents are never soluble in water. (T/F)
5. Monoterpenes are found in large quantities in the essential oils from these plants: (a) flowers, (b) woods and resins, (c) citruses and needles of trees, (d) roots.
6. Essential oils high in monoterpenes and aldehydes deteriorate quickly because they react with _____.
7. Alcohols are generally: (a) very skin irritating, (b) hepatotoxic, (c) to be avoided during pregnancy, (d) very mild in all cases.
8. Phenols are strong antiseptics and safe on the skin as well. (T/F)
9. Many aldehydes smell like: (a) turpentine, (b) lemon, (c) antiseptics (d) flowers.

10. Esters are: (a) antispasmodic and sedative, (b) antiseptic and stimulating, (c) analgesic and skin irritating.

11. Coumarins are phototoxic; in other words, they cause the skin to _____.

12. 1,8 cineole is an _____ commonly found in eucalyptus and rosemary.

Notes

1. These books include: Bowles J. The Basic Chemistry of Aromatherapeutic Essential Oils. St. Leonards, Australia: Allen & Unwin, 2003; Price S. Aromatherapy Workbook. London, UK: Thorsons, 1998; Clarke S. Essential Chemistry for Safe Aromatherapy. Edinburgh UK: Churchill Livingstone, 2002.

2. Mills S. The Essential Book of Herbal Medicine. London, UK: Arkana, 1993.

3. Dewick P. Medicinal Natural Products—A Biosynthetic Approach, 2nd Ed. Hoboken, NJ: John Wiley and Sons, 2002:8.

4. Harris B, Harris R. Advanced clinical aromatherapy. Course notes, Essential Oil Resource Consultants, La Martre, France, September 2002.

5. Takayama K, Nagai T. Limonene and related compounds as potential skin penetration promoters. Drug Dev Ind Pharm 1994;20(4):677–684.

6. Raphael TJ, Kuttan G. Immunomodulatory activity of naturally occurring monoterpenes carvone, limonene, and perillic acid. Immunopharmacol Immunotoxicol 2003;25(2):285–294.

7. Szőke E, Máthé I, Blunden G, et al. Constituents and biological activity of *Citrus aurantium amara* L. essential oil. Acta Horticulturae 2003; 597:115–117.

8. Guenther E. The Essential Oils, Vol. 1. New York: Van Nostrand, 1948:377.

9. Igimi H, Tamura R, Toraishi K, et al. Medical dissolution of gallstones. Clinical experience of *d*-limonene as a simple, safe and effective solvent. Dig Dis Sci 1991;36(2):200–208.

10. Ariyoshi T, Arakaki M, Ideguchi K, et al. Studies on the metabolism of *d*-limonene. Effects of *d*-limonene on the lipids and drug-metabolising enzymes in rat livers. Xenobiotica 1975;5(1):33–38.

11. Lorensetti BB, Souza GE, Sarti SJ, et al. Myrcene mimics the peripheral analgesic activity of lemongrass tea. J Ethnopharmacol 1991; 34(1):43–48.

12. Carle R, Gomaa K. The medicinal use of *Matricariae* flos. Brit J Phytother 1992;2(4):147–153.

13. Parke DV, Rahman KMQ, Walker R. The absorption, distribution and excretion of linalool in the rat. Biochem Soc Transact 1974;2: 612–615.

14. Megalla SE, El-Keltawi NEM, Ross SA. A study of antimicrobial action of some essential oil constituents. Herba Polonica 1980;26(3): 181–186.

15. Kalemba D, Kusewicz D, Swiader K. Antimicrobial properties of the essential oil of *Artemisia asiatica* Nakai. Phytother Res 2002;16(3): 288–291.

16. Elisabetsky E, Coelho de Souza GP, Dos Santos MAC, et al. Sedative properties of linalool. Fitoterapia 1995;66(5):407–414.

17. Taddei I, Giachetti D, Taddei E, et al. Spasmolytic activity of peppermint, sage and rosemary essences and their major constituents. Fitoterapia 1988;59(6):463–468.

18. Carle R, Gomaa K. The medicinal use of *Matricariae* flos. Brit J Phytother 1992;2(4):147–153.

19. Achterrath-Tuckermann U, Kunde R, Flaskamp E, et al. Pharmacological investigations with compounds of chamomile. Investigations on the spasmolytic effect of compounds of chamomile and *Kamillosan* on the isolated guinea pig ileum. Planta Medica 1980;39:38–50.

20. Okugawa H, Ueda R, Matsumoto K, et al. Effect of α-santalol and β-santalol from sandalwood on the central nervous system in mice. Phytomedicine 1995;2(2):119–126.

21. Deans SG, Noble RC, Hitunen R, et al. Antimicrobial and antioxidant properties of *Syzygium aromaticum* (L.) Merr. & Perry: impact upon bacteria, fungi and fatty acid levels in ageing mice. Flavor Fragrance J 1995;10(5):323–328.

22. Boonchird C, Flegel TW. *In vitro* antifungal activity of eugenol and vanillin against *Candida albicans* and *Cryptococcus neoformans*. Can J Microbiol 1982;28:1235–1241.

23. Wagner H, Wierer M, Bauer R. *In vitro* inhibition of prostaglandin biosynthesis by essential oils and phenolic compounds. Planta Medica, 1986;52(3):184–187.

24. Wagner H, Wierer M, Bauer R. *In vitro* inhibition of prostaglandin biosynthesis by essential oils and phenolic compounds. Planta Medica, 1986;52(3):184–187.

25. Deans SG, Noble RC, Hitunen R, et al. Antimicrobial and antioxidant properties of *Syzygium aromaticum* (L.) Merr. & Perry: impact upon bacteria, fungi and fatty acid levels in ageing mice. Flavor Fragrance J 1995;10(5):323–328.

26. Kurita N, Miyaji M, Kurane R, et al. Antifungal activity and molecular orbital energies of aldehyde compounds from oils of higher plants. Agriculture Biol Chem (Tokyo) 1979;43(11):2365–2371.

27. Onawunmi GO, Yisak WA, Ogunlana EO. Antibacterial constituents in the essential oil of *Cymbopogon citratus*. J Ethnopharmacol 1984; 12(3):279–286.

28. Orafidiya LO. The effect of autoxidation of lemongrass oil on its antibacterial activity. Phytother Res 1993;7(3):269–271.

29. Hayashi K, Kamiya M, Hayashi T. Virucidal effects of the steam distillate from *Houttuynia cordata* and its components on HSV-1, influenza virus and HIV. Planta Medica 1995;61(3):237–241.

30. Jager W, Buchbauer G, Jirovetz L, et al. Evidence of the sedative effects of neroli oil, citronellal and phenylethyl actetate on mice. J Essential Oil Res 1992;4:387–394.

31. Calnan CD. Cinnamon dermatitis from an ointment. Contact Dermatitis 1976;2:167–170.

32. Toaff ME, Abramovici A, Sporn J, et al. Selective oocyte degeneration and impaired fertility in rats treated with the aliphatic monoterpene, citral. J Reprod Fertility 1979;55:347–352.

33. Sandbank M, Abramovici A, Wolf R, et al. Sebaceous gland hyperplasia following topical application of citral. Am J Dermatopathol 1988;10(5):415–418.

34. Howes MJR, Houghton PJ, Barlow DJ, et al. Assessment of estrogenic activity in some common essential oil constituents. J Pharm Pharmacol 2002;54(11):1521–1528.

35. Inouye S, Takizawa T, Yamaguchi H. Antibacterial activity of essential oils and their major constituents against respiratory tract pathogens by gaseous contact. J Antimicrob Chemother 2001;47(5):565–573.

36. Millet Y, Jouglard J, Steinmetz MD, et al. Toxicity of some essential plant oils. Clinical and experimental study. Clin Toxicol (New York) 1981;18(12):1485–1498.

37. Moorthy B. Toxicity and metabolism of R-pulegone in rats: its effects on hepatic cytochrome P-450 *in vivo* and *in vitro*. Ind Institute Sci 1991;71(1):76–78.

38. Tisserand R, Balacs T. Essential Oil Safety. London, UK: Churchill Livingstone, 1999.

39. Jirovetz J, Jager W, Buchbauer G, et al. Investigations of animal blood samples after fragrance drug inhalation by gas chromatography/mass spectrometry with chemical ionization and selected ion monitoring. Biol Mass Spectr 1991;20:801–803.

40. Peana AT, D'Aquila PS, Panin F, et al. Anti-inflammatory activity of linalool and linalyl acetate constituents of essential oils. Phytomedicine 2002;9(8):721–726.

41. Ribnicky DM, Poulev A, Raskin I. The determination of salicylates in *Gaultheria procumbens* for use as a natural aspirin alternative. J Nutraceuticals Functional Med Foods 2002;4(1):39–52.

42. Tisserand R, Balacs T. Essential Oil Safety. London, UK: Churchill Livingstone, 1999.

43. Van Ketel WG. Allergy to *Matricaria chamomilla*. Contact Dermat 1982;8(2):143.

44. Neerman MF. Sesquiterpene lactones: a diverse class of compounds found in essential oils possessing antibacterial and antifungal properties. Int J Aromather 2003;13(2/3):114–120.

45. Clark SM, Wilkinson SM. Phototoxic contact dermatitis from 5-methoxypsoralen in aromatherapy oil. Contact Dermat 1998;38: 289–290.

46. Saleh M, Hashem F, Grace. Volatile oil of Egyptian sweet fennel (*Foeniculum vulgare var. dulce* Alef.) and its effects on isolated smooth muscles. Pharm Pharmacol Lett 1996; 6(1):5–7.

47. Alber-Puleo M. Fennel and anise as estrogenic agents. J Ethnopharmacol 1980;2(4):337–344.

48. Liu T Y, Chen CC, Chen CL, et al. Safrole-induced oxidative damage in the liver of Sprague-Dawley rats. Food Chem Toxicol 1999; 37(7):697–702.

49. Von Frohlich E. A review of clinical, pharmacological and bacteriological research into *Oleum spicae*. Weiner Medizinische Wochenschrift 1968;15:345–350.

50. Kovar KA, Gropper B, Friess D, et al. Blood levels of 1,8 cineole and locomotor activity of mice after inhalation and oral administration of rosemary oil. Planta Medica 1987;53(4):315–318.

51. Cornwell PA, Barry BW, Bouwstra JA, et al. Modes of action of terpene penetration enhancers in human skin: differential scanning calorimetry, small angle X-ray diffraction and enhancer uptake studies. Int J Pharm 1996;127:9–26.

52. Gamez MJ, Jimenez J, Navarro C, et al. Study of the essential oil of *Lavandula dentata* L. Pharmazie 1990;45:69.

53. Southwell IA, Freeman S, Rubel D. Skin irritancy of tea tree oil. J Essential Oil Res 1997;9:47–52.

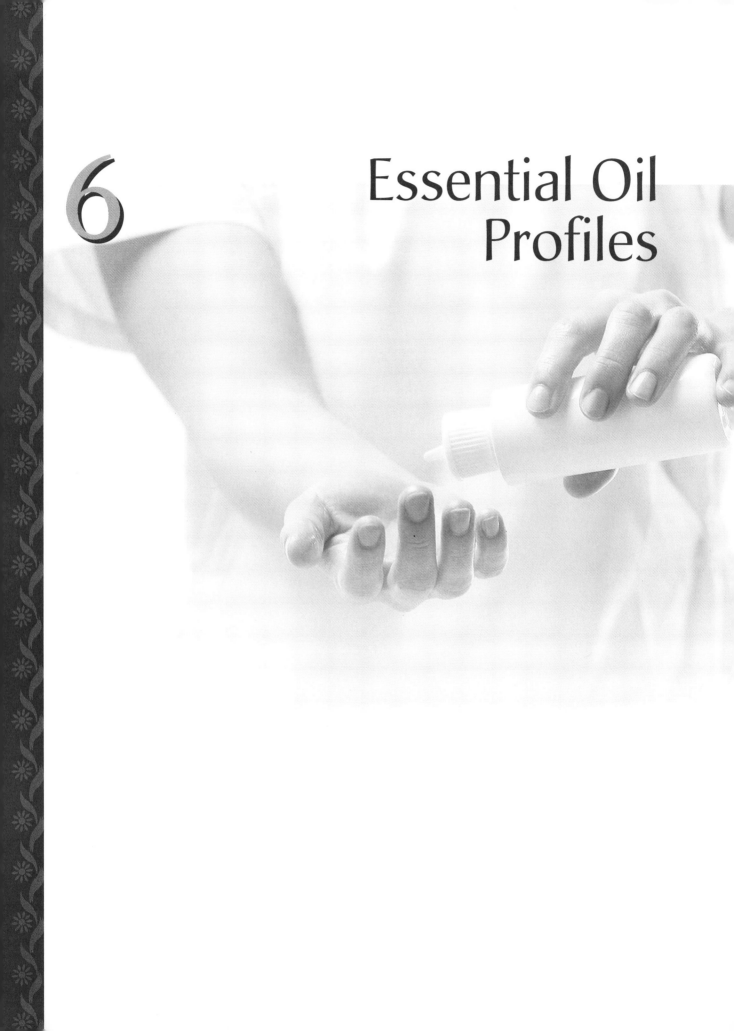

6

Essential Oil Profiles

If you look at a specialist aromatherapy supplier's price list you will probably see well over 100 essential oils. Some names will be familiar, such as ginger and lavender; others, such as zedoary root and kewda, probably will be unfamiliar. All of them have their own distinct aromas, colors, textures, and therapeutic effects. It was not possible to write about all of them in a book of this size, so I included those that I consider to be most valuable for massage and bodywork of all kinds. Profiles of 50 essential oils are included, presented in alphabetical order. The chapter is intended as a reference and guide. Each profile includes two illustrations: one of the whole plant and one of the part of the plant used for extraction.

The botanical families listed may be slightly confusing because several have recently been changed, and both the older and the newer names are commonly and interchangeably used. The families that are known by more than one name are Lamiaceae (Labiatae), Gramineae (Poaceae), Asteraceae (Compositae), and Apiaceae (Umbelliferae).

The extraction method listed is the one most commonly used to produce the oil for aromatherapy use. Most oils can be extracted in several ways, but all types of extract might not be readily available to aromatherapists. For example, absolutes of many oils are produced, but they are almost always sold to the perfume industry. Although various CO_2 extracts are now widely available, many are produced experimentally and in such small amounts that they are not sold commercially.

The descriptions of color, consistency, and odor of the oils are given as baselines to help distinguish an authentic essential oil from a possible adulteration. Only the major chemical constituents are listed. Essential oils are complex, and many oils contain several hundred components. Occasionally minor components are also named if they are considered

particularly important. The constituents of essential oils are extremely variable depending on the country or the year in which the plant is grown, the extraction methods used, and the exact species or variety of species. For these reasons I have generalized a typical chemical breakdown of the main constituents after looking at several analyses of each essential oil.

The section on therapeutic effects lists several effects of each essential oil, followed by one or more asterisks. The asterisks are used to indicate the relative strength of the effects, from mild (one asterisk) to extremely powerful (four asterisks). For example, tea tree (*Melaleuca alternifolia*) is often cited as being antifungal, but this effect is quite mild compared with its strong antibacterial effects. Therefore, in the list, antifungal has two asterisks and antibacterial has four. Any unfamiliar words in this section will either be explained in the text under "main uses in massage" or can be found in the glossary.

In the sections on therapeutic effects and main uses in massage, for the sake of simplicity and ease of reference I have concentrated on the properties that are most representative of that essential oil and that will be most useful to the massage practitioner. As most massage therapists would never treat tropical malaria, head lice, or severe psychological disturbances in their professional lives, information on these kinds of conditions is not included. Also, some effects of the essential oils are apparent only when they are taken internally, for example, the French medical use of oils to treat diabetes, cancer, and acute bacterial diseases. Because it is outside the scope of practice of massage practitioners, internal use is excluded.

I have chosen essential oils that I have found to be generally useful in massage. For some of these oils, there is not much research available and, as a result, the sections on main uses are correspondingly short.

BASIL

Botanical name: *Ocimum basilicum.*

Family: Lamiaceae.

Native to: India.

Part of plant used: Flowering tops.

Extraction method: Steam distillation.

Color of oil: Clear to pale yellow, or sometimes pale green.

Consistency: Thin.

Odor: Varies greatly, depending on the chemotype, though often it has an aniseed or liquorice smell. It can be extremely delicate and sweet, or harsh and pungent.

Chemistry: The main chemotypes are:

(a) Exotic basil: Chemotype (CT) methyl chavicol (or estragole), which contains 75–85% methyl chavicol (phenolic ether) and up to 20% linalol (alcohol).

(b) French basil: CT linalol, which contains up to 55% linalol (alcohol), about 15% eugenol (phenol), and small amounts of methyl chavicol and 1,8 cineole (oxide).[1]

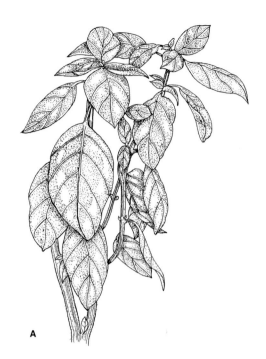

A

Precautions: The linalol chemotype is generally regarded as safe for external use, but the safe use of the methyl chavicol chemotype is much debated. Tisserand and Balacs say it "should not be used in therapy, either internally or externally" because of studies showing the carcinogenic and hepatotoxic nature of methyl chavicol.[2] However, research in Germany into the toxicology of methyl chavicol states: "It is concluded that no dangers exist for human health, as long as normal intake of these products takes place. Many of the data used by the SCF (EU Scientific Committee for Food) were from laboratory studies with rats and mice, consuming high doses."[3]

History and Traditional Uses: Basil is native to India, where according to the Ayurvedic doctors Frawley and Lad, "next to the Lotus, Basil is perhaps the most sacred plant of India."[4] They add that it should be kept in every house for its purifying influence. In many countries, including Egypt and Greece, it is associated with death and mourning,[5] and among older herbalists it seems to have a mixed reputation. Culpeper says that "this is the herb which all authors are together by the ears about and rail at one another (like lawyers)." He ends mysteriously: "I dare write no more of it."[6]

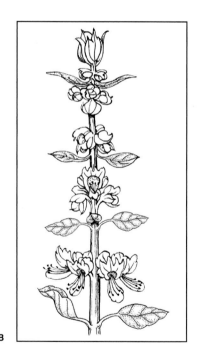

B

Main Uses in Massage

The most notable aspect of basil is its extremely powerful antispasmodic action on smooth muscle.[7] It can be used effectively in abdominal massage for irritable bowel syndrome, colic, and any other spasm of the digestive tract. Experiments have shown that basil has a beneficial effect on gastric ulcer,[8] and it is also helpful in cases of diarrhea.[9] It may be useful in lower back or abdominal application for dysmenorrhea or applied to the chest or upper back for respiratory spasms, such as from whooping cough or asthma.

Therapeutic Effects

Antibacterial ***
Antifungal **
Anti-inflammatory **
Antispasmodic ****
Digestive tonic ***

** = mild   **** = extremely powerful

I have observed that basil seems to have a stimulating effect on digestion and may be helpful in treating low appetite and nausea, either used in massage or diffused.

Experiments using EEG measurements of brain wave patterns show basil to be stimulating to the brain,[10,11] which corresponds with its traditional use in aromatherapy as a **cephalic.** It often is used as an antidepressant, when the client is lethargic and tired and complains of an inability to concentrate or think clearly. It is both physically relaxing and mentally stimulating, making it useful for stressful situations such as exams or interviews.

Notes

1. Essential Oil Resource Consultants. Essential Oil Database. Available at: http://www.essentialoilresource.com. Accessed October 10, 2004.
2. Tisserand RB, Balacs T. Essential Oil Safety. London, UK: Churchill Livingstone, 1999:120.
3. Düshop L. Toxicological evaluation of estragole and methyl eugenol in fennel, basil and other products or consumer protection against natural products. Zeitschrift für Arznei- & Gewürzpflanzen, 2003; 8(1):37–38.
4. Frawley D, Lad V. The Yoga of Herbs. Twin Lakes, WI: Lotus Press, 2001:103.
5. McIntyre A. Flower Power. New York: Henry Holt, 1996:165.
6. Culpeper N. Culpeper's Complete Herbal. Ware, UK: Wordsworth Editions Ltd, 1995:24.
7. Reiter M, Brandt W. Relaxant effects on tracheal and ileal smooth muscles of the gut. Arznermittelforschung 1985;35(1A):408–414.
8. Singh S. Evaluation of gastric anti-ulcer activity of fixed oil of *Ocimum basilicum* Linn. and its possible mechanism of action. Ind J Exp Biol 1999;37(3):253–257.
9. Singh S. Mechanism of action of anti-inflammatory effect of fixed oil of *Ocimum basilicum* Linn. Ind J Exp Biol 1999;37(3):248–252.
10. Manley C H. Psychophysiological effect of odor. Crit Rev Food Sci Nutr 1993;33(1):57–62.
11. Son-KiCheol, Song-JongEun, Um-SuJin, et al. Effect of absorption of essential oils on the changes of arousal and antistress. J Korean Soc Horticult Sci 2001;42(5):614–620.

BAY LAUREL

Botanical name: *Laurus nobilis.*

Family: Lauraceae.

Native to: Mediterranean region.

Part of plant used: Leaves.

Extraction method: Steam distillation.

Color of oil: Greenish-yellow.

Consistency: Thin to medium.

Odor: Warm, spicy, slightly citrusy.

Chemistry: 1,8 cineole (oxide) 26–50%, α-terpinyl acetate (ester) 9–11%, sabinene (monoterpene) 8%, α-pinene (monoterpene) 6.5%, β-pinene (monoterpene) 6%.

Precautions: May be skin sensitizing. Cases of allergic dermal reactions to the oil have been reported.[1] Use it in low doses (1%) on sensitive skin.

History and Traditional Uses: Bay laurel is traditionally believed to ward off evil spirits; as Culpeper says, "neither witch nor devil, thunder nor lightning will hurt a man in the place where a Bay tree is."[2] As evil spirits were regarded as the cause of sickness, this could mean that people previously recognized the prophylactic uses of bay. The leaves were used to crown athletes, poets, and generals in Roman times, hence the expressions "resting on one's laurels," "poet laureate," and "baccalaureate."

Main Uses in Massage

As seen from its traditional use to keep away sickness, bay laurel is regarded as an excellent antiviral[3] and antibacterial[4] agent. In clinical tests it has been shown to have a much stronger antimicrobial effect than many other essential oils.[5] It is extremely useful during cold and flu season to help keep clients (and therapists) healthy and to head off an infection at the first sign.

Bay laurel feels warming and comforting when used on the skin, but it has a strong anti-inflammatory effect.[6] Thus, it is ideal for the treatment of chronic inflammation, for which applied heat feels soothing and helps in tissue softening and range-of-motion work. It may be sensitizing to the skin and therefore should not be used neat or in very strong dilutions, even over restricted areas such as a knee or elbow joint.

Bay laurel is used as an antiepileptic remedy in traditional Iranian medicine, and clinical tests have shown that it provides protection against convulsions.[7] It may be useful as a regular topical remedy in those in whom convulsions and spasm are likely to occur, such as people with epilepsy and Parkinson's disease.

I use bay laurel with clients who feel emotionally weary, shut down, and depressed. Its warming, tonic qualities help strengthen and uplift, while at the same time it seems to be calming and soothing to the nervous system.

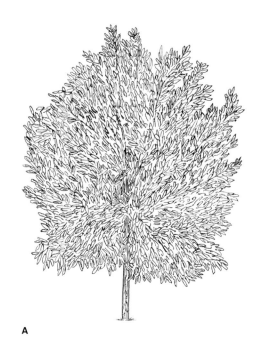

A

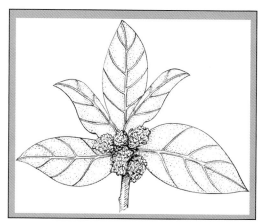

B

Therapeutic Effects

Analgesic ***
Antibacterial **
Anti-inflammatory **
Antiviral ****

** = mild   **** = extremely powerful

Notes

1. Özden MG, Özta P, Öztas MO, et al. Allergic contact dermatitis from Laurus nobilis (laurel) oil. Contact Dermatitis 2001;45(3):178.

2. Culpeper N. Culpeper's Complete Herbal. Ware, UK: Wordsworth Editions Ltd, 1995:24–25.

3. May G, Willuhn G. Antiviral activity of aqueous extracts from medicinal plants in tissue cultures. Arzneimittel-Forschung/Drug Res 1978;28:1–7.

4. Deans SG, Ritchie G. Antibacterial properties of plant essential oils. Int J Food Microbiol 1987;5:165–180.

5. Friedman M, Henika PR, Mandrell RE. Bactericidal activities of plant essential oils and some of their isolated constituents against *Campylobacter jejuni*, *Escherichia coli*, *Listeria monocytogenes*, and *Salmonella enterica*. J Food Protect 2002;65(10):1545–1560.

6. Sayyah M, Saroukhani G, Peirovi A, et al. Analgesic and anti-inflammatory activity of the leaf essential oil of *Laurus nobilis* Linn. Phytother Res 2003;17(7):733–736.

7. Sayyah M, Valizadeh J, Kamalinejad M. Anticonvulsant activity of the leaf essential oil of *Laurus nobilis* against pentylenetetrazole and maximal electroshock-induced seizures. Phytomedicine 2002;9(3):212–216.

BERGAMOT

Botanical name: *Citrus aurantium* subsp. *bergamia* (often written *Citrus x bergamia*).

Family: Rutaceae.

Native to: All citruses originally come from southern and Southeast Asia, and it is not known where bergamot was originally hybridized and grown. Today it is cultivated mostly in Italy, the Ivory Coast, and Brazil.

Part of plant used: Rind of the fruit, which is often picked when still green.

Extraction method: Cold expression.

Color of oil: Pale green or yellowish-green.

Consistency: Very thin.

Odor: Citrusy, with an almost perfumelike undertone.

Chemistry: Limonene (monoterpene) 26–45%, linalyl acetate (ester) 23–32.5%, linalol (alcohol) 7–29%. Bergamot also contains up to 3% of bergapten, a furocoumarin that is strongly photosensitizing at these levels. A rectified oil, which is bergapten-free, can be obtained, but the fragrance is definitely inferior to the untreated oil.

Precautions: Photosensitizing. Do not use on skin for 12 hours prior to sunbathing, either in sunlight or on a tanning bed.[1] Many cases of skin reaction because of sunbathing after using bergamot have been reported.[2]

History and Traditional Uses: Grown historically in Italy, it is named after the city of Bergamo and has been used in Italian folk medicine mostly to treat fevers and parasites. It also provides the flavoring for Earl Grey tea.

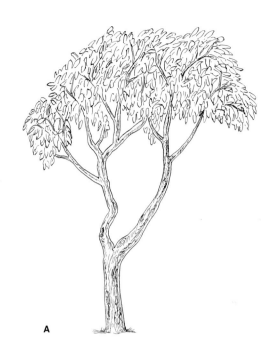

A

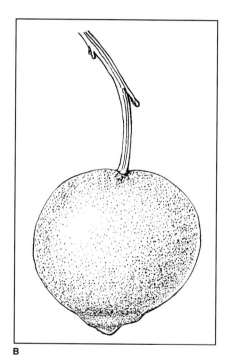

B

Main Uses in Massage

The main traditional use of bergamot oil in aromatherapy has been as a calming antidepressant. Rovesti did extensive work on the uses of essential oils for psychotherapeutic work in the 1950s in Italy and was particularly impressed by bergamot's beneficial effects on anxiety and depression. EEG tests measuring brain wave patterns show that bergamot is relaxing,[3] and clinical tests in mental health patients suggest that citrus fragrances in general improved their mood and allowed them to reduce their medication.[4] The essential oil is frequently used in blends to help with nervous tension, fear and anxiety, depression, and stress-related problems.

Chronic stress has been shown to have drastic effects on resistance to illness. It has been suggested that using essential oils such as bergamot, which help with depression or lower a heightened sympathetic nervous response, may also boost immunity, and this effect seems to be borne out by certain studies.[5] Like most citrus oils, bergamot is a good antibacterial and antifungal,[6] and these qualities, together with its antidepressant effect, make it useful for clients who tend to catch infections when they feel low and disheartened. I frequently use the citrus oils, especially bergamot, in the winter here in the Pacific Northwest, where many people suffer from a mild form of seasonal affective disorder (SAD), which

Therapeutic Effects

Antibacterial and antifungal **
Antidepressant and anxiolytic ***
Antispasmodic **
Digestive tonic and appetite stimulant **

** = mild   **** = extremely powerful

makes them feel lethargic and depressed, thereby lowering their immune function.

In my aromatherapy practice, I have found bergamot useful as an appetite stimulant, especially for clients who feel nauseous—for example, when undergoing chemotherapy for cancer. The most effective application method is inhalation, either sniffing the oil out of a bottle or from a tissue, or diffusing it in the air.

Notes

1. Tisserand RB, Balacs T. Essential Oil Safety. London, UK: Churchill Livingstone, 1999:121.

2. Meyer J. Accidents due to tanning cosmetics with a base of bergamot oil. Bulletin Societe Francaise de Dermatologie et de Syphiligraphie 1970;77(6):881–884.

3. Manley CH. Psychophysiological effect of odor. Crit Rev Food Sci Nutr 1993;33(1):57–62.

4. Komori T, Fujiwara F, Tanida M, et al. Effects of citrus fragrance on immune function and depressive states. Neuroimmunomodulation 1995;2:174–180.

5. Komori T, Fujiwara F, Tanida M, et al. Effects of citrus fragrance on immune function and depressive states. Neuroimmunomodulation 1995;2:174–180.

6. Maudsley F, Kerr KG. Microbiological safety of essential oils used in complementary therapies and the activity of these compounds against bacterial and fungal pathogens. Support Care Cancer 1999;7:100–102.

BLACK PEPPER

Botanical name: *Piper nigrum.*

Family: Piperaceae.

Native to: India. Today it is cultivated in many tropical countries, especially India, China, and Madagascar.

Part of plant used: Fruit (peppercorns). White, green, black, and pink peppercorns are all fruit from *Piper nigrum*, picked at different stages of ripeness or preserved in different ways. Essential oils from both green pepper and black pepper are commercially available.

Extraction method: Steam distillation.

Color of oil: Clear to very pale green.

Consistency: Very thin.

Odor: Dry, spicy, woody, peppery.

Chemistry: β-caryophyllene (sesquiterpene) 9–46%, limonene (monoterpene) 9–23%, sabinene (monoterpene) 0.1–27%, β-pinene (monoterpene) 3.8–15%.[1]

Precautions: Black pepper is a hot oil. Use in moderation generally, and in low doses on sensitive skin.

History and Traditional Uses: Used extensively in Ayurvedic medicine as a digestive stimulant and for respiratory infections.[2] In traditional Chinese medicine, white pepper is used to treat digestive problems and fevers, such as malaria.

Main Uses in Massage

I have found black pepper to be one of the most useful oils for work on skeletal muscles. Its anti-inflammatory and analgesic properties,[3] together with its warming and antispasmodic[4] qualities, make it an ideal remedy for chronic inflammation accompanied by stiffness and limited range of motion. It is one of the essential oils that is used most often in aromatherapy in localized treatments for painful, overworked muscles, osteoarthritis, rheumatoid arthritis, and fibromyalgia.

Because of its warming nature, I frequently include it in blends for people with poor circulation who have cold hands and feet and a general feeling of chilliness. It can be used in small amounts (up to 2%) in a full-body massage, or in higher amounts (3–4%) for a hand or foot massage. Bear in mind that although there are no contraindications for use, this is a hot oil. Children and other people with sensitive skin will be more aware of the feeling of heat it gives and may need milder dilutions to be comfortable.

Black pepper is traditionally regarded in aromatherapy as a stimulating oil, and this effect has been confirmed in clinical testing.[5] It often is used in a more vigorous massage for clients who feel tired and lethargic, perhaps because of a lack of exercise, low blood pressure, or poor circulation.

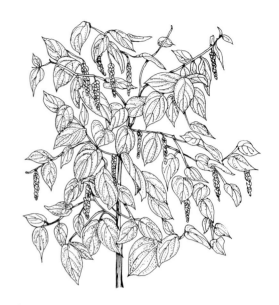

A

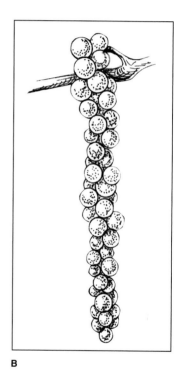

B

Therapeutic Effects

Analgesic ***
Anti-inflammatory ***
Antispasmodic **
Stimulant ***
Warming ***

** = mild   **** = extremely powerful

Notes

1. Menon AN, Padmakumari KP, Jayalekshmy AJ. Essential oil composition of four major cultivars of black pepper. J Essential Oil Res 2002;14(2):84–86.
2. Frawley D, Lad V. The Yoga of Herbs. Twin Lakes, WI: Lotus Press, 2001:105.
3. Park J, Choi H, Jung S, et al. Analgesic and anti-inflammatory activities of some oriental herbal medicines. Kor J Pharmacog 2001;32(4): 257–268.
4. Chakma TK, Choudhuri MSK, Shaila J, et al. Effect of some medicinal plants and plant parts used in Ayurvedic system of medicine on isolated guinea-pig ileum preparations. Hamdard Medicus 2001; 44(2):70–73.
5. Haze S, Sakai K, Gozu Y. Effects of fragrance inhalation on sympathetic activity in normal adults. Jpn J Pharmacol 2002;90(3): 247–253.

BLUE CYPRESS

Botanical name: *Callitris columellaris* var. *intratropica.*

Family: Cupressaceae.

Native to: Northern Australia.

Part of plant used: Essential oils have been extracted from the leaves, the wood, and the heartwood. The wood oil is the one most available outside of Australia and is the one discussed here.

Extraction method: Steam distillation.

Color of oil: The wood oil is a deep blue. The heartwood oil, known in Australia as Cypressance clear, is a clear, colorless liquid.[1]

Consistency: Slightly thick and sticky.

Odor: Smoky, woody, deep, and very slightly sweet. The odor is long-lasting.

Chemistry: Guaiol (sesquiterpene alcohol) 20–30%, guaiazulene (sesquiterpene) percentage unknown.[2]

Precautions: None known. As a new oil in the aromatherapy field, it has not undergone extensive testing, but the chemistry and anecdotal evidence suggest that it is mild and safe.

History and Traditional Uses: According to Webb, blue cypress has been used by indigenous people in the Northern Territories of Australia to soothe cuts, sores, and insect bites and to treat abdominal cramps.[3]

Main Uses in Massage

This oil is just being discovered by the aromatherapy community outside of Australia, and thus far it has been used primarily as an anti-inflammatory. It is significantly cheaper than the other well-known blue oil, German chamomile (*Matricaria recutita*). It seems to be very effective, especially for localized "spot" treatments in strong dilutions, because it is so mild on the skin. I have used it extensively with clients in lotions for carpal tunnel syndrome, muscle sprains and strains, and rheumatoid arthritis. I have also used it in undiluted form for small burns and acne.

According to Webb, it also is effective as a treatment for warts, shingles, diaper rash, and erythema[4]—all conditions that require an anti-inflammatory remedy. I have not tried it as a treatment for respiratory or dermal allergies, but its anti-inflammatory quality would probably be helpful as an antiallergenic. (**Note**: With all clients who have allergies, essential oils should be used with care and in extremely mild dilutions.)

I also use blue cypress as a remedy for clients who seem anxious, emotionally upset, or particularly ungrounded. Its deep, tenacious scent seems to bring clients "down to earth" and calms them.

Notes

1. Webb MA. Bush Sense. Adelaide, Australia: Griffin Press, 2000:35.
2. Webb MA. Bush Sense. Adelaide, Australia: Griffin Press, 2000:35.
3. Webb MA. Bush Sense. Adelaide, Australia: Griffin Press, 2000:36.
4. Webb MA. Bush Sense. Adelaide, Australia: Griffin Press, 2000:36.

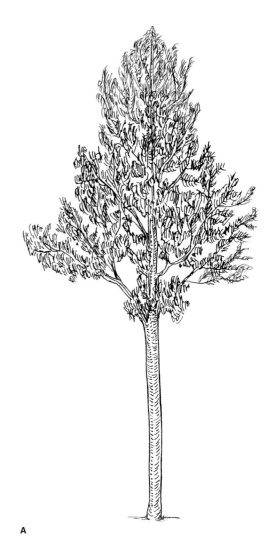

A

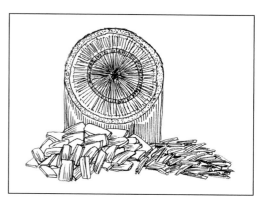

B

Therapeutic Effects

Antiallergenic ***
Anti-inflammatory ***
Antiviral **

** = mild   **** = extremely powerful

CARDAMON

Botanical name: *Elettaria cardamomum.*

Family: Zingiberaceae.

Native to: Southern India and Sri Lanka. Most of the Indian production is used for the large domestic demand. Also grown in Guatemala, mostly for export.

Part of plant used: Seeds.

Extraction method: Steam distillation. A CO_2 extract is also widely available.

Color of oil: Clear to very pale yellow.

Consistency: Thin.

Odor: Very fresh, sweet-spicy, slightly lemony or minty. However, because of its very variable chemistry, some oils also have a strong camphoraceous note if the 1,8 cineole content is higher.

Chemistry: (Variable) α-terpineol (alcohol) up to 45%, α-terpinyl acetate (ester) up to 30%, myrcene (monoterpene) up to 27%, limonene (monoterpene) 2–14%, 1,8 cineole 2–50%.[1]

Precautions: None known.

History and Traditional Uses: Cardamon (or cardamom) is widely used in Indian cooking, in both spicy dishes and sweets, and in Ayurvedic medicine as a carminative and digestive remedy.[2] It has been exported to Europe since Roman times and is particularly traditional in many Scandinavian dishes.

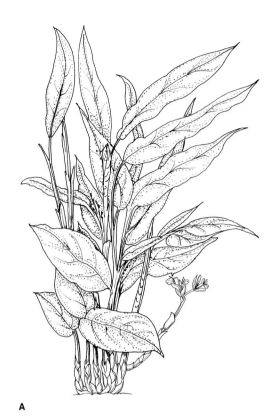

A

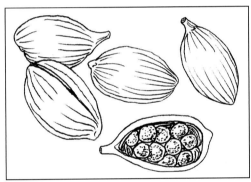

B

Main Uses in Massage

Cardamon is an unknown oil to many massage therapists. Because of its extensive beneficial properties and extreme mildness, it deserves to be more widely used. I have used this oil with no ill effects with very small children, with very old and frail people, and with those who have sensitive skin.

It is a highly effective digestive remedy, with antispasmodic, carminative, and anti-inflammatory qualities,[3] making it useful in cases of irritable bowel syndrome, colic, and general digestive pain and discomfort. I have also frequently used cardamon with great success with clients who have nausea or lack of appetite, perhaps as a result of prolonged illness or chemotherapy. Its light, minty aroma seems to stimulate appetite without the danger of causing further nausea.

Another accepted use in aromatherapy is for respiratory problems; the cardamon oils that are higher in 1,8 cineole seem to be particularly effective in this area. Cardamon can be used in a chest rub for colds, asthma, or other respiratory conditions, such as sinus congestion or wheezing.

I also find cardamon extremely useful as an antidepressant, especially for clients who are lethargic and cold and appear to see the world in tones of grey. It seems to have a gently warming and stimulating action, similar to its relative, ginger, but in much milder terms. It also seems to have an

---

Therapeutic Effects

Antidepressant ***
Antispasmodic ***
Appetite stimulant ****
Carminative ****
Expectorant ***

** = mild   **** = extremely powerful

uplifting, almost sparkly character, which helps clients when everything looks gloomy and uninteresting.

Notes

1. Essential Oil Resource Consultants. Essential Oil Database. Available at: http://www.essentialoilresource.com. Accessed February 11, 2004.

2. Frawley D, Lad V. The Yoga of Herbs. Twin Lakes, WI: Lotus Press, 2001:109.

3. al-Zuhair H, el-Sayeh B, Ameen HA, et al. Pharmacological studies of cardamom oil in animals. Pharmacol Res 1996;34(1–2):79–82.

CARROT

Botanical name: *Daucus carota.*

Family: Apiaceae.

Native to: Europe, Southwest and Central Asia, and North Africa. Now grows wild in the United States.

Part of plant used: Seeds.

Extraction method: Steam distillation. (An oil is also solvent extracted from the root of the cultivated carrot, *Daucus carota* subsp. *sativa*.)

Color of oil: Clear to yellow.

Consistency: Thin.

Odor: Dry, musty, spicy, woody.

Chemistry: Carotol (sesquiterpene alcohol) up to 75%, daucol (sesquiterpene alcohol) 1–5%, daucene (sesquiterpene) about 6%, β-bisabolene (sesquiterpene) 4–8%.

Precautions: None known.

History and Traditional Uses: According to the seventeenth-century herbalist Culpeper, carrots "break wind, and remove stitches in the sides, provoke urine and women's courses, and help to break and expel the stone."[1] The grated root is a folk remedy in Europe for sores, wounds, and tumors.

Main Uses in Massage

Carrot seed essential oil is a remarkably effective, yet mild, detoxifier. It can be used in full-body massages or in detox wraps, or given to clients in blends to use in the bath at home. It has a gentle diuretic quality, helping to move toxins out of the body via the urine. The essential oil has been used for some time in French internal medicine to support and tone the liver.[2] There is no evidence that it has any of the same effects when used externally, but given its results, it is reasonable to assume that it does something similar, even if in a mild form. This purifying effect can be used for edema, accumulation of toxins, arthritis, and gout.

It is also traditionally used in aromatherapy to revitalize the skin—not an unusual idea, since any toxins in the system tend to manifest as skin problems. It is an ideal oil in blends for dermatitis, psoriasis, rashes, and boils. According to Kenner and Requena, it is used "in France in skin care to promote skin elasticity and tone."[3]

Notes

1. Culpeper N. Culpeper's Complete Herbal. Ware UK: Wordsworth Editions Ltd, 1995:58.
2. Kenner D, Requena Y. Botanical Medicine. Brookline, MA: Paradigm Publications, 2001:243.
3. Kenner D, Requena Y. Botanical Medicine. Brookline, MA: Paradigm Publications, 2001:243.

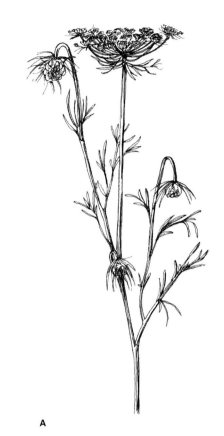

A

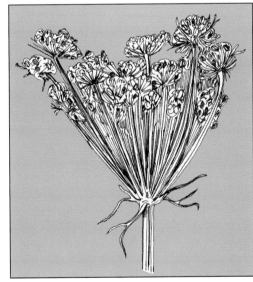

B

Therapeutic Effects

Diuretic ***
General tonic and stimulant **
Liver regenerator ***
Skin tonic ***

** = mild   **** = extremely powerful

CEDAR

Botanical name: *Cedrus atlantica.* Various woods are referred to as cedar, including the Atlas cedar (*Cedrus atlantica*), the Himalayan cedar (*Cedrus deodara*), and the cedar of Lebanon (*Cedrus libani*), which is now nearly extinct. These three are closely related as species and are similar in use. However, trees from other unrelated families are also commonly called cedar, for example, the Virginian cedar (*Juniperus virginiana*), Western red cedar (*Thuja plicata*), or the Japanese cedar (*Cryptomeria japonica*), to name only a few. These are also distilled for their essential oils but have very different properties and contraindications than the *Cedrus* genus.

Family: Pinaceae.

Native to: The region stretching from North Africa to Asia.

Part of plant used: Wood.

Extraction method: Distillation.

Color of oil: Pale yellow to deep amber.

Consistency: Viscous and slightly sticky, especially when exposed to air for some time.

Odor: Freshly cut sawmill timber, may be very sweet, may have a slight cat urine odor.

Chemistry: α-, β-, and γ-himachalene (sesquiterpene) about 70%, δ-cadinene (sesquiterpene) 2%.

Precautions: None known.

History and Traditional Uses: Mention of the cedars of Lebanon is found in some of the most ancient texts, including Egyptian writings. The oil was used by the Egyptians for incense, cosmetics, and embalming,[1] and the wood (as can be read in the book of Solomon in the Bible) was prized as a building material because of its resistance to insects. The resin is still valued in Tibet as an incense and is used in Tibetan medicine.

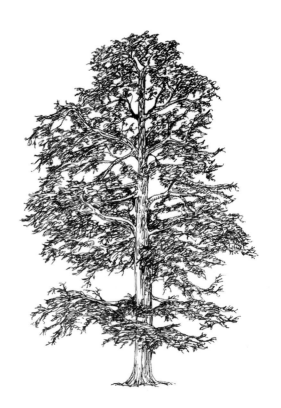

Main Uses in Massage

Cedarwood essential oil is commonly used in aromatherapy to calm clients and to treat the effects of stress. Cedrol, one of the components of cedarwood oil, has been shown in clinical trials to decrease blood pressure, reduce mental tension, and shift subjects into the parasympathetic mode.[2] It is probably useful for clients with heightened blood pressure and other stress-related issues, including insomnia, and adrenal burnout, especially when used in a relaxation massage.

In my experience, it is an extremely useful oil for chronic respiratory problems, especially those involving a lot of mucus in the lungs. Because of its mildness, it can be used in quite strong concentrations (probably up to 25%) over the chest and upper back, or given to clients in a respiratory blend to use at home in a steam inhalation. It also appears to have a good effect on allergic respiratory problems, possibly as a result of its stabilization of mast cells, a contributor to allergic responses.[3]

It has been shown clinically to be a strong anti-inflammatory and analgesic when given orally,[4] but whether it has these effects when applied topically is less clear.

Therapeutic Effects

Anti-inflammatory ***
Expectorant ***
Sedative ***

** = mild   **** = extremely powerful

Notes

1. Fischer-Rizzi S. The Complete Incense Book. New York: Sterling, 1998:75–76.
2. Yada Y. The psychological analysis for the sedative effect of cedrol. Aroma Res 2003;4(3):213–223.
3. Shinde UA, Kulkarni KR, Phadke AS, et al. Mast cell stabilizing and lipoxygenase inhibitory activity of Cedrus deodara (Roxb.) Loud. wood oil. Ind J Exp Biol 1999;37(3):258–261.
4. Shinde UA, Phadke AS, Nair AM, et al. Studies on the anti-inflammatory and analgesic activity of Cedrus deodara (Roxb.) Loud. wood oil. J Ethnopharmacol 1999;65(1):21–27.

CHAMOMILE, GERMAN

Botanical name: *Matricaria recutita*.

Family: Asteraceae.

Native to: Mediterranean region.

Part of plant used: Flowers.

Extraction method: Steam distillation.

Color of oil: Inky blue, occasionally deep greenish-blue.

Consistency: Thick.

Odor: Strong, warm, earthy, deep

Chemistry: β-farnesene (sesquiterpene) 30–41%, α-bisabolol (sesquiterpene alcohol) up to 25%, bisabolol oxide (oxide) up to 25%, bisabolone oxide (oxide) about 6%, chamazulene (sesquiterpene) 4–6%.

Precautions: None known.

History and Traditional Uses: See Chamomile, Roman.

Main Uses in Massage

Blue chamomile is as cooling as its color suggests. German chamomile is the best essential oil remedy I know of for inflammation in any form. It excels at treating acute inflammation, and I have frequently used it undiluted as a first aid remedy for sprained wrists and ankles, and for massage therapists' overworked thumbs and wrists. It also works very well on irritated skin, helping to soothe dermatitis and rashes of almost any kind. One study compared it with nonsteroidal anti-inflammatories in its benefits,[1] and another concluded that oils with a higher content of α-bisabolol and chamazulene had a stronger anti-inflammatory effect.[2]

Research shows that German chamomile strongly inhibits histamine, which is part of the body's anti-inflammatory process.[3] Thus, it is an effective remedy for any kind of allergic response. It has good results on allergic dermatitis, hayfever, asthma, and food sensitivity reactions.

Other dermatological effects include wound-healing properties. The oil was studied in trials in Germany, where it was tested on patients after dermabrasion of tattoos.[4] Healing time was significantly shortened. It also has moisturizing properties,[5] useful for clients who have extremely dry, inflamed, and flaking skin.

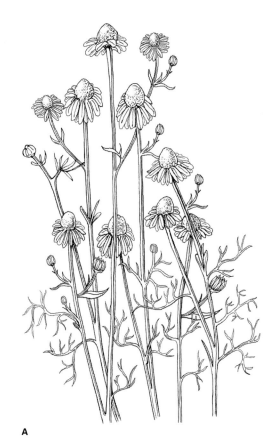

A

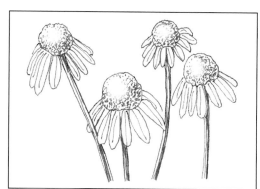

B

Notes

1. Tubaro A, Zilli C, Redaelli C, et al. Evaluation of anti-inflammatory activity of a chamomile extract topical application. Planta Medica 1984;50(4):359.
2. Jakovlev V, Isaac O, Thiemer K, et al. Pharmacological investigations with compounds of chamomile. Planta Medica 1979;35:125–140.
3. Miller TM, Wittstock U, Lindequist U, et al. Effects of some components of the essential oil of chamomile, *Chamomilla recutita*, on histamine release from rat mast cells. Planta Medica 1996;62(1):60–61.
4. Glowania HJ, Raulin C, Swoboda M. Effect of chamomile on wound healing—a clinical double-blind study. Zeitschrift fur Hautkrankheiten (Berlin) 1987;62(17):1267–1271.
5. Monges P, Joachim G, Bohor M, et al. Comparative *in vivo* study of the moisturizing properties of three gels containing essential oils: mandarin, German chamomile, orange. Nouveau Dermatologie 1994;13:470–475.

Therapeutic Effects

Anti-allergenic ***
Anti-inflammatory ****
Carminative ***
Sedative **

** = mild   **** = extremely powerful

CHAMOMILE, ROMAN

Botanical name: *Chamaemelum nobile* (also sometimes referred to as *Anthemis nobilis*).

Family: Asteraceae.

Native to: Mediterranean region; also cultivated in the United States.

Part of plant used: Flowers.

Extraction method: Steam distillation.

Color of oil: Very pale blue when first distilled; soon changes to pale yellow.

Consistency: Thin to medium.

Odor: Very strong. It needs to be highly diluted in a carrier to bring out the delicate, sweet, slightly fruity character.

Chemistry: Isobutyl angelate (ester) 13–38%, isoamyl angelate (ester) 5–21%, and other esters, totaling up to 85% of esters.

Precautions: None known.

History and Traditional Uses: This was an herb known to the ancient Egyptians and used medicinally for thousands of years in the Mediterranean region. It is widely used as a children's remedy in the forms of an herb, an essential oil, and a homeopathic remedy. It has also frequently been planted in place of grass—the famous "chamomile lawn" of the Victorian age in Britain—and gives off a sweet scent when walked on. The tea is often drunk as a mild sedative or digestive remedy.

Main Uses in Massage

Roman chamomile's extremely high ester content shows that it is likely to have antispasmodic and sedative qualities. It is best known in folk medicine for these effects, and they have been confirmed in laboratory and clinical studies.[1] It is frequently used in aromatherapy as a children's sedative because of its mildness, although it works equally effectively with adults. It is good for any stress-related disorder, but especially when there is a spasmodic component, such as digestive pain, constipation, or headache. A study of the use of the essential oil in a palliative care setting showed that "there was a statistically significant reduction in anxiety after each aromatherapy massage."[2]

Roman chamomile has a soothing effect on colic and on mild aches and pains, making it an ideal essential oil for almost any baby's issues. I often give a mild dilution (perhaps 0.5–1%) to mothers of newborns, telling them that they can use it topically for almost any of the minor ailments that infants get, from teething to colic to sleeplessness.

Like its relative German chamomile, Roman chamomile has an anti-inflammatory quality. Although not as strong as *Matricaria*, it is still very effective, especially in skin care.

Notes

1. Rossi T, Melegari M, Bianchi A, et al. Sedative, anti-inflammatory and anti-diuretic effects induced in rats by essential oils of varieties of *Anthemis nobilis*: a comparative study. Pharmacol Res Comm 1988;20(Suppl. 5):71–74.
2. Wilkinson S. An evaluation of aromatherapy massage in palliative care. Palliat Med 1999;13:409–417.

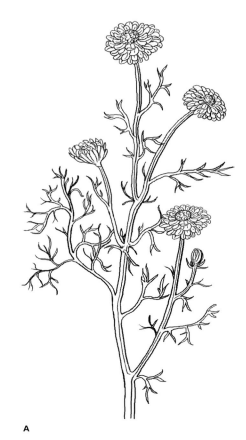

A

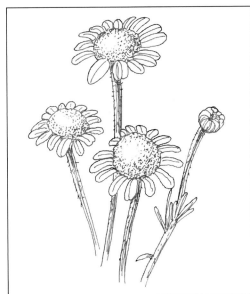

B

Therapeutic Effects

Analgesic **
Anti-inflammatory **
Antispasmodic ***
Sedative ****

** = mild   **** = *extremely powerful*

CINNAMON

Botanical name: *Cinnamomum verum.* Also commonly called *C. zeylanicum.* Other species of cinnamon used in aromatherapy, cassia (*Cinnamomum cassia*) and camphor (*Cinnamomum camphora*), have different uses and contraindications.

Family: Lauraceae.

Native to: India and Sri Lanka.

Part of plant used: Bark or leaves.

Extraction method: Steam distillation.

Color of oil: Yellow to light brown.

Consistency: Thin to medium.

Odor: Leaf and bark oil both have the typical cinnamon smell, though the bark oil is much sweeter and smoother.

Chemistry: Bark: Cinnamaldehyde (phenylpropanoid aldehyde) 55–77%, β-caryophyllene (sesquiterpene) 5–7.5%, linalol (monoterpene alcohol) 4–8%, eugenol (phenol) 2.5–10%. Leaf: Eugenol (phenol) 73–85%, β-caryophyllene (sesquiterpene) 3%, linalol (monoterpene alcohol) 1–2%.

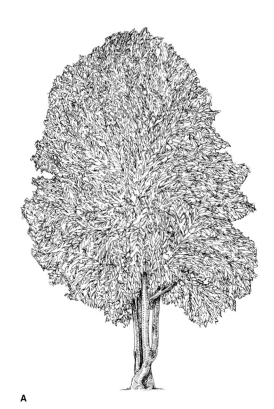

A

Precautions: Cinnamaldehyde, found in large amounts in the bark oil, has a widespread reputation as a skin and mucous membrane irritant and skin sensitizer.[1] Even workers processing the raw cinnamon before distillation have a high incidence of asthma, skin and eye irritation, and loss of hair.[2] According to Tisserand and Balacs, the International Fragrance Association (IFRA) recommends that "cinnamon bark oil should not be used as a fragrance ingredient at a level over 1% in a fragrance compound (equivalent to 0.2% in the final product) due to its sensitizing potential. As a recommended maximum use level, this percentage seems high."[3] They recommend a maximum use level of 0.1%. The leaf oil is much less irritating and not considered to be sensitizing at all,[4] but should still be used with some care topically.

History and Traditional Uses: Cinnamon has been used traditionally as both an incense and a medicine at least from the time of the ancient Egyptians, as well as in the Middle East, India, China, and Japan. In Ayurvedic medicine it is regarded as "almost a universal medicine"[5] and is used extensively as a pain reliever, for colds and coughs, and to strengthen the heart.

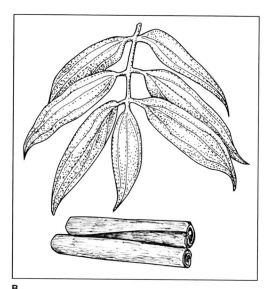

B

Main Uses in Massage

Cinnamon bark oil has been extensively tested as being extremely antimicrobial.[6] However, it can also be very skin irritating, which makes it difficult to use as a topical application on athlete's foot, for example. The IFRA recommends that equal amounts of δ-limonene, found in citrus oils like grapefruit (*Citrus paradisii*), be used with it to lessen the skin-irritating effects of the cinnamaldehyde.[7] Another possible way to use it is diffused in the air, in small enough amounts to avoid irritation of the eyes and throat.

Therapeutic Effects

Antibacterial ****
Antifungal ***
Antirheumatic ***
Antiviral ****
Tonic ***

** = mild   **** = extremely powerful

The leaf oil is known to strongly inhibit the synthesis of prostaglandins, a class of chemicals produced by the body during the inflammatory response, probably because of its high eugenol content.[8] This makes it extremely useful in blends for rheumatoid arthritis, fibromyalgia, and other problems causing inflammation of the joints. The leaf oil, being milder on the skin, can be used in dilutions of up to 3%.

Both oils are generally regarded in aromatherapy as being warming and stimulating, useful for people with low blood pressure or for those who feel cold, tired, and lethargic. Cinnamon has traditionally been used in both Chinese medicine and Ayurvedic medicine as a tonic for those who are tired or recovering from illness.

Notes

1. Tisserand R, Balacs T. Essential Oil Safety. London, UK: Churchill Livingstone, 1999:129–130.
2. Uragoda CG. Asthma and other symptoms in cinnamon workers. Br J Indust Med 1984;41(2):224–227.
3. Tisserand R, Balacs T. Essential Oil Safety. London, UK: Churchill Livingstone, 1999:129.
4. Tisserand R, Balacs T. Essential Oil Safety. London, UK: Churchill Livingstone, 1999:130.
5. Frawley D, Lad V. The Yoga of Herbs. Twin Lakes, WI: Lotus Press, 2001:112.
6. Chao SC, Young DG, Oberg CJ. Screening for inhibitory activity of essential oils on selected bacteria, fungi and viruses. J Essential Oil Res 2000;12(5):639–649.
7. Clarke S. Essential Chemistry for Safe Aromatherapy. London, UK: Churchill Livingstone, 2002:115.
8. Wagner H, Wierer M, Bauer R. *In vitro* inhibition of prostaglandin biosynthesis by essential oils and phenolic compounds. Planta Medica 1986;52(3):184–187.

CLARY SAGE

Botanical name: *Salvia sclarea.*

Family: Lamiaceae.

Native to: Northern Mediterranean region. Today it is cultivated extensively in England, the United States, Russia, and Morocco.

Part of plant used: Flowering tops.

Extraction method: Steam distillation.

Color of oil: Clear to very pale yellow.

Consistency: Thin.

Odor: Sweet, herbaceous, often floral, very heady, slightly woody.

Chemistry: Linalyl acetate (ester) 52–72%, linalol (monoterpene alcohol) 10–30%, Germacrene D (sesquiterpene) 2.4–8%, β-caryophyllene (sesquiterpene) 1–3.1%.

Precautions: None known. Clary sage is often contraindicated during pregnancy because it is an **emmenagogue,** encouraging menstrual flow. However, there is no evidence that emmenogogues cause any problem during pregnancy, and Tisserand and Balacs regard clary sage as safe.[1] Some clients may become very drowsy after a massage with clary sage, so it may not be suitable for certain situations or times of day. It definitely intensifies dreaming, making dreams more vivid and active, and this may not be desirable for certain people.

History and Traditional Uses: An ancient medicinal herb used by the ancient Egyptians for infertility. Hildegard of Bingen, the renowned medieval healer, recommends clary sage as a stomach tonic.[2] It was the most popular "tea" in Britain before black tea was imported, and it was used in the Middle Ages to flavor wine in Germany, and in England to flavor beer instead of using hops.

Main Uses in Massage

Because of the high content of the spasmolytic ester linalyl acetate, clary sage is an extremely useful oil to help relieve spasms of both smooth and skeletal muscle.[3] It can be used in massage or warm compresses on the low back or abdomen to help with menstrual cramping or backache, or in upper back or chest massage for symptoms of asthma. It also is used in abdominal massages for many spasmodic digestive problems, including colic pains and irritable bowel syndrome.

The oil also is regularly used in aromatherapy for the relief of stress. A blend containing clary sage was shown in tests to reduce systolic blood pressure and stress,[4] and it seems to have a good effect on clients who are both tired and tense. It appears to both relax and strengthen the nervous system, as well as being an effective antidepressant. This makes it very helpful in massage work for any kind of stress-related problem, for depression, or for the weak tiredness that often occurs after illness.

Clary sage is an oil that is sometimes quoted as being useful during childbirth. A recent evaluation of aromatherapy in Britain involving 8058 mothers in childbirth over an 8-year period concluded that clary sage was effective in alleviating pain and may also be useful in reducing anxiety and

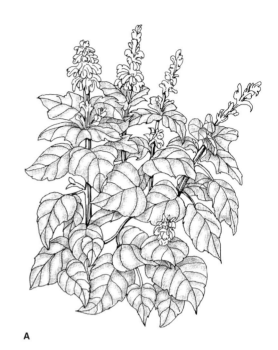

A

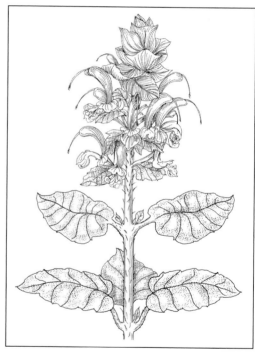

B

Therapeutic Effects

Antidepressant and euphoric ****
Antispasmodic ****
Nervine/tonic **
Sedative ***

** = mild   **** = extremely powerful

fear during labor.[5] The essential oils were applied via skin absorption and inhalation. Low-back massage is excellent for any massage therapist to perform if present during labor.

The essential oil is also frequently used in aromatherapy to help with the symptoms of menopause, and it can be included in massage for leg cramps, irritability, and mood swings. It can be used in a spritzer to help with hot flashes. There is no direct evidence that clary sage is a hormonal balancer, but it does contain the unusual diterpene alcohol sclareol. According to Clarke, diterpene alcohols "have structural similarities to human steroid hormones and may have a balancing effect on the endocrine system."[6] This would obviously also be helpful for symptoms of PMS and for menstrual problems.

Notes

1. Tisserand R, Balacs T. Essential Oil Safety. London, UK: Churchill Livingstone, 1999:110.
2. Strehlow W, Hertzka G. Hildegard of Bingen's Medicine. Santa Fe, NM: Bear & Co, 1988:55.
3. Lis-Balchin M, Hart S. A preliminary study of the effect of essential oils on skeletal and smooth muscle *in vitro*. J Ethnopharmacol 1997; 58(3):183–187.
4. Son K, Song J, Um S, et al. Effect of absorption of essential oils on the changes of arousal and antistress. J Korean Soc Horticult Sci 2001;42(5):614–620.
5. Burns E, Blamey C, Ersser SJ, et al. The use of aromatherapy in intrapartum midwifery practice: an observational study. Complement Ther Nursing Midwifery 2000;6(1):33–34.
6. Clarke S. Essential Chemistry for Safe Aromatherapy. London, UK: Churchill Livingstone, 2002:56–57.

CLOVE

Botanical name: *Syzygium aromaticum* (sometimes called *Eugenia caryophyllus*).

Family: Myrtaceae.

Native to: The Molucca Islands. Today it is cultivated in many tropical areas, especially Indonesia, Madagascar, and Brazil.

Part of plant used: Different essential oils are extracted from the bud, leaves, or stems.

Extraction method: Steam distillation

Color of oil: Bud and stem oils are pale yellow, while the leaf oil can be brown.

Consistency: Medium.

Odor: The bud oil has the finest aroma, with sweet, spicy, penetrating notes. The leaf and stem oils also have the characteristic clove odor but are much harsher and rougher.

Chemistry: Eugenol (phenol) 70-83%, β-caryophyllene (sesquiterpene) 5.8–20%. (The bud oil also contains eugenyl acetate [ester] 2.7–11.6%.)

Precautions: A dermal and a mucous membrane irritant in high concentrations, it is not advisable to apply any of the clove oils neat, because of the high eugenol content. Cases have been reported of permanent desensitization and lack of sweating after accidental neat spillage on the skin.[1] The oils do not seem to be sensitizing. The bud oil seems to be the gentlest, although it would probably be best not to use any of the clove oils on sensitive skin or with children.

History and Traditional Uses: Cloves were used in the Middle Ages to ward off the plague, and the oranges studded with cloves that we use for decoration date from that time. Cloves are used worldwide as a food flavoring and to scent cigarettes in Southeast Asia. In Chinese and Ayurvedic medicine, they are widely used to treat digestion and respiratory conditions of the lungs. Hildegard of Bingen recommends cloves as part of her remedy for gout.[2]

Main Uses in Massage

Clove oil is an excellent anti-inflammatory and **anesthetic,** or numbing agent, because of both the eugenol and the β-caryophyllene it contains.[3,4] It is an ideal addition to a massage blend for rheumatoid arthritis, overworked muscles, and other inflammations of the joints or tissues.

The essential oil is highly antimicrobial, with a useful action against bacteria, fungi, and viruses, and can be incorporated into a massage blend to help the immune system fight against any of these infections. It is also reported to be active against the herpes simplex virus,[5] making it a useful addition to take-home remedies for cold sores or for the relief of shingles.

Its traditional use in digestive remedies is supported by research showing that eugenol produces smooth muscle relaxation.[6] This effect makes it useful in abdominal massage designed to relieve abdominal bloating, pain, and a sluggish digestion, resulting from spasm in the digestive tract, as in irritable bowel syndrome.

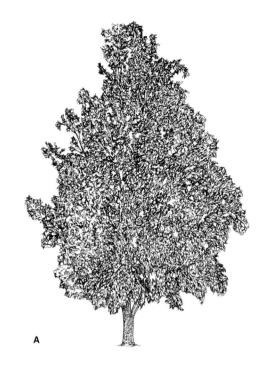

A

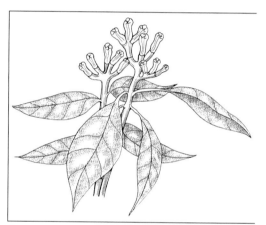

B

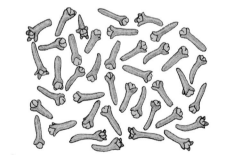

C

Therapeutic Effects

Anesthetic ****
Antibacterial, antifungal, antiviral ***
Anti-inflammatory ***
Antispasmodic **
Aphrodisiac ***

** = mild   **** = extremely powerful

Notes

1. Isaacs G. Permanent local anaesthesia and anhidrosis after clove oil spillage. Lancet 1983;16:882.
2. Strehlow W, Hertzka G. Hildegard of Bingen's Medicine. Santa Fe, NM: Bear & Co, 1988:106.
3. Ghelardini C, Galeotti N, Di Cesare Mannelli L, et al. Local anaesthetic activity of beta-caryophyllene. Farmacologia 2001;56(5–7): 387–389.
4. Kim H M, Lee E H, Hong S H, et al. Effect of Syzygium aromaticum extract on immediate hypersensitivity in rats. J Ethnopharmacol 1998;60(2):125–131.
5. Benencia F, Courreges MC. *In vitro* and *in vivo* activity of eugenol on human herpes virus. Phytother Res 2000;14:495–500.
6. Damiani CEN, Rossoni LV, Vassallo DV. Vasorelaxant effects of eugenol on rat thoracic aorta. Vascul Pharmacol 2003;40(1):59–66.

CUMIN

Botanical name: *Cuminum cyminum.*

Family: Apiaceae.

Native to: Mediterranean region, North Africa, and Central Asia.

Part of plant used: Seeds.

Extraction method: Steam distillation.

Color of oil: Yellow.

Consistency: Thin.

Odor: Warm, soft, spicy, and lingering.

Chemistry: Cuminaldehyde (aldehyde) 20–38%, γ-terpinene (monoterpene) 17.25–21%, β-pinene (monoterpene) 10–13%, other aldehydes 14–34%.

Precautions: Cumin oil is strongly phototoxic and should not be used in concentrations of higher than 0.4% for 12 hours prior to exposure to sun or sunbed tanning.[1]

History and Traditional Uses: Cumin has been cultivated since the time of the Minoans, in about the thirteenth century B.C., and used to flavor liqueurs, cakes, cheeses, and curry. It is used extensively in Ayurvedic medicine, mostly for digestive problems.

Main Uses in Massage

Cumin is a very good essential oil to use with abdominal massage for spasmodic problems of the digestive system. Its antispasmodic[2] and anti-inflammatory properties make it an ideal addition to a blend for irritable bowel syndrome or Crohn's disease, though it can be used for any kind of digestive pain or bloating.

Cumin oil also seems to be an extremely potent antifungal agent,[3,4] active against many different forms of fungus, and may be included in take-home blends for athlete's foot, for example.

Notes

1. Tisserand R, Balacs T. Essential Oil Safety. London, UK: Churchill Livingstone, 1999:134.
2. Sayyah M, Mahboubi A, Kamalinejad M. Anticonvulsant effect of the fruit essential oil of *Cuminum cyminum* in mice. Pharm Biol 2002;40(6):478–480.
3. Shetty RS, Shinghai RS, Kulkarni PR. Antimicrobial properties of cumin. World J Microbiol Biotechnol 1994;10(2):232–233.
4. Garg SC, Siddiqui N. Antifungal activity of some essential oil isolates. Pharmazie 1992;47(6):467–468.

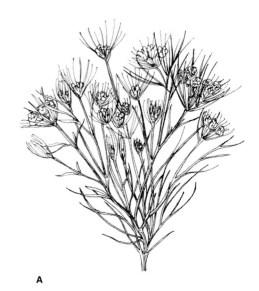

A

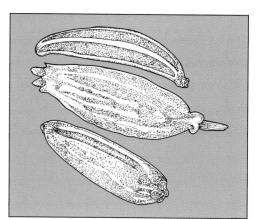

B

Therapeutic Effects

Antifungal ***
Anti-inflammatory ***
Antispasmodic ***
Carminative ****

** = mild   **** = extremely powerful

CYPRESS

Botanical name: *Cupressus sempervirens*. Many unrelated plants are commonly known as cypress, so it is important to check the botanical name.

Family: Cupressaceae.

Native to: Eastern Mediterranean regions, both Europe and the Middle East.

Part of plant used: Needles and twigs. (The tiny cones are also included.)

Extraction method: Steam distillation.

Color of oil: Clear to pale yellow or very pale green.

Consistency: Very thin.

Odor: Clean, piney, sour, lingering.

Chemistry: α-pinene (monoterpene) 28–78%, δ-3-carene (monoterpene) 9–32%, limonene (monoterpene) 1.5–10%.

Precautions: None known. As with other essential oils that are very high in monoterpenes, it is probably best to use cypress when it is as fresh as possible because monoterpenes, especially α-pinene, have the reputation of being more skin sensitizing when oxidized.[1]

History and Traditional Uses: The word *sempervirens* means ever-living, reflecting not just that cypress is an evergreen tree that can live up to 2000 years but also its ancient connection with death and the afterlife. The Egyptians built their sarcophagi of the tough wood, and they (and the Greeks and Romans after them) dedicated the tree to their god of the underworld. It is still planted in cemeteries in southern Europe and in New Orleans.

Main Uses in Massage

Cypress is one of several essential oils that are more useful for chronic conditions than for acute problems. In France it is known as a "terrain" remedy; in other words, it supports the health of the whole body, bringing it back gently to homeostasis. According to the French aromatherapist Mailhebiau, "*Cupressus* is rebalancing and nervine; it is suitable for people who are unbalanced, weary from nerves due to a lack of stability and exhausted as a result of a poor diet."[2] I add it to take-home blends for longer-term use for these kinds of clients, as well as using it in massage.

The essential oil has a well-earned reputation for being a regulator of fluids. It is a lymphatic stimulant and is useful with manual lymphatic drainage for the treatment of edema. It is also recommended by Valnet for excessive sweating of the feet[3]—a great oil to add to footbaths in the summertime, before doing foot massage or reflexology. It can also be used in longer-term remedies for this problem, or in cooling spritzers or baths for the excessive sweating experienced during perimenopause. The **astringent,** or tissue-tightening, quality of cypress, which helps it move fluids, also makes it an effective vasoconstrictor, and it is frequently used in lotions for varicose veins.

Because of its anti-inflammatory, antispasmodic, and antibacterial properties,[4] cypress is a good treatment oil for chronic problems of the lower respiratory system, such as chronic bronchitis, asthma, or any kind

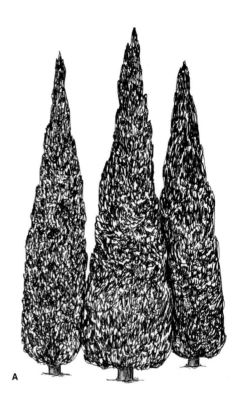

A

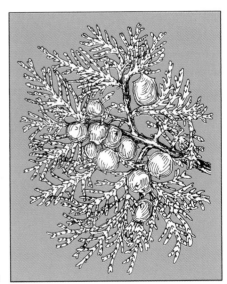

B

Therapeutic Effects

Antibacterial **

Anti-inflammatory **

Antitussive ***

Astringent ***

Lymphatic stimulant and fluid regulator ***

Nervine ***

Vasoconstrictor ****

** = mild   **** = extremely powerful

of spasmodic coughing. It can be used in chest rubs or in inhalations.

Notes

1. Tisserand R, Balacs T. Essential Oil Safety. London, UK: Churchill Livingstone, 1999:197.

2. Mailhebiau P. Portraits in Oil. Saffron Walden, UK: CW Daniel, 1995:51.

3. Valnet J. The Practice of Aromatherapy. Saffron Walden, UK: CW Daniel, 1992:120–121.

4. Chanegriha N, Foudil-Cherif Y, Baailouamer A, et al. Antimicrobial activity of Algerian Cyprus and eucalyptus essential oils. Rivista Italiana EPPOS 1998;25:11–16.

EUCALYPTUS

Botanical name: There are more than 450 different species of eucalyptus plants, and most produce essential oil. Only a few of these are distilled commercially and made widely available, although Australian aromatherapists are experimenting with more and more of this useful genus. The most easily available oils are *Eucalyptus globulus* and *Eucalyptus radiata*, which are very similar in chemistry and use, and these are the species discussed here. For information on other species, refer to Mark Webb's book on Australian aromatherapy, which discusses nine species in depth.[1]

Family: Myrtaceae.

Native to: Australia, although *E. globulus* has naturalized in Spain and California and is widely cultivated in many other countries.

Part of plant used: Leaves and twigs. (All parts of the plant have such a high yield of essential oil that a fire chief in California recently warned the public against building near eucalyptus trees, as they are highly flammable because of the essential oil content.)

Extraction method: Steam distillation.

Color of oil: Clear.

Consistency: Thin and watery.

Odor: High, penetrating, medicinal, camphoraceous, like a mentholated vapor rub. The aroma of the *radiata* species is slightly sweeter and more appealing.

Chemistry: Both species: 1,8 cineole (oxide) 47–70%. *Globulus*: α-pinene (monoterpene) 10–29%. *Radiata*: α-terpineol (alcohol) 8.5%, limonene (monoterpene) 6%.

Precautions: None known for external use. Eucalyptus has been reported as being highly toxic internally and carries an S4 poison warning in Australia. However, it seems to be no more toxic when taken orally than any other commonly used essential oil.[2] It has probably gained its reputation because it is kept in so many home medicine kits in Australia, and there is a high potential that it will be drunk accidentally by young children.[3]

History and Traditional Uses: Various species of eucalyptus were probably used medicinally by the Australian aboriginal people, but no written record remains. However, it is likely that they taught its use to the early settlers, who smoked the leaves like tobacco for respiratory ailments and also used the smoke as an insect repellant.

Main Uses in Massage

Eucalyptus is known primarily as a remedy for respiratory ailments. Because of its high 1,8 cineole content, it is highly antiviral and thus useful at the beginning of a viral respiratory infection. It also is a strong expectorant for mucus in the lungs and **antitussive,** or soothing for unproductive coughs.[4] It can be added in high concentrations (up to 20% for an acute treatment) to blends for chest rubs or upper back massage, diffused in the massage room to clear sinuses and lungs, or sent home

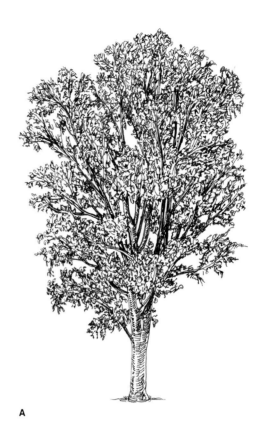

A

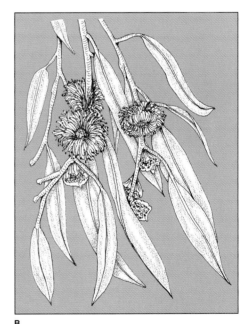

B

> **Therapeutic Effects**
>
> Anti-inflammatory **
> Antitussive ***
> Antiviral ***
> Expectorant ****

** = mild   **** = extremely powerful

with clients to use in steam inhalation or baths. It seems to be effective for any respiratory infection or problem, from mild winter colds to many asthmatic symptoms, bronchitis, sinusitis, and even tuberculosis.[5]

It also is a useful addition to massage blends for painful or overworked muscles, partly because it helps the blend permeate tissue more quickly[6] and partly because of its ability to increase blood flow and muscle temperature.[7] It can be used in sports massage, either as a passive warm-up for athletes or after exercise to relax muscles. It also is useful for ailments that include muscle fatigue and pain, such as chronic fatigue syndrome and fibromyalgia.

For massage therapists who treat clients who have allergies to dust mites, eucalyptus essential oil is much more effective than detergent in killing these mites. A study showed that 100 mL of eucalyptus oil added to 15 mL of detergent and then to 50 L of warm water killed 99.4% of dust mites, as opposed to 2.4% killed with detergent alone.[8] Therapists may want to consider washing sheets for these particular clients in a combination of eucalyptus essential oil and regular detergent.

Another species of eucalyptus that is fairly common in aromatherapy circles, but which has a very different chemical composition to *globulus* and *radiata*, is *E. citriadora*. This oil has high amounts of citronellal (aldehyde) and citronellol (alcohol) and is highly antibacterial and antifungal; it is particularly effective against staphylococcus infections and *Candida* yeast infections (candidiasis).

Notes

1. Webb M. Bush Sense. Adelaide, Australia: Griffin Press, 2000.
2. Tisserand R, Balacs T. Essential Oil Safety. London, UK: Churchill Livingstone, 1999:206.
3. Tibballs J. Clinical effects and management of eucalyptus oil ingestion in infants and young children. Med J Aust 1995;163:177–180.
4. Penoel D. *Eucalyptus smithii* essential oil and its use in aromatic medicine. Br J Phytother 1992;2(4):154–159.
5. Kazarinova NV, Tkachenko KG. Medicinal plants in treatment of different forms of tuberculosis (review of Russian-language literature). Rastitel'nye Resursy 2000;36(1):92–106.
6. Williams AC, Barry BW. Essential oils as novel human skin penetration enhancers. Int J Pharm 1989;57:7–9.
7. Hong C-Z, Shellock FG, Shellock MD. Effects of a topically applied counterirritant (*Eucalyptamint*) on cutaneous blood flow and on skin and muscle temperatures. Am J Phys Medi Rehab 1991;70:29–33.
8. Tovey ER, McDonald LG. A simple washing procedure with eucalyptus oil for controlling house dust mites and their allergens in clothing and bedding. J Allergy Clin Immunol 1997;100(4):464–466.

FENNEL

Botanical name: *Foeniculum vulgare.*

Family: Apiaceae.

Native to: Mediterranean.

Part of plant used: Seeds.

Extraction method: Steam distillation.

Color of oil: Clear to very pale yellow.

Consistency: Thin.

Odor: Aniselike, very sweet, slightly spicy.

Chemistry: Trans-anethole (phenolic ether) 36–76%, fenchone (ketone) 4.5–13%, methyl chavicol (phenolic ether) 3–23.5%.

Precautions: None in normal therapeutic dosages.

History and Traditional Uses: Used by both Roman soldiers and Christians on fasting days to decrease appetite and increase stamina, fennel has a long history of use as a digestive remedy and as a tonic. It is often eaten in India after meals and is used in Ayurvedic medicine as a stimulant to digestion and to calm the nerves.[1] Culpeper lists many beneficial properties, stating that it helps to break up kidney stones, promotes lactation and urination, eases shortness of breath, aids weight loss, and is an antidote for poisons.[2]

Main Uses in Massage

Fennel essential oil is one of the best remedies in aromatherapy for many kinds of issues involving the female reproductive system. It reduces spasm in smooth muscle, making it an ideal treatment for dysmenorrhea or menstrual cramping.[3] It also has marked estrogenic action, with possible uses for PMS and menopausal problems.[4] One study found good results when fennel oil was used topically in a cream to treat unusually heavy hair growth in women possibly resulting from hormonal imbalances.[5]

The antispasmodic qualities of fennel can also be used to ease spasmodic coughing, as in asthma or whooping cough, or any spasms of the digestive system, such as infantile colic[6] or irritable bowel syndrome. In various European countries, weak fennel tea often is given to babies to prevent colic, and the essential oil, in a dilution of 0.5%, is also effective when massaged over the abdomen.

Fennel is a good general digestive aid, stimulating the release of bile from the liver and therefore helping with the breakdown of fats.[7] This gives fennel the reputation of being an excellent cleanser for the body, and it is often used in aromatherapy to treat conditions that sometimes respond well to detoxification, such as gout, rheumatoid arthritis, kidney stones, and cellulite.

Clinical testing shows that the essential oil is a mild stimulant to the sympathetic nervous system.[8] Fennel oil also seems to reduce fatigue and mental stress.[9] These effects support its reputation as a strengthening remedy, suitable for clients who are generally low in energy from illness or overwork.

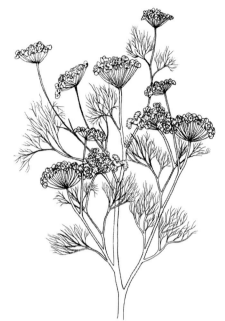

A

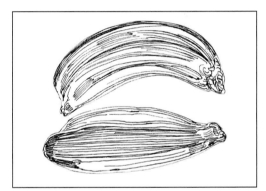

B

Therapeutic Effects

Antispasmodic ***
Carminative, choleretic,
   digestive stimulant ****
Detoxifier ***
Estrogenic ***
Tonic ***

** = mild   **** = extremely powerful

Notes

1. Frawley D, Lad V. The Yoga of Herbs. Twin Lakes, WI: Lotus Press, 2001:117.

2. Culpeper N. Culpeper's Complete Herbal. Ware, UK: Wordsworth Editions, 1995:103–104.

3. Ostad SN, Soodi M, Shariffzadeh M, et al. The effect of fennel essential oil on uterine contraction as a model for dysmenorrhoea, pharmacology and toxicology study. J Ethnopharmacol 2001;76:299–304.

4. Albert-Puleo M. Fennel and anise as estrogenic agents. J Ethnopharmacol 1980;2(4):337–344.

5. Javidnia K, Dastgheib L, Mohammadi Samani S, et al. Antihirsutism activity of fennel (fruits of *Foeniculum vulgare*) extract; a double-blind placebo controlled study. Phytomedicine 2003;10(6/7):455–458.

6. Alexandrovich I, Rakovitskaya O, Kolmo E, et al. The effect of fennel (*Foeniculum vulgare*) seed oil emulsion in infantile colic; a randomized placebo-controlled study. Altern Ther Health Med 2003;9(4): 58–61.

7. Rangelov A. An experimental characterization of cholagogic and cholesteric activity of a group of essential oils. Folia Medica 1989;31(1): 46–53.

8. Haze S, Sakai K, Gozu Y. Effects of fragrance inhalation on sympathetic activity in normal adults. Jpn J Pharmacol 2002;90(3): 247–253.

9. Nagai H, Nakagawa M, Nakamura M, et al. Effects of odors on humans (II). Reducing effects of mental stress and fatigue. Chem Senses 1991;16:198.

FIR

Botanical name: Several species of fir are used in aromatherapy. The main ones are *Abies alba*, *Abies balsamea*, and *Abies sibirica*, and they have similar properties and uses.

Family: Pinaceae.

Native to: Europe and North America.

Part of plant used: Needles.

Extraction method: Steam distillation.

Color of oil: Clear.

Consistency: Thin.

Odor: Clean, piney, sharp.

Chemistry: α-pinene (monoterpene) 31–34%, β-pinene (monoterpene) 18%, camphene (monoterpene) 16%, limonene (monoterpene) 15–17%, bornyl acetate (ester) 3–5%.

Precautions: None known. However, there is some evidence that α-pinene, which is a major component, may be more irritating to the skin when it is oxidized.[1] Fresh essential oil should therefore always be used.

History and Traditional Uses: Fir is the main source of Christmas trees, and it is used in construction work and for telegraph poles. It is the source of turpentine, which was used medicinally for respiratory problems.

Main Uses in Massage

Fir oil is mostly used in aromatherapy because of its good all-around action on the respiratory system. It is a useful addition to blends to help with unproductive, irritating coughs and can be combined with lavender and clary sage for this purpose. It is also a mild, easily tolerated antiseptic for the lower respiratory tract, when a cold has progressed to the stage of becoming a bacterial infection, with a lot of congestion in the lungs.

It also is useful for painful tight muscles and aching joints and is often added to sports massage blends and to remedies for arthritis and fibromyalgia.

Notes

1. Tisserand R, Balacs T. Essential Oil Safety. London, UK: Churchill Livingstone, 1999:197.

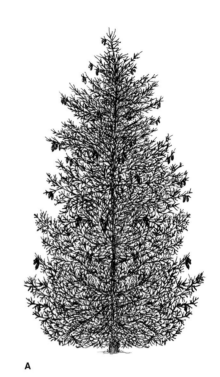

A

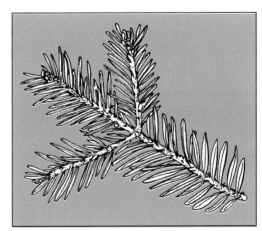

B

Therapeutic Effects

Antidepressant **
Antiseptic **
Antitussive ***
Expectorant **

** = mild   **** = extremely powerful

FRANKINCENSE

Botanical name: *Boswellia carteri* or *B. sacra*. There are various species of *Boswellia*, several of which are sold as frankincense, including *B. thurifera* and *B. frereana*. They appear to be similar in effect and aroma.

Family: Burseraceae.

Native to: Northeast Africa.

Part of plant used: Resin.

Extraction method: Steam distillation and CO_2 extraction.

Color of oil: Clear to pale yellow.

Consistency: Thin to medium.

Odor: Fresh, dry, top note, with a sweet, warm, lingering bottom note.

Chemistry: α-pinene (monoterpene) 3–30%, *p*-cymene (monoterpene) 5–10%, α-terpinene (monoterpene) 5–8%. Also small amounts of sesquiterpenes and esters.

Precautions: None known.

History and Traditional Uses: Frankincense is an aromatic plant with an extremely ancient and well-recorded history. It has been in continuous use for at least 5000 years in many different cultures. It was used by the ancient Egyptians in their famous perfume Kyphi[1] and has been used as a sacred incense by Jews, Christians, and Buddhists. Avicenna claimed that it strengthened the wit and the understanding, and Culpeper states that "it strengthens the memory exceedingly, comforts the heart, expels sadness and melancholy, strengthens the heart, helps coughs, rheums and pleurisies."[2]

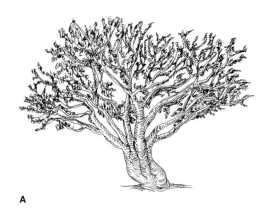

A

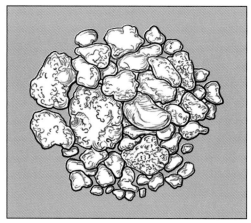

B

Main Uses in Massage

Frankincense is a very interesting essential oil because of its long use in many religious and spiritual settings. The smoke from the burnt resin has been shown to contain tetrahydrocannabinol, a "consciousness-expanding substance," and this is obviously one of the reasons why it has been used as an incense, for meditation and worship. The essential oil does not contain this chemical, but personal experience and general aromatherapy usage support the idea that the oil is ideal for calming and focusing the mind. Obviously this has many applications, including stress-related symptoms, inability to concentrate, mild attention-deficit hyperactivity disorder (ADHD), mental fatigue, anxiety, and fear. It can be used in a diffuser or spritzer, or as part of a massage blend for this purpose.

Frankincense is one of my favorite essential oils to use for asthma. The anxiety-reducing qualities mentioned above have a particularly good effect on stress-triggered asthmatic symptoms, and its well-proven antispasmodic properties also benefit these clients.[3] The antiseptic and mild expectorant nature of frankincense also helps, since asthmatics often develop bacterial infections in the lungs from a tendency toward shallow breathing. Many other respiratory conditions, such as bronchitis and laryngitis, can be helped by the anti-inflammatory effects of frankincense.[4]

Therapeutic Effects

Antidepressant and calmative ***
Anti-inflammatory **
Antispasmodic ***
Expectorant **
Immunostimulant ***
Vulnerary ****

** = mild   **** = extremely powerful

Studies have shown that frankincense is also useful in the treatment of other inflammatory problems, such as chronic colitis and phlebitis.[5,6] It would probably be helpful for any type of tissue inflammation.

Resins were frequently used as **vulneraries** (substances that help in tissue healing) in the ancient world, the rationale being that since they were produced by the tree to seal cuts in its bark, they would be equally successful in healing wounds in people. Certainly, the antiseptic, anti-inflammatory quality of frankincense would help damaged tissue, and laboratory studies show that the essential oil speeds up fibrinolysis, one of the initial processes in wound healing after clotting.[7] The essential oil can be used diluted in a carrier oil (probably about 3%) to apply to closed wounds after surgery or accidents.

One of the most important uses of frankincense essential oil for massage work is its marked ability to boost immune function. Lowered immunity is a common side effect of chronic stress and various diseases, and the ability of essential oils to reduce stress and increase resistance to illness is extremely hopeful. Researchers at Mansoura University in Egypt state that "biologically, the oil exhibited a strong immunostimulant activity (90% lymphocyte transformation)."[8]

It can be used in massage and take-home blends to help clients who develop infections frequently or who have lowered immunity from HIV infection or in response to chemotherapy.

Notes

1. Manniche L. Perfume of the Pharaohs. In Essence 2002;1(2):20–24.
2. Culpeper N. Culpeper's Complete Herbal. Ware, UK: Wordsworth Editions, 1995:386.
3. Lis-Balchin M, Hart S. A preliminary study of the effect of essential oils on skeletal and smooth muscle *in vitro*. J Ethnopharmacol 1997;58(3):183–187.
4. Duwiejua M, Zeitlin IJ, Waterman PG, et al. Anti-inflammatory activity of resins from some species of the plant family Burseraceae. Planta Medica 1993;59(1):12–16.
5. Gupta I, Parihar A, Malhotra P, et al. Effects of gum resin of *Boswellia serrata* in patients with chronic colitis. Planta Medica 2001;67(5): 391–395.
6. Wang T, Wang L. Using Huoxuetongluo lotion (HXTLL) to treat phlebitis in tumor patients treated with chemotherapy. Chin J Infor Trad Chin Med 2002;9(2):47.
7. Sumi H. Fibrinolysis-accelerating activity of the essential oils and Shochu aroma. Aroma Res 2003;4(3):264–267.
8. Mikhaeil BR, Maatooq GT, Badria FA, et al. Chemistry and immunomodulatory activity of frankincense oil. Z Naturforsch 2003; 58(3–4):230–238.

GERANIUM

Botanical name: *Pelargonium graveolens* or *P. x asperum.* (The x indicates a hybrid between two other species of *Pelargonium.*)

Family: Geraniaceae.

Native to: South Africa. Today it is cultivated for its oil in China, Egypt, and Morocco. The finest essential oil is supposed to come from the Reunion Islands (near Madagascar, off the southeastern coast of Africa), and this oil is traditionally called Bourbon Geranium, although care is needed when buying, as Geranium oils from other countries are now labeled Bourbon.

Part of plant used: Leaves and flowers.

Extraction method: Steam distillation.

Color of oil: Pale green.

Consistency: Thin.

Odor: Sweet, roselike, with citrus overtones.

Chemistry: Citronellol (alcohol) 23–30%, geraniol (alcohol) 18%, linalol (alcohol) 9–12%, citronellyl formate (ester) 10%.

Precautions: None known.

History and Traditional Uses: The pelargonium, or scented geranium, does not have a long history of medicinal or therapeutic use. It was brought to Europe in the late seventeenth century and was used for perfumery from the mid-nineteenth century.

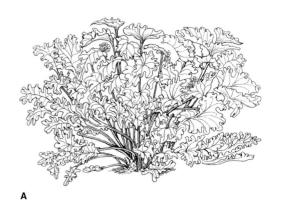

A

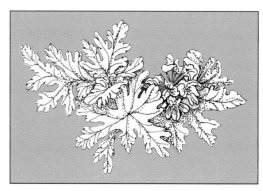

B

Main Uses in Massage

Geranium oil is one of the most useful remedies in aromatherapy massage because of its wide range of action, its mildness on the skin, and its reasonable cost. It is an extremely effective antidepressant and hypotensive, and some sources claim that it is a stimulant, while others say that it is a sedative. Geranium probably has some **adaptogenic** qualities, helping the body cope with stress, making it suitable both for calming and uplifting. One researcher states that after using Geranium essential oil, "the changes observed after treatment for 2 months resembled those obtained with meditation."[1] With its floral, slightly citrusy smell, it makes a pleasant addition to most blends for relaxation massage.

It is an oil I frequently use with good results with clients who are both tired and mentally overstimulated. Valnet recommends it for adrenal cortex deficiency,[2] in other words, for the tiredness that results from chronic stress, leading to adrenal burnout.

This hormonal action has been observed by other aromatherapists, and its action on the adrenal glands is thought to help balance fluctuating levels of hormones during menopause. Holmes suggests that it may encourage regular ovulation,[3] and I have used geranium successfully with several clients to decrease the effects of PMS. Simply smelling the essential oil was enough in most cases to produce a beneficial change in symptoms, especially in mood swings.

With its high levels of alcohols, geranium oil is a highly effective antifungal that is well tolerated by the skin.[4] It is useful for clients with

---

Therapeutic Effects

Antidepressant ***
Antifungal ***
Antispasmodic ***
Astringent ****
Hypotensive ***

** = mild   **** = extremely powerful

Candida yeast infections (candidiasis) and possibly for athlete's foot.

For such a gentle oil, geranium is extremely astringent and is used in aromatherapy for tightening and firming the skin and underlying tissue. It is also anti-inflammatory for the skin and mildly antibacterial, making it an excellent remedy for acne, dermatitis,[5] rosacea, shingles, and other skin problems, as well as for varicose veins.

Notes

1. Nozaki Y. Clinical studies of essential oil of *Pelargonium graveolens*. Aroma Res 2001;2(1):61–65.
2. Valnet J. The Practice of Aromatherapy. Saffron Walden, UK: CW Daniel, 1992:133.
3. Holmes P. The Energetics of Western Herbs, Vol. 1. Boulder, CO: Snow Lotus Press, 1997:321.
4. Chaumont JP, Bardey I. The *in vitro* antifungal activities of seven essential oils. Fitoterapia 1989;60(3):263–266.
5. Allan R. Seborrhoeic dermatitis. Int J Aromather 2003;13(1):47–48.

GINGER

Botanical name: *Zingiber officinale.*

Family: Zingiberaceae.

Native to: India, East Asia, and tropical Australia. Today it is also cultivated in Jamaica, China, and parts of Africa.

Part of plant used: Rhizome, usually described as the root (it is actually an underground stem).

Extraction method: Steam distillation or CO_2 extraction.

Color of oil: Distilled oil is clear to pale yellow; CO_2 extract is dark yellow to brown.

Consistency: Distilled oil is medium consistency; CO_2 extract is very thick and sticky.

Odor: The distilled oil smells most like the dried ground ginger spice—dry, spicy, and woody; the CO_2 resembles the fresh grated rhizome—sharp, warm, and very spicy.

Chemistry: Essential oil: α-zingiberene (sesquiterpene) 30–40%, β-sesquiphellandrene (sesquiterpene) 10–15%, camphene (monoterpene) 6–10%, β-bisabolene (sesquiterpene) 0.5–12%, Ar-curcumene (sesquiterpene) 7%. CO_2 extract: Gingerol, shogaol, and zingerone (phenyl propanoids) 25–33%.[1]

Precautions: None known.

History and Traditional Uses: Both a popular cooking spice and a medicinal plant, ginger has been used in a large proportion of prescriptions in both Ayurvedic and traditional Chinese medicine for at least 2000 years. In Ayurvedic medicine it is referred to as *vishwabhesaj*, the "universal medicine."[2] It had arrived in Europe at least by the time of Alexander the Great (around 356 B.C.) and was used in cooking and for digestive problems. In medieval Italy, its rejuvenating and aphrodisiac qualities provoked a popular saying: "Eat ginger and you will love and be loved as in your youth."[3]

Main Uses in Massage

Ginger is an excellent essential oil to use with any kind of work—massage or hydrotherapy—for painful muscles and joints because of its anti-inflammatory and analgesic effects.[4] It has been widely used traditionally and investigated clinically for rheumatoid arthritis and other inflammatory conditions of the musculoskeletal system.[5] It has a deeply penetrating, comforting warmth that soothes pain.

Because of its warmth and painkilling effect and its antispasmodic properties, ginger is one of the best topical remedies for dysmenorrhea. Use with a warm compress or massage on the low back and/or lower abdomen to relieve menstrual pain and cramping. The deep warmth of ginger is also useful for clients with chronically cold hands and feet as a result of poor circulation, or for clients who feel as if they are on the edge of catching a viral infection such as the flu, with the shivering and aching that accompany it. Ginger footbaths are effective in both these situations.

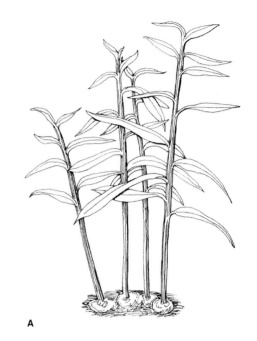

A

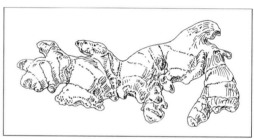

B

Therapeutic Effects
Antiemetic **
Anti-inflammatory and analgesic ***
Antirheumatic ***
Antispasmodic ***
Cardiostimulant **
Digestive tonic, appetite stimulant, cholagogue ***

** = mild   **** = extremely powerful

Ginger has long been used in Asian medicine as a cardiac tonic and mild stimulant, but it is not known whether it has much effect on the heart when used either topically or inhaled. However, I have noticed it has a marked stimulating effect on most people, and I use it with clients who find it hard to get going in the wet cold of our Pacific Northwest winters. Mojay recommends this stimulating yet grounding essential oil for clients who have a lot of creative ideas but lack the energy or optimism to carry out their projects.[6]

For a long time ginger has been used as a stimulant of the appetite and digestive tract, and studies show that it stimulates bile secretion from the liver, making digestion, especially of fats, more efficient.[7] Its antiemetic properties have also been exhaustively researched for relief from nausea during motion sickness, chemotherapy, and pregnancy, and it is clear that ingestion of the spice itself is effective for this problem.[8] However, smelling the essential oil does also seem to have some antinausea effect, though it is not as effective as peppermint essential oil in this situation. I have used the essential oil successfully in blends for clients who have lost their appetite.

Notes

1. Guba R. The modern alchemy of carbon dioxide extraction. Int J Aromather 2002;12(3):120–126.
2. Frawley D, Lad V. The Yoga of Herbs. Twin Lakes, WI: Lotus Press, 2001:121–122.
3. McIntyre A. Flower Power. London, UK: Henry Holt, 1996: 243–244.
4. Thomson M, Al-Qattan KK, Al-Sawan SM, et al. The use of ginger (*Zingiber officinale* Rosc.) as a potential anti-inflammatory and antithrombotic agent. Prostaglandins Leukot Essent Fatty Acids 2002; 67(6):475–478.
5. Sharma JN, Ishak FI, Yusef APM, et al. Effects of eugenol and ginger oil on adjuvant arthritis and kallikreins in rats. Asia Pac J Pharmacol 1997;12(1–2): 9–14.
6. Mojay G. Aromatherapy for Healing the Spirit. London, UK: Gaia, 1996:78–79.
7. Ozaki Y, Soedigdo S. Cholagogic effect of Zingiber plants obtained from Indonesia. Shoyakugaku Zasshi 1988;42(4):333–336.
8. Vishwakarma SL, Pal SC, Kasture VS, et al. Anxiolytic and antiemetic activity of *Zingiber officinale*. Phytother Res 2002;16(7):621–626.

GRAPEFRUIT

Botanical name: *Citrus x paradisii* (The x indicates a hybrid between two other species of citrus, probably *C. maxima* and *C. x aurantium*.)

Family: Rutaceae.

Native to: Southeast Asia. Today it is cultivated in Israel, South Africa, and the United States.

Part of plant used: Rind of fruit; the peel.

Extraction method: Cold expression.

Color of oil: Yellow to pale green.

Consistency: Very thin and watery.

Odor: Fresh, bright, citrusy, slightly bitter.

Chemistry: Limonene (monoterpene) up to 97%. (Trace components such as nootkatone and octanal give grapefruit its characteristic aroma.)

Precautions: Slightly phototoxic. Tisserand and Balacs recommend that it be used at 4% dilution or less if the skin is going to be exposed to direct sunlight or a tanning bed (UV light) within the following 12 hours.[1] Cases of allergic contact dermatitis to δ-limonene, the largest component in grapefruit oil, have been reported but they occurred only with oxidized limonene, showing the need for freshness in the citrus expressed oils.[2]

History and Traditional Uses: The origin of grapefruit is uncertain, although it is thought to be a hybrid of the sweet orange and the pomelo. It is mostly grown for its juice, although the expressed oil is popular in aromatherapy. Pink grapefruit essential oil is also commonly available.

Main Uses in Massage

Grapefruit is well known in aromatherapy massage work as an excellent lymphatic stimulant and cholagogue, helping the body move excess fluid and break down fats.[3] It is often used for fluid retention, cellulite, and arthritis, all of which often benefit by decongesting the body. It is a useful addition to a manual lymphatic drainage treatment. Its major component, δ-limonene, has been shown to help break down gallstones,[4] making it a possible choice for relief from other similar problems such as gout and kidney stones.

Grapefruit has long been promoted in diet books as an ideal food for weight loss. Some evidence shows that even smelling grapefruit may help suppress weight gain, by activating sympathetic nerves that innervate adipose tissue.[5] Grapefruit oil could be an interesting essential oil to use with clients as part of a weight loss program. This impact on the sympathetic nervous system is also reflected in the use of grapefruit oil as a refreshing, mild stimulant, suitable for clients who want to relax but not be sedated by a massage.

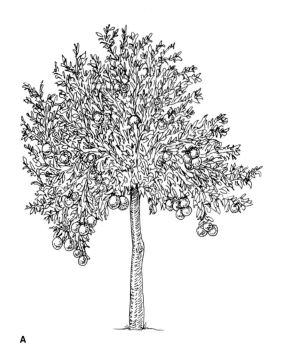

A

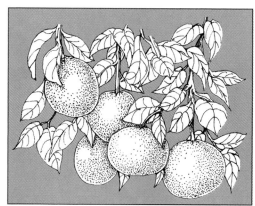

B

Therapeutic Effects

Cholagogue ***
Coolant ***
Detoxifier ***
Lymphatic stimulant ***
Stimulant **

** = mild   **** = extremely powerful

Notes

1. Tisserand R, Balacs T. Essential Oil Safety. London, UK: Churchill Livingstone, 1999:138.
2. Chang YC, Karlberg AT, Maibach HI. Allergic contact dermatitis from oxidized *d*-limonene Contact Dermatitis 1997;37:308–309.
3. Trabace L, Avato P, Mazzocoli M, et al. Choleretic activity of some typical components of essential oils. Planta Medica 1992;52 (Supplement 1):650–651.
4. Igimi H, Tamera R, Toraishi K, et al. Medical dissolution of gallstones. Clinical experience of *d*-limonene as a simple, safe and effective solvent. Dig Dis Sci 1991;36(2):200–208.
5. Sakata T, Yoshimatsu H, Woods SC, et al. Effect of olfactory stimulation with flavor of grapefruit oil and lemon oil on the activity of sympathetic branch in the white adipose tissue of the epididymis. Exp Biol Med 2003;228(10):1190–1192.

HELICHRYSUM

Botanical name: *Helichrysum italicum* (sometimes called *H. angustifolium*). Also has the common names of immortelle and everlasting.

Family: Asteraceae.

Native to: Mediterranean region. The best oil is reputed to come from Corsica.

Part of plant used: Flowers and flowering tops.

Extraction method: Distillation.

Color of oil: Yellow to red.

Consistency: Medium.

Odor: Very medicinal, deep, sweet, with turpentine overtones.

Chemistry: Neryl acetate (ester) 35–42%, γ-curcumene (sesquiterpene) 12–28%, limonene (monoterpene) 7%, neryl propanoate (ester) 5%. Also contains up to 10% di-ketones, which are unusual compounds in essential oils.

Precautions: None known.

History and Traditional Uses: Helichrysum does not have a long history of use as an essential oil. It was practically unknown in aromatherapy circles until the 1980s, when French aromatic physicians Pénoël and Franchomme publicized its benefits.

Main Uses in Massage

Most aromatherapists are enthusiastic about helichrysum. It is an effective remedy for a large range of problems, and yet it appears to have no side effects at all, being mild enough to use undiluted in large amounts if necessary. Not much clinical or laboratory testing has been done yet on this essential oil, but as Schnaubelt remarks, "its effects are so convincing that it has never met with any kind of criticism despite the absence of data on its effectiveness."[1]

Helichrysum is a successful anti-inflammatory.[2] It is one of the first oils I turn to for pain relief from arthritis, fibromyalgia, or injury—sprains or strains—because it eases the inflammation and helps edema. It can be applied undiluted to acute injuries until other help is available. As an **antihematomic,** it is the best remedy to resolve bruising, either mild or severe. John Steele, an aromatherapy consultant and teacher in California, was badly bitten by a dog while traveling, and although the skin was unbroken, the underlying tissue was torn and bruised. He applied neat helichrysum liberally during the course of the evening and found that the injury was almost completely gone the following day.[3]

Helichrysum is also frequently used on recent cuts and surgical wounds, as it both disinfects the area and helps new tissue to form, speeding up healing and reducing scarring noticeably. It can also be effective on older scars, and its **cicatrizant,** or skin-regenerating, properties (possibly deriving from the unusual di-ketones), together with its anti-inflammatory effects, make it ideal for many kinds of dermal issues, such as acne and dermatitis.

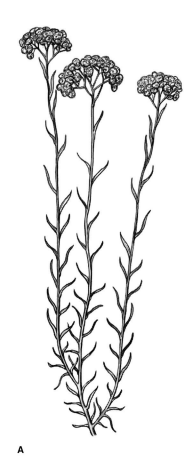

A

B

Therapeutic Effects

Antihematomic ****
Anti-inflammatory ***
Antiviral ***
Cicatrizant ****
Mucolytic ****
Sedative **

** = mild   **** = extremely powerful

It is a good astringent, both tightening tissue and providing support for structures below the superficial tissue. I regularly add helichrysum to blends for varicose veins. The results are excellent, if the oil is used consistently.

It also is an amazingly potent remedy for the respiratory system, especially as a **mucolytic,** to break down thick, sticky mucus in the lungs or sinuses. Used in a steam inhalation, it provides almost immediate relief, and its anti-inflammatory effects also help those in whom the problem starts with an allergic reaction, as in hay fever or asthma.

Evidence suggests that helichrysum may also be a strong antiviral agent, with studies showing significant activity against the herpes virus.[4]

Notes

1. Schnaubelt K. Medical Aromatherapy. Berkeley, CA: Frog Ltd, 1999:240.
2. Sala A, del Carmen Recio M, Giner RM, et al. Anti-inflammatory and antioxidant properties of *Helichrysum italicum.* J Pharm Pharmacol 2002;54(3):365–371.
3. Personal communication from John Steele.
4. Nostro A, Cannatelli MA, Marino A, et al. Evaluation of antiherpesvirus-1 and genotoxic activities of *Helichrysum italicum* extract. Microbiologica 2003;26(1):125–128.

HYSSOP

Botanical name: *Hyssopus officinalis.*

Family: Lamiaceae.

Native to: Southern Europe.

Part of plant used: Flowering tops.

Extraction method: Steam distillation.

Color of oil: Clear to pale yellow.

Consistency: Thin.

Odor: Medicinal herbaceous aroma, with camphoraceous overtones.

Chemistry: Pinocamphone and isopinocamphone (ketones) 20–43%, camphor (ketone) 16%, β-pinene (monoterpene) 11–20%.

Precautions: Neurotoxic. Avoid during pregnancy and with epilepsy. It is best not to use this oil with children. The ketone content of *Hyssopus officinalis* is cause for concern, as various case studies and animal studies show that the essential oil can cause convulsions because of its neurotoxic effects.[1] Many aromatherapists substitute creeping hyssop (*Hyssopus officinalis* var. *decumbens*) because it does not have the toxic effects of hyssop.

History and Traditional Uses: The name derives from the ancient Hebrew word *ezob*, and hyssop was used by the Hebrews for cleansing sacred places. It has often been used as a purifying aromatic herb, used to fumigate sick-houses (hospitals), and spread on the floor during the Middle Ages.[2] It is also used to flavor liqueurs. Hippocrates recommended it for pleurisy and Dioscorides for asthma.

Main Uses in Massage

Hyssop is an oil to be used with caution. However, if used in normal therapeutic doses with clients who are not contraindicated, it should not present any risk. I have found it to be useful for respiratory problems, and it can be used in chest rubs and inhalations for asthma, chronic bronchitis, and respiratory allergies, as well as to relieve bronchial spasms and decrease mucus buildup.

It is an excellent nerve tonic, warming, gently stimulating, and strengthening, making it a good choice for clients who tend to get exhausted because of nervous tension and worry, or for people recovering from an illness. According to Tisserand, "it strengthens and warms the nerves, bringing a feeling of relaxation."[3]

It is one of the best remedies for bruising, and Valnet also recommends it in the treatment of eczema.[4]

Notes

1. Millet Y, Tognetti P, Lavaire-Perlovisi M, et al. Experimental study of the toxic convulsant properties of commercial preparations of essences of sage and hyssop. Revue d'E.E.G. Neurophysiologie 1979;9(1):12–18.
2. McIntyre A. Flower Power. London, UK: Henry Holt, 1996:133.
3. Tisserand R. The Art of Aromatherapy. Saffron Walden, UK: CW Daniel, 1994: 235–236.
4. Valnet J. The Practice of Aromatherapy. Saffron Walden, UK: CW Daniel, 1992: 137–139.

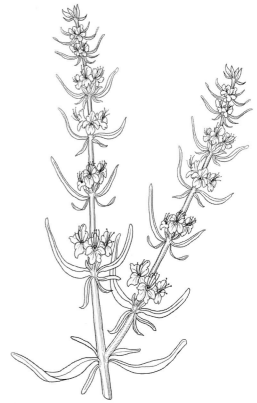

A

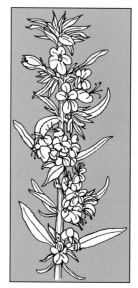

B

Therapeutic Effects

Antiseptic **
Antispasmodic ***
Expectorant ***
Nervine ***

** = mild   **** = extremely powerful

INULA

Botanical name: *Inula graveolens.* (Not to be confused with *Inula helenium*, commonly known as elecampane, a severe dermal sensitizer.)

Family: Asteraceae.

Native to: Mediterranean region.

Part of plant used: Flowering plant.

Extraction method: Steam distillation.

Color of oil: Clear emerald green.

Consistency: Slightly thick.

Odor: Penetrating, sweet, with deep balsamic undertones.

Chemistry: Bornyl acetate (ester) 48%, T-cadinol (sesquiterpene alcohol) 11%, borneol (monoterpene alcohol) 9%.

Precautions: None known.

History and Traditional Uses: None known for this particular species. Its relative, the herb elecampane, was used by the Romans and Greeks as a cure-all and by the Anglo-Saxons for skin diseases.[1]

Main Uses in Massage

Inula is an oil with a relatively narrow range of use, but it is very powerful in its effects. It is probably the most powerful mucolytic to be found among the essential oils, liquefying dense, sticky mucus in the sinuses and lungs, thereby making it easier to expel from the body. Although it is expensive, so little needs to be used that it is actually quite economical. Inula is at its most effective when used in a steam inhalation, although it is also effective when used in massage on the chest. Although it has a peculiar aroma, I have found by experience that people who need this oil love its smell.

It is also recommended by Badoux as a cardiac tonic, helpful in cases of tachycardia, arrhythmia, and cardiac fatigue.[2]

Notes

1. Ody P. The Complete Medicinal Herbal. London, UK: Dorling Kindersley, 1993:70.
2. Badoux D. L'Aromathérapie. Anglet, France: Éditions atlantica, 2001:152–153.

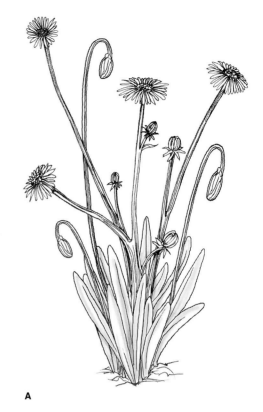

A

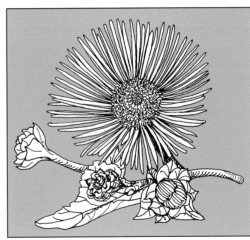

B

Therapeutic Effects

Antitussive **
Cardiac tonic **
Expectorant **
Mucolytic ****

** = mild   **** = extremely powerful

JASMINE

Botanical name: Various species of jasmine are used in aromatherapy, the most common being *Jasminum grandiflorum, J. officinale,* and *J. sambac.*

Family: Oleaceae.

Native to: China, India, and the Middle East.

Part of plant used: Flowers.

Extraction method: Solvent extraction. Jasmine cannot be extracted by steam distillation because the aroma tends to be destroyed by heat. In India you can occasionally obtain jasmine rhu, a water-distilled jasmine oil, but it is rare and expensive.[1]

Color of oil: Amber to dark reddish-brown.

Consistency: Quite thick.

Odor: Heavy, intensely sweet, warm, floral aroma.

Chemistry: Benzyl acetate (ester) 60–65%, linalol (monoterpene alcohol) 15%, linalyl acetate (ester) 7%, jasmone (ketone) 3%, indole (a nitrogen-containing compound) 3%. Jasmone and indole are the constituents with the strongest aroma, even though they make up only about 6% of the absolute.

Precautions: Jasmine should be avoided by lactating mothers.

History and Traditional Uses: Jasmine is a sacred flower in India, used in bridal wreaths, as hair decorations, and in hair oil. Because the flower opens in the dark, it is known in India as the "Queen of the Night." The Indian god of love, Kama, is supposed to tip his arrows with the oil, and the flower has been associated with love and fertility in various traditions. It is used in Ayurvedic medicine to calm the nerves and for menstrual difficulties.

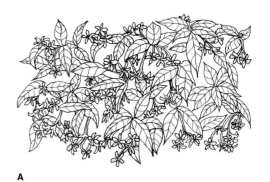

A

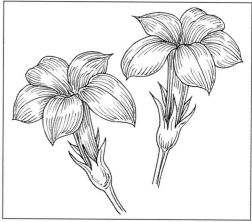

B

Main Uses in Massage

Because of its high price, jasmine tends to be reserved for psychotherapeutic use, as its other functions can be carried out by much less expensive oils. It is one of the best antidepressants among essential oils—comforting, warming, and joyous. It has a definite stimulating effect, confirmed by various clinical and laboratory studies,[2,3] and it may be best not to use it late in the evening for that reason. However, this does give it a strengthening quality, making it useful for clients who are both depressed and tired.

It is an extremely sensuous aroma, and one I like to use with clients who tend to dissociate from their body and live in their intellect, or those who are afraid of their physical nature and dislike being touched. It is also a wonderful treat for anyone who needs pleasure and delight.

Jasmine has been shown in several studies to be an **antigalactagogue,** an agent that suppresses the production of breast milk,[4] and it is traditionally used for this purpose in India. One study suggests that "both tactile and olfactory stimuli of the flowers were responsible for suppression of lactation and that the olfactory route mediated suppression of serum prolactin."[5] If this is the case, the use of jasmine should be avoided with breast-feeding mothers, as even the smell may disrupt

Therapeutic Effects

Antidepressant ****
Antigalactagogue ***
Stimulant **

** = mild   **** = extremely powerful

the production of milk. However, it could be useful to women who are ready to wean their baby.

Notes

1. For further information on jasmine rhu, see www.whitelotusaromatics.com.
2. Kikuchi A, Tsuchiya T, et al. Stimulant-like ingredients in absolute jasmine. Chem Senses 1989;14(2):304.
3. Sugano H. Effects of odours on mental function. Chem Senses 1989;14(2):303.
4. Abraham M, Devi, NS, Sheela R. Inhibiting effect of jasmine flowers on lactation. Ind J Med Res 1979;69:88–92.
5. Shrivastav P, George K, Balasubramaniam N, et al. Suppression of puerperal lactation using jasmine flowers (*Jasminum sambac*). Aust N Z J Obstet Gynaecol 1988;28:68–71.

JUNIPER

Botanical name: *Juniperus communis*. Several other *Juniperus* species are distilled for essential oils, such as *J. virginiana* (Virginian cedar), *J. sabina* (savin), and *J. oxycedra* (cade), all of which have very different properties and contraindications.

Family: Cupressaceae.

Native to: All parts of the northern hemisphere.

Part of plant used: Fruit. (An essential oil is also made from the branches, but it is considered less desirable in aromatherapy than the oil from the ripe berries.)

Extraction method: Steam distillation.

Color of oil: Clear.

Consistency: Thin.

Odor: Sharp, clear, penetrating, reminiscent of gin.

Chemistry: α-pinene (monoterpene) 33–40%, myrcene (monoterpene) 5–11%, sabinene (monoterpene) 5–15%.

Precautions: None known. Juniper has often been contraindicated during pregnancy and in cases of kidney disease. Various studies show that juniper is nontoxic, even at fairly high oral doses,[1] and Tisserand and Balacs state that "there is no reason to regard juniper oil as being hazardous in any way."[2]

History and Traditional Uses: Juniper has been used medicinally at least as far back as the ancient Egyptians, and very possibly much earlier. It has been referred to in shamanistic traditions as "the tree of life"[3] and was burnt in temples during purification rituals. The oil has been used in central Europe as a folk remedy for typhoid, cholera, and dysentery.[4] It is also used to flavor gin.

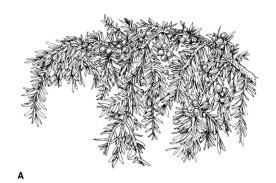

A

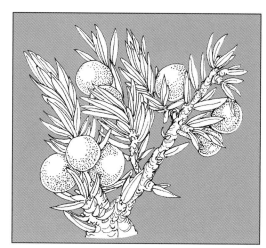

B

Main Uses in Massage

Juniper oil is a very effective skin cleanser. Because of its high percentage of monoterpenes, it has a strong antiseptic and astringent quality. It can be used for oily and congested skin, for acne, and, in small doses, for certain types of eczema.

This decongesting quality is important in other ways. Juniper is frequently used as part of a detoxifying blend, especially in cases of gout or arthritis, where its warming nature is also helpful. Studies show that it is a mild analgesic, which is also useful for these conditions.[5]

The antiseptic, warming yet anti-inflammatory[6] nature of Juniper makes it a good choice for urinary tract infections, and it can be used in massage on the lower abdomen or low back, or put into a blend for clients to use at home in the bath.

Notes

1. Schilcher H, Leuschner F. Studies of potential nephrotoxic effects of essential juniper oil. Arzneimittel-forschung 1997;47(7):855–858.
2. Tisserand R, Balacs T. Essential Oil Safety. London, UK: Churchill Livingstone, 1999:142.

Therapeutic Effects

Antiseptic ***
Astringent ***
Stimulant ***
Warming ***

** = mild   **** = extremely powerful

3. Fischer-Rizzi S. The Complete Incense Book. New York: Sterling, 1998:28–29.
4. Ody P. The Complete Medicinal Herbal. London, UK: Dorling Kindersley, 1993:72.
5. Wakame K, Wagatsuma C, Miura T. Sedative, analgesic and sleep-prolonging effects to the mouse of commercial essential oils. Aroma Res 2003;4(3):249–252.
6. Mascolo N, Autore G, Capasso F. Biological screening of Italian medicinal plants for anti-inflammatory activity. Phytother Res 1987;1:28–31.

LAVENDER

Botanical name: Several species of lavender are used in aromatherapy, the most common being *Lavandula angustifolia* ("true" lavender, often called *L. vera* or *L. officinalis*); *L. latifolia* ("spike" lavender); and *L. x intermedia* (a natural hybrid of *angustifolia* and *latifolia*, often called lavandin). Lavandin is the "lavender" most often used in soaps, lotions, and detergents.

Family: Lamiaceae.

Native to: Europe, North Africa, and India. Today it is cultivated worldwide.

Part of plant used: Flowering tops.

Extraction method: Steam distillation.

Color of oil: Clear.

Consistency: Thin.

Odor: The smell of *angustifolia* species varies depending on the altitude and location where it is grown. Its aroma is generally light-floral and sweet, with either a buttery or a minty note. The *latifolia* has a more camphoraceous smell, and the *intermedia* smells like either parent species, depending on its chemistry.

Chemistry: Lavender grown at high altitudes has a higher percentage of esters. The major chemical components of the different *Lavandula* species are listed in the table below.

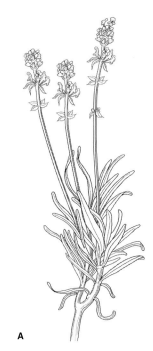

A

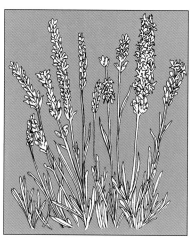

B

Major components				
	Linalyl acetate (ester)	Linalol (monoterpene alcohol)	Camphor (ketone)	1,8 cineole (oxide)
L. angustifolia	22–53%	18–49%	1–3%	1–3%
L. latifolia	–	19–43%	6–19%	20–43%
L. intermedia	19–47%	24–38%	4–12%	3–12%

Precautions: None known.

History and Traditional Uses: The word lavender comes from the Latin *lavare*, to wash, indicating its long use as a bath and laundry aromatic. During the Middle Ages it was a favorite herb to spread on the floors of houses, place in linen closets, and hang in rooms to keep away flies. It was popularly used in France as a wound healer and as a **vermifuge,** a remedy for intestinal worms.

Main Uses in Massage

L. angustifolia has so many uses that it is almost indispensable to an aromatherapist. It is also so mild that it can be used safely with anyone and used in high concentrations. It is best known as a sedative, and many studies confirm this property.[1] One interesting point that emerged in a clinical study was that the subjects not only slept better when using lavender, but they also reported having a better day subsequently, with more alertness.[2]

Therapeutic Effects

angustifolia:
Analgesic ★★★★
Antidepressant ★★★
Anti-inflammatory ★★★★
Cicatrizant ★★★
Sedative and hypotensive ★★★

latifolia:
Analgesic, antirheumatic ★★★
Detoxifier ★★★
Expectorant ★★★

★★ = mild   ★★★★ = extremely powerful

Lavender also has good potential as an antidepressant; studies show that people feel less depressed and can perform tasks better after smelling it.[3] This finding suggests that it leads to a more relaxed, less anxious, and therefore more efficient state of being. It is extremely useful for most stress-related issues.

The anti-inflammatory and analgesic effects of lavender are well known and have also been thoroughly researched,[4] and there is some evidence to suggest that it may also be a mild local anesthetic.[5] This makes the essential oil a good addition to a blend for any kind of pain, including headaches, arthritis, or overworked muscles. Its anti-inflammatory effect also indicates its use in soothing allergic reactions,[6] whether respiratory or dermal.

Lavender is a wonderful remedy for minor burns of all kinds, kitchen burns as well as sunburn, because of its cicatrizant, or tissue-healing, properties. It is also useful for the same reason for acne, dermatitis, rosacea, and any other inflammatory skin conditions. Scars that have been treated with lavender are much less noticeable than those that have not, and even old scars can benefit from its application.

Studies show lavender oil's strong anticonvulsive effects, even when simply inhaled, making it ideal for all kinds of spasmodic issues, such as muscle cramping, dysmenorrhea, irritable bowel syndrome, and asthma.

Spike lavender (*Lavandula latifolia*) has quite different qualities. It is a strong expectorant[7] with a soothing effect, and it works well in cases of bronchitis, laryngitis, and sinusitis. It is my favorite oil, along with eucalyptus, for a viral respiratory infection. It also is useful for muscular aches and pains, and in studies of its use with chronic joint pain it reduced both pain and swelling.[8]

Lavandin (*Lavandula x intermedia*) shares the properties of its parent plants, some clones being closer in chemistry to the *angustifolia*, others to the *latifolia*. If a lavandin has a high percentage of esters, it can make an extremely good substitute for true lavender, at a fraction of the cost. A study by Buckle shows that lavandin may actually be superior to lavender in reducing anxiety after surgery.[9]

Notes

1. Buchbauer G, Jirovetz L. Aromatherapy: evidence for sedative effects of the essential oil of lavender after inhalation. Zeitschrift fur Naturforschung 1991;46(11–12):1067–1072.
2. Hudson R. The value of lavender for rest and activity in the elderly patient. Complement Ther Med 1996;4:52–57.
3. Diego MA, Jones NA, Field T, et al. Aromatherapy positively affects mood, EEG patterns of alertness and math computations. Int J Neurosci 1998;96:217–224.
4. Hajhashemi V, Ghannadi A, Badie S. Anti-inflammatory and analgesic properties of the leaf extracts and essential oil of *Lavandula angustifolia* Mill. J Ethnopharmacol 2003;89(1):66–71.
5. Ghelardini C, Galeotti N, Salvatore G, et al. Local anaesthetic activity of the essential oil of *Lavandula angustifolia*. Planta Medica 1999;65:700–703.
6. Kim H-M, Cho S-H. Lavender oil inhibits immediate-type allergic reaction in mice and rats. J Pharm Pharmacol 1999;51:221–226.
7. Von Frohlich E. A review of clinical, pharmacological and bacteriological research into *Oleum spicae*. Weiner Medizinische Wochenschrift 1968;15:345–350.
8. Von Frohlich E. A review of clinical, pharmacological and bacteriological research into *Oleum spicae*. Weiner Medizinische Wochenschrift 1968;15:345–350.
9. Buckle J. Aromatherapy. Does it matter which lavender essential oil is used? Nurs Times 1993;89(20):32–35.

LEMON

Botanical name: *Citrus limon.*

Family: Rutaceae.

Native to: Southern and Southeast Asia. Today it is cultivated commercially worldwide, including North and South America, Israel, South Africa, and Italy.

Part of plant used: Rind of fruit.

Extraction method: Cold expression.

Color of oil: Very pale yellow.

Consistency: Very thin.

Odor: Clear, sharp, light, very citrusy.

Chemistry: Limonene (monoterpene) 60–76%, β-pinene (monoterpene) 10–13%, γ-terpinene (monoterpene) 5–10%.

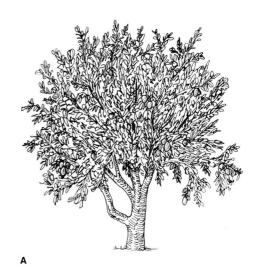

A

Precautions: Slightly phototoxic.[1] Tisserand and Balacs recommend using it at less than 2% if there will be exposure to sunlight or a tanning bed (UV light) within the next 12 hours.[2] Also, limonene (a major constituent of lemon oil) can cause allergic contact dermatitis if oxidized.[3] All expressed citrus oils should be used as fresh as possible.

History and Traditional Uses: Originating in Asia, the lemon was not used much in the West until at least A.D. 1100, when it was mentioned in Arabic herbal books. European herbalists later recognized it as a good blood cleanser, and it was used by the British navy to counteract scurvy during long journeys by sailing ship. It has been widely used in Europe as a folk remedy for colds and fevers.[4]

Main Uses in Massage

Lemon oil has a strong effect on the immune system, by both strengthening and supporting it. It is not as highly antiviral or antibacterial as some other oils, but its medium antimicrobial action,[5] together with its ability to enhance the activity of white blood cells,[6] makes it a potent support to immunity.

In various studies, this increase in immune functioning was linked to a heightening of positive mood in the client. In one study, most patients in the group exposed to a citrus blend (which included lemon) were able to reduce their antidepressant drug intake to zero, while those in the control group still needed their usual doses of antidepressants.[7] The levels of the stress chemicals noradrenaline and adrenaline in their bodies were also lower, and natural killer cell activity was higher than in the control group. The connection between chronic stress and a lowered immune function has been thoroughly explored, and the antidepressant properties of lemon and of other citruses can only have a beneficial effect on both mood and immunity.

Another study on the antidepressant effects of lemon oil observed that fewer health symptoms were reported by patients after exposure to the essential oil,[8] suggesting that lemon may also have a positive effect on how people perceive themselves and their health.

Lemon has been classified as a stimulant in various studies.[9] It is useful to clear and focus the mind. It seems to be more mentally refreshing

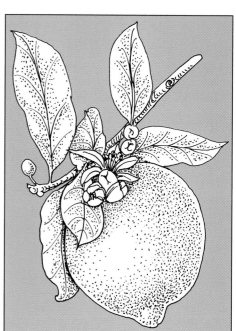

B

Therapeutic Effects

Antibacterial **
Antidepressant ***
Antiviral **
Astringent ***
Immunostimulant ***
Stimulant **

** = mild   **** = extremely powerful

rather than strongly stimulating to the body, and I have used it with clients who tend to think obsessively or who have a lot of decisions or worries.

Like grapefruit, it has a strong ability to decongest and detoxify, partly because of its astringent action, which helps move lymphatic fluid. It has been used (sometimes successfully) as part of a cellulite regimen, and also for edema. The effect of tightening tissue also has a good effect on circulation and blood vessels, making it appropriate for varicose veins and broken capillaries. Some studies suggest that it may also be helpful for weight loss.[10]

Like grapefruit, its major chemical component is limonene, which has been shown to help break down gallstones.[11] Lemon juice has long been used in folk medicine for this purpose.[12] It has potential uses even when used topically for various types of stones and for gout.

Notes

1. Naganuma M, Hirose S, Nakayama Y, et al. A study of the phototoxicity of lemon oil. Arch Dermatol Res 1985;278(1):31–36.
2. Tisserand R, Balacs T. Essential Oil Safety. London, UK: Churchill Livingstone, 1999:146.
3. Chang YC, Karlberg AT, Maibach HI. Allergic contact dermatitis from oxidized d-limonene. Contact Dermatitis 1997;37:308–309.
4. de Bairacli Levy J. Common Herbs for Natural Health. Woodstock, NY: Ash Tree Publishing, 1997:95–96.
5. Kivanc M, Akgul A. Antibacterial action of essential oils from Turkish spices and citrus. Flavor Frag J 1986;1:175–179.
6. Fujiwara R, Komori T, Noda Y, et al. Effects of a long-term inhalation of fragrances on the stress-induced immunosuppression in mice. Neuroimmunomodulation 1998;5:318–322.
7. Komori T, Fujiwara R, Tanida M, et al. Effects of citrus fragrance on immune function and depressive states. Neuroimmunomodulation 1995;2:174–180.
8. Knasko S C. Ambient odor's effect on creativity, mood and perceived health Chem Senses 1992;17:27–35.
9. Kikuchi A, Tanida M, Venoyamas S, et al. Effect of odors on cardiac response patterns in a reaction time task. Chem Senses 1991;16:183.
10. Sakata T, Yoshimatsu H, Woods SC, et al. Effect of olfactory stimulation with flavor of grapefruit oil and lemon oil on the activity of sympathetic branch in the white adipose tissue of the epididymis. Exp Biol Med 2003;228(10):1190–1192.
11. Igimi H, Tamura R, Toraishi K, et al. Medical dissolution of gallstones. Clinical experience of δ-limonene as a simple, safe and effective solvent. Dig Dis Sci 1991;36(2):200–208.
12. Valnet J. The Practice of Aromatherapy. Saffron Walden, UK: CW Daniel, 1982:151.

MANDARIN

Botanical name: *Citrus reticulata*. Tangerine and satsuma are other varieties of the same species, although they do not seem to have certain trace components, such as *n*-methyl methyl anthranilate, that exist in mandarin oil, and do not have such a full aroma.

Family: Rutaceae.

Native to: Southeast Asia. Today it is cultivated extensively in Brazil and Italy.

Part of plant used: Peel or rind.

Extraction method: Cold expression.

Color of oil: Yellowish orange.

Consistency: Thin.

Odor: Very sweet, rich, slightly floral.

Chemistry: Limonene (monoterpene) 72–82%, γ-terpinene (monoterpene) 11–20%, methyl-*n*-methyl anthranilate (ester that contains nitrogen) less than 1%. (Compounds that contain nitrogen or sulphur have a much stronger smell than other essential oil components, so the methyl-*n*-methyl anthranilate has a considerable influence on the aroma of mandarin oil. This component is also found in neroli, bergamot, and ylang ylang essential oils and in jasmine absolute.[1])

Precautions: None known.

History and Traditional Uses: The name is said to derive from the one-time rulers of China, the Mandarins, for whom the fruit was considered a suitable gift.

Main Uses in Massage

Mandarin is an extremely useful essential oil for clients who are tense and stressed to the point that they find it difficult to sleep, or to relax at all. More than any of the other citruses, it seems to have a marked sedative quality, which derives from a calming influence rather than a soporific one. As the French aromatherapist Baudoux remarks, it has almost a "slightly hypnotic" effect.[2] It is often used to help small children sleep, when they have gotten to that overtired, hyperactive, slightly hysterical state with which parents are so familiar. It works equally well with adults who are in a similar state.

Schnaubelt cites it as a "useful antispasmodic for cardiovascular, digestive and respiratory systems."[3] It is appropriate in massage blends for asthmatic coughing, colic, irritable bowel syndrome, and palpitations. It may be most useful in this way for children, who enjoy its candylike aroma.

Mandarin oil is also frequently used in aromatherapy as a moisturizing agent, and studies have confirmed its hydrating effects on the skin.[4] It is often added to rich creams to apply to the abdomen during pregnancy, to minimize stretch marks.

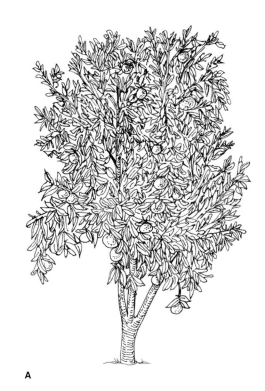

A

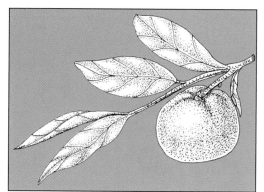

B

Therapeutic Effects

Antidepressant **
Antispasmodic **
CNS sedative and relaxant ****
Cicatrizant ***

** = mild   **** = extremely powerful

Notes

1. Tisserand R, Balacs T. Essential Oil Safety. London, UK: Churchill Livingstone, 1999:194.
2. Badoux D. L'Aromathérapie. Anglet, France: Éditions atlantica, 2001: 168–169.
3. Schnaubelt K. Medical Aromatherapy. Berkeley, CA: Frog Ltd, 1998:185.
4. Monges PH, Joachim G, Bohor M, et al. Comparative *in vivo* study of the moisturizing properties of three gels containing essential oils: mandarin, German chamomile, orange. Nouveau Dermatologie 1994;13:470–475.

MARJORAM

Botanical name: *Origanum majorana*. It is important not to confuse this essential oil with that of oregano (*Origanum vulgare*), or with other "marjorams" or "oreganos." There is confusion between the common names of these plants, even in scientific studies, and they have very different properties and contraindications.

Family: Lamiaceae.

Native to: Mediterranean region.

Part of plant used: Flowering tops.

Extraction method: Steam distillation.

Color of oil: Clear to pale amber.

Consistency: Thin.

Odor: Herbaceous, woody, slightly camphoraceous.

Chemistry: Terpinen-4-ol (monoterpene alcohol) 20–31%, *Cis*-thujan-4-ol (monoterpene alcohol) 5–19%, linalol (monoterpene alcohol) 2–19%, γ-terpene (monoterpene) 12–15%.

Precautions: None known. Some sources contraindicate this oil for pregnancy, but no evidence suggests that this is necessary.

History and Traditional Uses: Marjoram is an herb with an ancient history. Cultivated by the Egyptians for both perfumes and medicines, it was dedicated to Osiris, god of the afterlife and agriculture. The seventeenth-century herbalist Culpeper recommends the oil for stiff joints and tight muscles, to make them softer and more supple.[1] The contemporary herbalist de Bairacli Levy suggests topical use for headaches, earache, toothache, and sore throat.[2]

Main Uses in Massage

Culpeper's observations of the effects of marjoram oil are still relevant today. This is one of the best essential oils for tight muscles, stiff joints, and muscular cramps and spasms. It is gently warming and antispasmodic and appears to be slightly analgesic, all helpful for various musculoskeletal conditions. It is one of the three essential oils used by Price in 1992 in a small project with patients who had Parkinson's disease.[3] The difference between the group who received the essential oil blend and the control group, who received only massage, was particularly striking in the area of muscular pain and stiffness. It is also useful for arthritis, sciatica, and low-back pain.

Marjoram also works well on smooth muscle, easing the pain and discomfort experienced with asthmatic coughing, whooping cough, colic, and stomach pains.

It is highly relaxing and hypotensive. One study showed that the application of only 0.05 mL (about 1–2 drops) of the essential oil on the wrist lowered heart rate, blood pressure, and levels of cortisol in subjects under stress. It is extremely good for nervous types of depression, anxiety, insomnia, and many stress-related issues. Mailhebiau is so impressed by its relaxant properties that he recommends its use for epilepsy.[4]

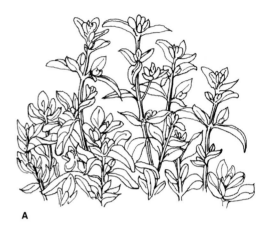

A

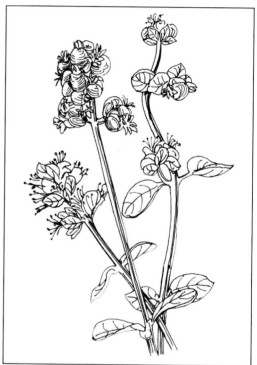

B

Therapeutic Effects

Antimicrobial **
Antispasmodic ***
Relaxant and hypotensive ****
Tonic ***

** = mild   **** = extremely powerful

Many writers on aromatherapy, ancient and modern, also comment on marjoram's tonic and strengthening qualities, and it seems to be an ideal oil for clients who are both tired and tense, for fibromyalgia and chronic fatigue syndrome, and for progressive diseases such as multiple sclerosis and rheumatoid arthritis. These properties also make it suitable for emotional support, and it is frequently used in aromatherapy for clients who are grieving or who feel isolated and lonely. According to Mojay, it helps to "promote the capacity for inner self-nurturing."[5]

Notes

1. Culpeper N. Culpeper's Complete Herbal. Ware, UK: Wordsworth Editions Ltd., 1995:160–161.
2. de Bairacli Levy J. Common Herbs for Natural Health. Woodstock, NY: Ash Tree Publishing, 1997:102–103.
3. Price S, Price L. Aromatherapy for Health Professionals. London, UK: Churchill Livingstone, 2001:171–173.
4. Mailhebiau P. Portraits in Oils. Saffron Walden, UK: CW Daniel, 1995:57–63.
5. Mojay G. Aromatherapy for Healing the Spirit. London, UK: Gaia Books Ltd, 1996:94–95.

MELISSA

Botanical name: *Melissa officinalis.* Other common names are balm and lemon balm.

Family: Lamiaceae.

Native to: Europe and Central Asia.

Part of plant used: Flowering tops.

Extraction method: Steam distillation, which gives a yield of only 0.01–0.13%, making this oil extremely expensive. As a result, it is often adulterated with lemongrass (*Cymbopogon citratus*) or citronella (*Cymbopogon nardus*), or completely imitated with various "lemony" smelling, cheaper oils.[1]

Color of oil: Clear or pale yellow.

Consistency: Thin.

Odor: Sweet, sharp, lemony.

Chemistry: Geranial (aldehyde) 25–47%, neral (aldehyde) 19–36%, β-caryophyllene (sesquiterpene) 2–11%, citronellal (aldehyde) 1–24%.

Precautions: As with other essential oils high in aldehydes, melissa can cause skin irritation and sensitization and should be used with caution when dealing with sensitive skin and/or people with allergies.[2] The high aldehyde content also makes melissa a rather unstable oil, so it is advisable to buy it in small amounts and use it within about a year.

History and Traditional Uses: Melissa is an herb with an ancient history. The name is derived from the Latin word for bee, as honeybees are very fond of the plant. According to the herbalist Evelyn, it is "sovereign for the brain, strengthening memory and powerfully chasing away melancholy."[3] The contemporary herbalist de Bairacli Levy states, "the plant is said to safeguard against early senility and impotency."[4]

Main Uses in Massage

Clinical investigations demonstrate that melissa is highly antimicrobial; in fact, one report stated that it "tended to exhibit higher activities against a battery of microorganisms (bacteria and fungi) than the other essential oils."[5] Its antiviral activity has been strongly documented against the herpes simplex virus,[6] and it seems to be able to both treat outbreaks and prolong the intervals between outbreaks.[7] It also appears to be extremely effective in treating the *Candida* yeast infection (candidiasis).[8] It can be given to clients in take-home blends to use in topical applications and baths, or used in massage sessions to alleviate symptoms or avoid outbreaks.

Melissa is also useful as a sedative; it has a calming effect on the central nervous system. This characteristic makes it a good remedy for any kind of stress-related condition, including generalized anxiety, hypertension, insomnia, tension headaches, and depression. It has also been used in several studies for the relief of agitation in dementia resulting from Alzheimer's disease and other illnesses.[9]

Its antispasmodic qualities, together with its sedative effect, make it ideal for spasms of the digestive system, such as irritable bowel syndrome, which are often triggered by stress.[10]

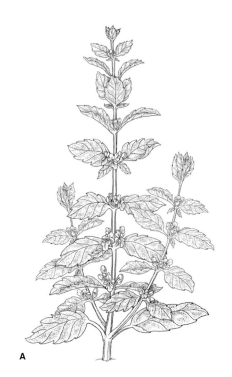

A

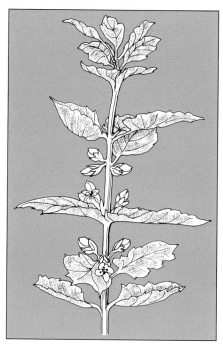

B

Therapeutic Effects

Antibacterial ***
Antifungal ***
Antispasmodic **
Antiviral ***
Sedative and anxiolytic ***

** = mild   **** = extremely powerful

Notes

1. Sorenson JM. Melissa officinalis. Int J Aromather 2000;10(1/2):7–15.
2. Tisserand R, Balacs T. Essential Oil Safety. London, UK: Churchill Livingstone, 1999:151.
3. McIntyre A. Flower Power. London, UK: Henry Holt, 1996:159.
4. de Bairacli Levy J. Common Herbs for Natural Health. Woodstock, NY: Ash Tree Publishing, 1997:20.
5. Larrondo JV, Agut M, Calvo-Torras MA. Antimicrobial activity of essences from labiates. Microbios 1995;82(332):171–172.
6. Dimitrova Z, Dimov B, Manolova N, et al. Antiherpes effect of *Melissa officinalis* L. extracts. Acta Microbiol Bulg 1993;29: 65–72.
7. Kotychev R, Alken RG, Dundarov S. Balm mint extract (Lo-701) for topical treatment of recurring herpes labialis. Phytomedicine 1999;6(4):225–230.
8. Larrondo JV, Calvo MA. Effect of essential oils on *Candida albicans*: a scanning electron microscope study. Biomed Lett 1991;46(184): 269–272.
9. Ballard CG, O'Brien JT, Reichelt K, et al. Aromatherapy as a safe and effective treatment for the management of agitation in severe dementia: the results of a double-blind, placebo-controlled trial with Melissa. J Clin Psychiatr 2002;63(7):553–558.
10. Sandraei H, Ghannadi A, Malekshahi K. Relaxant effect of essential oil of *Melissa officinalis* and citral on rat ileum contractions. Fitoterapia 2003;74(5):445–452.

MYRRH

Botanical name: *Commiphora myrrha*. It is sometimes called *C. molmol* in older literature, but this is not a valid name.

Family: Burseraceae.

Native to: Northeast Africa and Southeast Asia, especially Oman, Somalia, Yemen, and Ethiopia.

Part of plant used: Resin.

Extraction method: Steam distillation and CO_2 extraction.

Color of the oil: Essential oil: clear or pale yellow; CO_2 extract: reddish brown.

Consistency: Essential oil: slightly thick; CO_2 extract: thick and sticky. Both tend to crystallize around the lip of the bottle, making them extremely difficult to open.

Odor: Dry, dusty, warm, slightly medicinal.

Chemistry: Furanoeudesma-1,3-diene (sesquiterpene) 12–37%, curzerene (sesquiterpene) 11–27%, lindestrene (sesquiterpene) 3–7%.

Precautions: None known.

History and Traditional Uses: The burning of myrrh resin as an incense goes back as far as recorded history. According to Egyptian mythology, it was created from the tears of Horus, the falcon god, and the ancient peoples of Arabia used it medicinally to heal wounds. It was dissolved in wine and given as a painkiller to condemned men before an execution.[1] The medieval healer Hildegard of Bingen recommended it for toothache.[2]

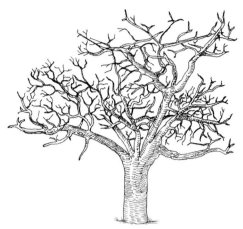

A

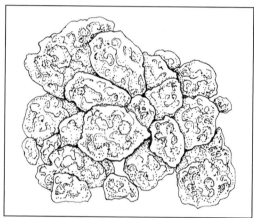

B

Main Uses in Massage

Myrrh has a gently calming effect on the nervous system, which, combined with its anesthetic aspects, makes it ideal for those in chronic pain, whose nervous system has become hypersensitive to any discomfort. A study showed that sesquiterpenes in myrrh bind to opioid receptors in the brain, probably easing pain and calming the nervous system through the same pathways as the opioids.[3] This is possibly also the origin of its reputation as a "meditation" oil, able to clear the mind of distractions and worries.

It is also a good anti-inflammatory[4] and therefore suitable for painful problems that include inflammation, such as sprains and strains, arthritis, gout, and sciatica.

Myrrh, like the other resins, has long been used as a folk remedy to assist in wound healing. It has been shown in studies to have cicatrizant[5] and antiseptic properties,[6] and it may be useful in treating scars, skin problems, and canker sores. It is one of the best essential oils for treating cracked skin on heels and hands, preferably in a heavy cream or salve.

Notes

1. Fischer-Rizzi S. The Complete Incense Book. New York: Sterling, 1998:139–140.
2. Strehlow W, Gottfried H. Hildegard of Bingen's Medicine. Santa Fe, NM: Bear & Co., 1988:17.

Therapeutic Effects

Analgesic ***
Anti-inflammatory **
Antimicrobial ***
Cicatrizant ***

** = mild   **** = extremely powerful

3. Dolara P, Moneti G, Pieraccini G, et al. Characterization of the action on central opioid receptors of furaneudesma-1,3-diene, as sesquiterpene extracted from myrrh. Phytother Res 1996;10(Supplement 1):S81–S83.

4. Atta AH, Alkofahi A. Anti-nociceptive and anti-inflammatory effects of some Jordanian medicinal plant extracts. J Ethnopharmacol 1998; 60(2):117–124.

5. Borrelli F, Izzo AA. The plant kingdom as a source of anti-ulcer remedies. Phytother Res 2000;14(8):581–591.

6. El-Ashry ES, Rashed N, Salama OM, et al. Components, therapeutic value and uses of myrrh. Pharmazie 2003;58(3):163–168.

NEROLI

Botanical name: *Citrus aurantium.* (Often called *C. aurantium* var. *amara.*) Neroli can also be made from the sweet orange (*Citrus sinensis*), but it is usually made from the bitter orange, as the flowers are larger and the yield slightly better.

Family: Rutaceae.

Native to: Southeast Asia. Today it is cultivated in Italy, Tunisia, Morocco, and France.

Part of plant used: Flowers.

Extraction method: Steam distillation.

Color of oil: Pale yellow.

Consistency: Medium.

Odor: Light, floral, powdery, slightly citrusy.

Chemistry: Linalol (monoterpene alcohol) 28–55%, limonene (monoterpene) 12–19%, linalyl acetate (ester) 2–17%, β-pinene (monoterpene) 3–16%.

Precautions: None known.

History and Traditional Uses: The essential oil from the blossoms of the bitter orange is not mentioned until the mid-sixteenth century, and the name is said to derive from the seventeenth-century Italian Princess of Nerola and her extreme fondness for the fragrance of this oil. It has been valued by the perfume industry since that time and is a key constituent of the classic perfume eau de Cologne, favored by Napoleon. The very expensive essential oil is often adulterated, and it is important to buy it from a reputable supplier.

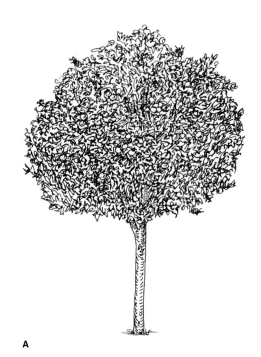

A

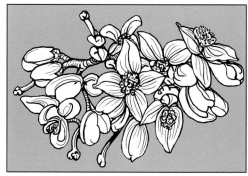

B

Main Uses in Massage

Neroli is mostly used in aromatherapy for its ability to relax and soothe. It seems to be particularly good at calming people after some kind of shock or trauma and in helping them to deal with anxiety or fear. Various studies show Neroli to be "sedating,"[1] but in my experience it is more calming, thereby giving people the strength to deal with crises. I have used it often to help clients with exam nerves, fear of flying, and anxiety before surgery. It is ideal for children or adults who tend to get overexcited or worried and as a result become exhausted.

Neroli has a small to medium amount of the ester linalyl acetate, which is antispasmodic. The antispasmodic effect, along with its calming nature, makes it helpful in blends for digestive problems caused by stress, such as abdominal pains, irritable bowel syndrome, and diarrhea.

Neroli oil is frequently used in aromatherapy as a skin remedy. It is added to blends for use in pregnancy to avoid stretch marks because of its **cytophylactic,** or cell-regenerating, properties.

Notes

1. Jager W, Buchbauer G, Jirovetz L, et al. Evidence of the sedative effects of neroli oil, citronellal and phenylethyl acetate on mice. J Essent Oil Res 1992;4:387–394.

> **Therapeutic Effects**
>
> Antispasmodic **
> Cicatrizant ***
> Hypotensive and anxiolytic ****

** = mild   **** = extremely powerful

NUTMEG

Botanical name: *Myristica fragrans*.

Family: Myristicaceae.

Native to: The Island of Run, East Indies. Today it is cultivated in Indonesia, the West Indies, and Sri Lanka.

Part of plant used: Seed. (Essential oil of mace is made from the red husk, or aril, from around the nutmeg seed, but mostly is used in flavoring food and drinks.)

Extraction method: Steam distillation.

Color of oil: Clear to pale yellow.

Consistency: Thin.

Odor: Light, warm, sweet, spicy aroma.

Chemistry: Sabinene (monoterpene) 15–50%, α-pinene (monoterpene) 10–26%, myristicin (phenolic ether) 0.5–14%. The myristicin content is considerably higher in the East Indian oil than in the West Indian one, whereas the sabinene content is much lower.

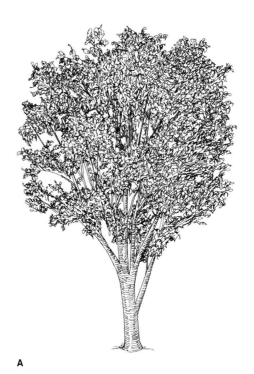

A

Precautions: It is advisable to avoid with pethidine, an analgesic drug, and otherwise use in moderation. Tisserand and Balacs recommend a maximum topical dilution of 2.25% for the East Indian oil, due to the possible carcinogenic effects of safrole and methyl eugenol (present in the East Indian oil in more than trace amounts). They also state that myristicin has been shown to be an MAO inhibitor, that oral doses or nutmeg oil should be avoided with pethidine, and that "the safety of non-oral dosages is uncertain."[1]

History and Traditional Uses: "The island can be smelled before it can be seen. From more than ten miles out to sea a fragrance hangs in the air . . . ." So begins Milton's story of the tiny island in the East Indies where nutmeg originally grew wild.[2] Men made fortunes in the seventeenth century by importing nutmeg to Europe, where it was used medicinally to treat the common cold, digestive problems, and even dysentery and the plague. It is used in Ayurvedic medicine for digestive spasms, for joint pains, and as an aphrodisiac.[3]

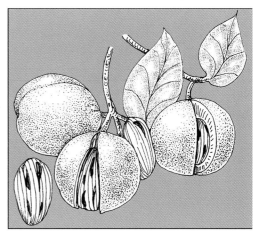

B

Main Uses in Massage

Nutmeg essential oil is a potent anti-inflammatory, suppressing the production of prostaglandins, chemicals produced by the body as part of the inflammatory response.[4] One study concluded that "nutmeg oil showed pharmacological activities similar to those of non-steroidal anti-inflammatory drugs."[5] It is particularly useful for acute inflammation in muscle injuries, arthritis, and overworked muscles.

Because it is also a good expectorant,[6] nutmeg has the potential for use in allergic respiratory problems, which always involve inflammation. Its antidiarrheal effects have also been researched,[7] and again, because of its anti-inflammatory properties, it may be most helpful for clients who suffer from allergic digestive problems.

Therapeutic Effects

Analgesic ****
Antidiarrheal ***
Anti-inflammatory ****
Expectorant ***

** = mild   **** = extremely powerful

Notes

1. Tisserand R, Balacs T. Essential Oil Safety. London, UK: Churchill Livingstone, 1999:152–153.
2. Milton G. Nathaniel's Nutmeg. London, UK: Hodder and Stoughton, 1999:1.
3. Farida I. The Magic of Ayurvedic Aromatherapy. West Pennant Hills, Australia: Subtle Energies, 2001:133.
4. Janssens J, Laekeman G M, Pieters L A, et al. Nutmeg oil: identification and quantitation of its most active constituents as inhibitors of platelet aggregation. J Ethnopharmacol 1990;29(2):179–188.
5. Olajide OA, Makinde JM, Awe SO. Evaluation of the pharmacological properties of nutmeg oil in rats and mice. Pharm Biol 2000;38(5):385–390.
6. Boyd EM, Sheppard P. Nutmeg oil and camphene as inhaled expectorants. Arch Otolaryngol (Chicago) 1970;92(4):372–378.
7. Olajide OA, Makinde JM, Awe SO. Evaluation of the pharmacological properties of nutmeg oil in rats and mice. Pharm Biol 2000;38(5):385–390.

PALMAROSA

Botanical name: *Cymbopogon martinii*. (Another variety *C. martinii* var. *sofia* yields the more unusual gingergrass essential oil.)

Family: Gramineae.

Native to: India. Today it is cultivated in India, Brazil, Indonesia, and the Comoros Islands.

Part of plant used: Grass.

Extraction method: Steam distillation.

Color of oil: Clear to pale green.

Consistency: Thin.

Odor: Intensely sweet, rather floral, with strong citrus overtones.

Chemistry: Geraniol (monoterpene alcohol) 60–83%, geranyl acetate (ester) 7–22%.

Precautions: None known.

History and Traditional Uses: Used in Ayurvedic medicine for skin problems and to relieve nerve pain. It is often used to adulterate rose oil. Commercially it is used to scent soaps and toiletry items.

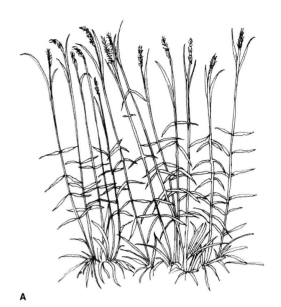

A

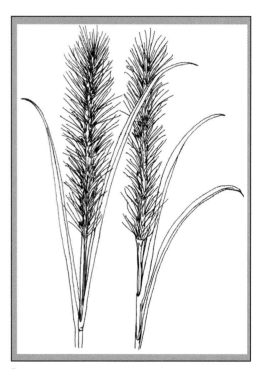

B

Main Uses in Massage

Palmarosa is extremely antimicrobial, yet very gentle on skin and mucous membranes. It can be compared with tea tree oil in this regard, but is a much stronger antifungal[1] than the Australian oil. Its mildness makes it useful for all kinds of chronic viral, bacterial,[2] and fungal infections, as it can be used for several weeks on a daily basis with no ill effects. Baudoux recommends it for sinusitis, any upper respiratory and ear infections, and urinary tract and reproductive system infections.[3] It is also useful in a take-home blend for athlete's foot and for long-term work with clients with candidiasis, a fungal yeast infection.

Palmarosa essential oil is much used in aromatherapy as a skin tonic, and this use along with its antibacterial and antiviral properties and a mild anti-inflammatory quality make it a good choice to treat acne, shingles, eczema/dermatitis, and any other inflammatory skin problem. A recent case of seborrheic dermatitis was helped by palmarosa as one of the essential oils added to a shampoo for treatment.[4] The problem was resolved within a few days, when even hydrocortisone cream or medicated shampoos had failed to improve the condition.

Various aromatherapy writers also recommend palmarosa as a uterine tonic, useful in the last few weeks of pregnancy, massaged into the lower back and abdomen, to support the uterus during this time. It also may be useful during childbirth, because of its rather relaxing yet nonsedative effects.[5] I have used it in regular aromatherapy massages for the same reason—with clients who want to relax but not become sleepy or disoriented.

Notes

1. Srivastava S, Naik SN, Maheshwari RC. *In vitro* studies on antifungal activities of palmarosa and eucalyptus oils. Ind Perfumer 1993;37(3):277–279.

Therapeutic Effects

Antibacterial **
Antiviral ***
Cicatrizant ***
Fungicidal ****
Nervine ***

** = mild   **** = extremely powerful

2. Pattnaik S, Subramanyam VR, Kole CR, et al. Antibacterial activity of essential oils from *Cymbopogon*: inter- and intra-specific differences. Microbios 1995;84:239–245.

3. Baudoux D. L'Aromathérapie. Anglet, France: Éditions atlantica, 2001:184–185.

4. Allan R. Seborrhoeic dermatitis. Int J Aromather 2003;13(1):47–48.

5. Franchomme P, Pénöel D. L'aromathérapie exactement, 347–402, quoted in Price S. Aromatherapy for Health Professionals. London, UK: Churchill Livingstone, 2001:182.

PATCHOULI

Botanical name: *Pogostemon cablin*. (Often called *P. patchouli*.)

Family: Lamiaceae.

Native to: Southeast Asia, especially Indonesia. Today it is also cultivated in China, India, and South America.

Part of plant used: Leaves, which are often fermented before distillation.

Extraction method: Steam distillation.

Color of oil: Dark brownish orange.

Consistency: Thick.

Odor: Earthy, sweet, dark, and very tenacious. There is a lot of extremely poor-quality patchouli oil on the market, which is possibly why many people strongly dislike the smell. The aroma of patchouli essential oil definitely improves with time; I have a 12-year-old patchouli oil that is soft, smooth, and beautiful—nothing like the raw, pungent smell of the inferior oil used in many cheap incenses and scents.

Chemistry: Patchoulol (sesquiterpene alcohol) 20–41%, α-guaiene (sesquiterpene) 14–18%. Patchouli from China has a higher sesquiterpene alcohol content than the oils from Indonesia and India.[1]

Precautions: None known.

History and Traditional Uses: It is traditionally used in India to scent clothes, linens, and carpets, as a protection against destructive insects. It was introduced to Europe in this way, in the mid-nineteenth century, in shipments of fine fabrics and shawls, and became popular as a base note in "Oriental" perfumes. It is also used in Indian medicine as an anti-inflammatory and antiseptic.

Main Uses in Massage

A highly valued skin remedy, patchouli combines anti-inflammatory and mildly antiseptic qualities to good effect. It is useful for acne, dermatitis, eczema, and dandruff, and is an excellent essential oil to add to a heavy cream or salve for cracked skin on heels and hands, perhaps in combination with myrrh oil. Patchouli has one of the strongest antifungal effects among essential oils, yet it is extremely gentle on the skin. One study on the antifungal and antibacterial properties of plant extracts stated that "only patchouli met the criteria of being an effective antifungal agent without affecting the commensal bacteria."[2]

In research on the effects of fragrance on sympathetic nervous system activity, it was found that patchouli had similar calming effects to rose, both oils decreasing activity in normal adults by 40%.[3] This makes it useful for insomnia, nervous tension, and anxiety.

Notes

1. Yang D, Michel D, Mandin, D, et al. Antifungal and antibacterial properties, *in vitro*, of three Patchouli essential oils of different origins. Acta Botanica Gallica 1996;143(1): 29–35.
2. Chaumont JP, Leger D, Marshall J. Differences among the anti-fungal and antibacterial properties of some products of plant origin. Activity on feet microflora. Bull Societe Française de Mycologie Medicale 1989;18(2):379–384.
3. Haze S, Sakai K, Gozu Y. Effects of fragrance inhalation on sympathetic activity in normal adults. Jpn J Pharmacol 2002;90(3):247–253.

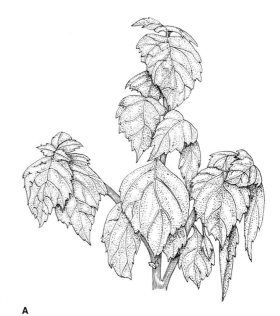

A

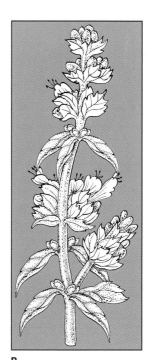

B

Therapeutic Effects

Antifungal ****
Anti-inflammatory ***
Sedative, calming ***

** = mild   **** = extremely powerful

PEPPERMINT

Botanical name: *Mentha x piperita*. There are many species of mint, probably derived from the wild watermint (*M. aquatica*). Some are used for food flavorings, toothpaste, candies, tea, and soaps. The most commonly used in aromatherapy are *M. piperita* and *M. spicata* (spearmint). Pennyroyal (*M. pulegium*) is also a member of the mint genus, though today it is not often used in aromatherapy.

Family: Lamiaceae.

Native to: Europe and the Middle East. Today it is naturalized (grows wild) worldwide, and it is cultivated for the oil in India, China, France, Russia, and the United States.

Part of plant used: Flowering tops.

Extraction method: Steam distillation.

Color of oil: Clear.

Consistency: Very thin.

Odor: Strong, penetrating, sharp, clean, minty. (Spearmint has a softer, sweeter aroma.)

Chemistry: Menthol (monoterpene alcohol) 35–50%, menthone (ketone) 19–24%, 1,8 cineole (oxide) 5%.

Precautions: Avoid all use with children and with people with cardiac fibrillation. *Mentha piperita* is an essential oil with extremely powerful results and, as with most potent remedies, should be approached with caution. Studies show that it can be neurotoxic or hepatotoxic in large oral doses, but does not tend to produce irritation or sensitization in normal adults with topical application.[1] However, it does seem to have a different effect on children and especially infants, with case studies of acute poisoning reported after topical application.[2] Also, tests with premature infants showed that "the inhalation of menthol fumes . . . caused transient respiratory arrest or a drop in the respiratory rate. The heart rate rose during chemical stimulation of the nasal mucosa."[3] It is therefore advisable to avoid peppermint essential oil, and any essential oil with a high menthol content, with young children, perhaps younger than 7 years, and to use it cautiously with older children. Spearmint, which has a very different chemical composition (mainly carvone), has much milder effects and is safer for use with children.

Tisserand and Balacs also advise against its use, in any way, with clients who have cardiac fibrillation, probably because of its strongly stimulating effects. They also state that it should not be used at a stronger dilution than 3% on mucous membranes.[4]

History and Traditional Uses: There are about 30 different species of mint, and they were used interchangeably until about the seventeenth century. Mint was used by the ancient Egyptians in ritual incense and by the Greeks and Romans for daily hygiene. The name is derived from the Latin *menthe*, meaning thought, reflecting its actions on the mind. Pliny states that the "very smell of it alone recovers and refreshes the spirit."[5]

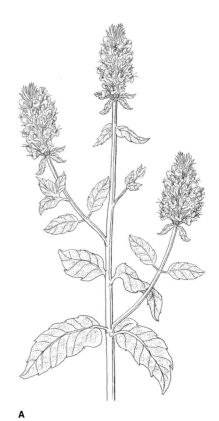

A

B

Therapeutic Effects

Analgesic and anesthetic ****
Antipruritic and cooling ****
Digestive tonic ***
Stimulant ***

** = mild   **** = extremely powerful

Main Uses in Massage

Peppermint is a wonder oil, with a seemingly endless list of properties and uses. It is extremely strong and excels when it is used for spot treatments on problem areas, rather than for full-body massage. Because of its high menthol content, peppermint has a cooling effect on the skin and mucous membranes as a result of its stimulation of nerve receptors (thermoreceptors) for cold.[6] Most people have experienced this sensation, at least through the refreshing feeling of toothpaste or chewing gum. The use of peppermint in full-body massage tends to make clients feel slightly chilly. However, this quality is useful in other ways, and it is frequently added to commercial products such as foot lotion. It is pleasant when used in foot baths or foot massage and is indispensable for any kind of **pruritis,**[7] or itching, such as insect bites, shingles, dermatitis, or allergic skin reactions. It does need to be highly diluted, except for insect bites, or it may make the itching worse (use at less than 1%).

Perhaps because of this intense cooling effect, peppermint has a quite strong anesthetic quality.[8] It can be used to treat headaches—a tiny drop of undiluted peppermint essential oil on the temples can give almost immediate relief, though it may make the user's eyes water. It can also be used for any kind of inflammatory pain, such as rheumatoid arthritis, neuralgia, or musculoskeletal injury, either diluted in a lotion or used with a compress. A case study from the Pain Clinic in a London hospital records the use of neat peppermint oil to treat the pain resulting from postherpetic neuralgia, which resulted in "almost immediate improvement" lasting for 4–6 hours after application.[9]

Peppermint is well known as a digestive aid, and mint tea or candies are often eaten after dinner. It has a proven choleretic effect,[10] stimulating bile flow to help with digestion, especially of fats. Studies show that the essential oil has an antispasmodic effect on the smooth muscle of the digestive tract,[11] and it is a standard remedy in medicine for irritable bowel syndrome. Even inhaling peppermint oil out of a bottle, or from a tissue, relieves nausea dramatically, and it is extremely useful for motion sickness, morning sickness during pregnancy, the nausea that happens with many chronic illnesses, or after chemotherapy or surgery. It also can be used in an abdominal massage.

The antispasmodic effect on smooth muscle is also helpful for bronchial spasms and coughing. Peppermint is frequently used in commercial remedies for respiratory problems—it has antibacterial[12] and antiviral[13] properties, and studies show its benefits for everything from chronic bronchitis[14] to tuberculosis.[15] The stimulation of cold receptors has an interesting implication for the upper respiratory system—it feels to someone inhaling peppermint oil as if it is having a decongestant effect, but, in fact, it simply reduces the discomfort associated with congestion. It is a useful addition to respiratory blends simply for this comfort factor.

Peppermint is also a powerful stimulant of the blood circulation when used in larger amounts. I had an opportunity to observe this effect in class, when a student, through a misunderstanding, put 36 drops of peppermint oil into her footbath. Although she stayed in the foot bath for only a few minutes, her feet quickly started feeling numb (the anesthetic effect), and then she felt cold (stimulation of cold receptors), but after about 30 minutes she appeared to be wearing pink socks, as the local blood vessels dilated. Her feet felt very warm and tingly, almost itchy, for several hours. Peppermint is thus regarded as a strong stimulant for the entire body and also the mind, helping to sharpen concentration and give energy. It should not be used late in the evening, as the stimulating effects may interfere with sleep.

Notes

1. Nair B. Final report on the safety assessment of Mentha Piperita (Peppermint) Oil, Mentha Piperita (Peppermint) Leaf Extract, Mentha Piperita (Peppermint) Leaf, and Mentha Piperita (Peppermint) Leaf Water. Int J Toxicol 2001;20(Suppl. 3):61–73.
2. Dupreyon JP, Quattrocchi F, Castaing H, et al. Acute poisoning of an infant by cutaneous application of a local counterirritant and pulmonary antiseptic salve. Eur J Toxicol Environ Hyg 1976;9(5):313–320.
3. Javorka K, Tomori Z, Zavarska L. Protective and defensive airway reflexes in premature infants. Physiol Bohemoslov 1980;29(1):29–35.
4. Tisserand R, Balacs T. Essential Oil Safety. London, UK: Churchill Livingstone, 1999:160–161.
5. Mojay G. Aromatherapy for Healing the Spirit. London, UK: Gaia, 1996:108.
6. Eccles R. Menthol and related cooling compounds. J Pharm Pharmacol 1994;46(8):618–630.
7. Burkhart EG, Burkhart HR. Contact irritant dermatitis and antipruritic agents: the need to address the itch. J Drugs Dermatol 2003; 2(2):143–146.
8. McCaffery M, Wolff M. Pain relief using cutaneous modalities, positioning and movement. Hospice J 1992;8(1–2):121–153.
9. Davies SJ, Harding LM, Baranowski AP. A novel treatment of postherpetic neuralgia using peppermint oil. Clin J Pain 2002;18(3): 200–202.
10. Rangelov A. An experimental characterization of cholagogic and cholesteric activity of a group of essential oils. Folia Medica (Plovdiv) 1989;31(1):46–53.
11. Hills JM, Aaronson PI. The mechanism of action of peppermint oil on gastrointestinal smooth muscle. Gastroenterology 1991;10(1):55–65.
12. Imai H, Osawa K, Yasuda H, et al. Inhibition by the essential oils of peppermint and spearmint of the growth of pathogenic bacteria. Microbios 2001;106(Suppl. 1):31–39.
13. Schuhmacher A, Reichling J, Schnitzler P. Virucidal effect of peppermint oil on the enveloped viruses herpes simplex virus type 1 and type 2 in vitro. Phytomedicine 2003;10(6–7):504–510.
14. Shubina LP, Siurin SA, Savchenko VM. Inhalations of essential oils in the combined treatment of patients with chronic bronchitis. Vrachebnoe Delo (Kiev) 1990;5:66–67.
15. Shkurupii VA, Kazarinova NV, Ogirenko AP, et al. Efficiency of the use of peppermint (Mentha piperita L) essential oil inhalations in the combined multi-drug therapy for pulmonary tuberculosis. Problemy Tuberkuleza 2002;4:36–39.

PETITGRAIN

Botanical name: *Citrus aurantium.* (Often called *C. aurantium* var. *amara.*) Technically, petitgrain essential oil can be made from any citrus tree; two examples are mandarin petitgrain and lemon petitgrain. However, the bitter orange petitgrain is the most common and is the one discussed here.

Family: Rutaceae.

Native to: Southeast Asia. Today it is cultivated in North Africa, France, and Paraguay.

Part of plant used: Leaves and twigs.

Extraction method: Steam distillation.

Color of oil: Clear to yellow.

Consistency: Thin.

Odor: Floral citrusy overtones, with a green, almost woody lower note.

Chemistry: Linalyl acetate (ester) 38–59%, linalol (monoterpene alcohol) 18–33%.

Precautions: None known.

History and Traditional Uses: Petitgrain was originally distilled from the tiny unripe fruits of the bitter orange, and it took its name from these "little grains" or "petits grains." It has been much used in perfumes, including the classic eau de Cologne.

Main Uses in Massage

Petitgrain has been compared with neroli for its calming and sedative effects, and it is significantly less expensive than the flower oil from the same plant. In a top-quality petitgrain with a high ester content, both the aroma and the properties are remarkably similar to neroli. It is often used in aromatherapy to balance the nervous system and help with stress or nervous tension. It is very helpful in cases of insomnia caused by stress, and for mental fatigue.

Because of its high level of esters, petitgrain is an extremely effective antispasmodic, for both smooth muscle and skeletal muscle. As it is so effective for nervous tension, it is particularly indicated for cramps and spasms triggered by stress, such as asthmatic coughing, digestive problems, or muscle cramps of any kind.

It is a mild antimicrobial agent and works successfully to treat fungal infections. One study on the antifungal properties of various essential oils states: "Petitgrain oil was particularly recommended for its action against yeasts."[1] It might be an especially useful oil in a blend for clients with candidiasis (*Candida* yeast infection).

Various aromatherapy writers, including Rose, mention the use of petitgrain for skin care.[2] It is certainly more astringent than the gentle neroli, but much less so than the expressed citrus oils. It may be a useful addition to a care routine for oily and congested skin.

Notes

1. Galal EE, Adel MS, El-Sherif S, et al. Evaluation of certain volatile oils for their antifungal properties. J Drug Res 1973;5(2):235–245.
2. Rose J. 375 Essential Oils and Hydrosols. Berkeley, CA: Frog Ltd, 1999:127.

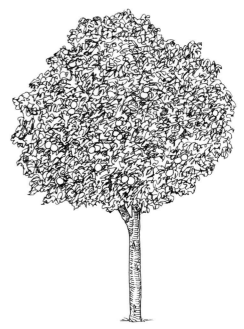

A

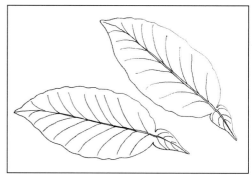

B

Therapeutic Effects

Antidepressant ***
Antispasmodic ***
Fungicidal ***
Sedative, calming ****

** = mild   **** = extremely powerful

PINE

Botanical name: *Pinus sylvestris*. There are about 93 species of pine, and several are distilled commercially to produce essential oils, including *P. mugo*, *P. palustris*, and *P. nigra*. *P. sylvestris*, the Scots pine, is the most common in aromatherapeutic use.

Family: **Pinaceae.**

Native to: **Northern Europe and Russia.** Other species of pine are found native worldwide.

Part of plant used: **Needles.**

Extraction method: **Steam distillation.**

Color of oil: **Clear.**

Consistency: **Thin.**

Odor: **Sweet, clear smell, reminiscent of sawmills and lumber yards.**

Chemistry: α-pinene (monoterpene) 18–33%, δ-3-carene (monoterpene) 9–25%

Precautions: None known. However, like other essential oils high in monoterpenes, it is best to use fresh oil only, as oxidized monoterpenes may irritate the skin.

History and Traditional Uses: Pine kernels have been an important food for thousands of years, and the resin and needles have been used for incense and medicine. The needles were used by Native Americans for ritual smudging and to make mattresses. Pine has been an important folk remedy in Europe for respiratory problems. The tree is extremely tall and straight and has been used to make masts for ships, telegraph poles, and railway sleepers.

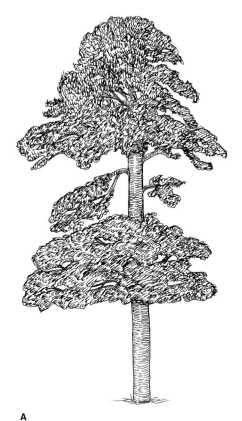

A

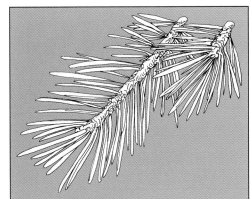

B

Main Uses in Massage

Pine is most often associated with treating infections of the respiratory system; syrup of pine and inhalations were used for such ailments in the medicine of many cultures. Pine essential oil is an effective expectorant,[1] helping rid the lungs of mucus, and a good antiseptic,[2] assisting in the fight against bacterial infections. It also stimulates the immune system.[3] The oil helps clients who are prone to frequent respiratory infections or whose immunity has been compromised by illness, depression, or chemotherapy.

Pine essential oil is also used in aromatherapy for the treatment of painful joints or muscles, and it is suitable for arthritis, sciatica, low-back pain, and similar conditions. It seems to have a slightly warming, penetrating quality, which makes it a good choice for loosening stiff joints and increasing range of motion.

Many writers in aromatherapy consider pine oil to have a stimulating effect on the adrenal cortex, and Mojay writes that it is "one of the most effective oils for fatigue and nervous debility."[4] Little clinical evidence exists to support this claim; I have found the essential oil to be definitely energizing without being strongly stimulating. I have used it extensively with clients who are in adrenal burnout, who have chronic fatigue syndrome, or who are generally overstressed.

Therapeutic Effects

Adrenal support ★★★★
Antiseptic ★★
Expectorant ★★★
Immunostimulant ★★★

★★ = mild   ★★★★ = extremely powerful

Notes

1. Schilcher H. Efficient phytotherapy. Herbal medicines in the upper respiratory tract for catarrh. Herba Polonica 2000;46(1):52–57.
2. Fanaki NH, El-Nakeeb MA. Antimicrobial activity of some essential oil components against multiresistant clinical isolates. Alexandria J Pharm Sci 1997;11(3):149–153.
3. Kedzia B, Jankowiak J, Holonska J, et al. Investigation of essential oils and components with immunostimulating activity. Herba Polonica 1998;44(2):126–135.
4. Mojay G. Essential Oils for Healing the Spirit. London, UK: Gaia, 1996:110–111.

ROSALINA

Botanical name: *Melaleuca ericifolia.* Closely related to *M. alternifolia* (tea tree).

Family: Myrtaceae.

Native to: Australia.

Part of plant used: Leaves and twigs.

Extraction method: Steam distillation.

Color of oil: Clear.

Consistency: Thin.

Odor: Sweet, clean, slightly spicy.

Chemistry: Linalol (monoterpene alcohol) 35–55%, 1,8 cineole (oxide) 18–26%, α-pinene (monoterpene) 5–10%.

Precautions: None known.

History and Traditional Uses: This is a very new essential oil in the aromatherapy field. It first received recognition as a valuable therapeutic remedy by the French naturopath Pénöel.[1]

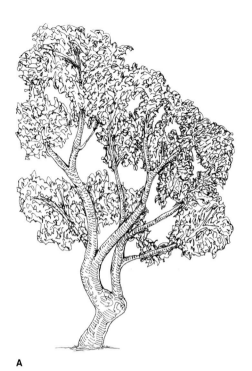

A

Main Uses in Massage

I have been searching for some time for an essential oil to replace rosewood (*Aniba roseadora*), because of the negative environmental implications of harvesting the rosewood tree. Rosalina seems to be a good choice, from the point of view of both therapeutic effects and aroma. The aroma is similar to that of rosewood, which is no surprise because both essential oils have linalol as their main chemical constituent.

Because of the significant amount of 1,8 cineole in the essential oil, rosalina is a good expectorant, and its mildness makes it particularly appropriate as a remedy for respiratory infections in very young children. Research shows it has clear antiviral and antibacterial effects.[2] Its ability to rid the body of mucus makes it useful for almost any kind of infection of the lungs or sinuses, including acute or chronic bronchitis, colds, influenza, and sinusitis. Pénöel particularly recommends it for infections of the ear, nose, and throat.[3] It is so gentle on the skin that it can be used in a massage blend on the chest or upper back on even very young children or infants.

The high linalol content means that rosalina is an effective sedative for both adults and children.[4] It can be used in massage for relaxation, to help calm emotions, or for stress-related hypertension. It can also be used in a take-home blend, and is particularly appropriate as a respiratory remedy to be used in the late evening or before bed. Unlike many other essential oils that help to decongest, it will not interfere with sleep.

The antibacterial property, combined with its gentleness on the skin, makes it ideal for acne, skin rashes, and dandruff, particularly for people with sensitive skin.

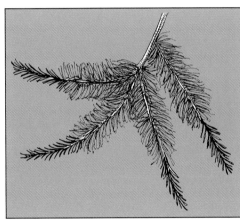

B

Therapeutic Effects

Antibacterial ***
Antispasmodic **
Antiviral ***
Expectorant **
Sedative ***

** = mild   **** = extremely powerful

Notes

1. Pénöel D, Pénöel R. Natural Home Health Care Using Essential Oils. La Drôme, France: Éditions Osmobiose, 1998:142–148.
2. Farag RS, Shalaby AS, El-Baroty GA, et al. Chemical and biological evaluation of the essential oils of different Melaleuca species. Phytother Res 2004;18(1):30–35.
3. Pénöel D, Pénöel R. Natural Home Health Care Using Essential Oils. La Drôme, France: Éditions Osmobiose, 1998:142–148.
4. Elisabetsky E, Coelho de Souza GP, Santos MA, et al. Sedative properties of linalool. Fitotherapia 1995;66(5):407–414.

ROSE

Botanical name: *Rosa x damascena* and *Rosa x centifolia* are the two species of rose most often used in aromatherapy. *R. x alba* (the white rose), *R. gallica*, *R. indica*, *R. rugosa* (a wild rose), and *R. rubiginosa* (usually for the extraction of rose hip seed oil, a carrier oil, not an aromatic oil) are also occasionally used.

Family: Rosaceae.

Native to: Most areas in the Northern Hemisphere. It is primarily cultivated for the oil in Bulgaria, Turkey, Egypt, Morocco, France, China, India, and Russia.

Part of plant used: Flowers.

Extraction method: Distillation and solvent extraction.

Color of oil: Essential oil: pale yellow. Absolute: reddish amber.

Consistency: Essential oil: medium to thick; often solidifies if kept in cold temperatures; it will reliquefy at room temperature or when held between the hands. Absolute: medium to thick.

Odor: Essential oil: sweet, honeylike aroma. Absolute: deep, rich, floral, lingering aroma.

Chemistry: Essential oil: citronellol (monoterpene alcohol) 18–50%, geraniol (monoterpene alcohol) 16–28%, nerol (monoterpene alcohol) about 8%, nonadecane 4–14%. Absolute: phenylethyl alcohol, citronellol (monoterpene alcohol), geraniol (monoterpene alcohol). Both oils are highly complex, with more than 300 components, many in trace amounts. The trace constituents are often those with the strongest aroma, especially those containing sulphur.

Precautions: None known. Some writers advise against using rose oil during pregnancy because of its mild emmenagogic effect. However, studies show that it does "not constitute a risk to pregnant women or their offspring in concentrations up to ten times higher than normal therapeutic doses."[1]

History and Traditional Uses: Rose has perhaps a longer, more complex recorded history than any other plant. It is an ancient plant, fossils having been found dating back 40 million years. There are more than 100 wild species and many thousands of cultivars, since it has been hybridized over many centuries. It is a central motif in many religions, a symbol of divine love for Christians, Sufis, and Hindus. It has been representative of human passion and longing for centuries. It is also an important medicinal remedy, used in Ayurvedic medicine and traditional Western herbalism for its cooling and regulating qualities. Rose is used in about 96% of all women's perfumes.

Main Uses in Massage

Because of the extremely high cost of rose oil, it is primarily used in aromatherapy for its effects on the emotions. It is extremely effective in the treatment of anxiety, one study concluding that "rose essential oil has a pharmacological activity similar to non-benzodiazepine anxiolytic drugs."[2] It can be used for nervous tension, worry, nervous palpitations,

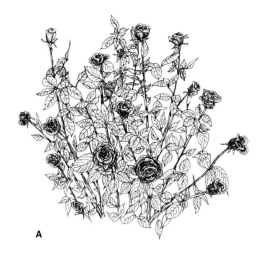

A

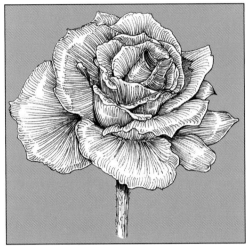

B

Therapeutic Effects
Anti-inflammatory for skin ***
Anxiolytic ****
Sedative ***

** = mild   **** = extremely powerful

and similar conditions. It has been traditionally used for grieving, and in my experience is unrivaled in its ability to soothe the pain of loss or rejection.

Research confirms its traditional use as a sedative.[3] I have found it to be most useful for the type of insomnia that results from emotional upset or anxiety, either temporary or long-term. I once did a foot massage using rose absolute on a friend who had just had an intense argument and was extremely distressed; she was asleep before the short massage was over.

It can also be used to promote relaxation with clients who have stress-related hypertension, or chronic pain. A case study related by Buckle tells of a 74-year-old woman with cancer, in intense pain. She had become withdrawn and depressed and her muscles were tight from the pain. Two drops of rose essential oil were given to her to inhale from a tissue, and the responses were an instant muscular relaxation and a reduction in her perception of the pain.[4]

It is cooling for the skin, recommended by the seventeenth-century herbalist Culpeper "to cool and heal flushes, wheals, and other red pimples rising in the face and other parts."[5] It can be added to creams or lotions to help with eczema or dermatitis of any kind, allergic rashes, acne, or any sensitive, inflamed skin.

Notes

1. Kirov M, Vergieva T, Spasovski M. Rose oil. Embryotoxic and teratogenic activity. Medico Biol Info 1988;3:15–17.
2. Umezu T. Anticonflict effects of plant-derived essential oils. Pharmacol Biochem Behav 1999;64(1):35–40.
3. Kikuchi A, Tanida M, Venoyama S, et al. Effect of odours on cardiac response patterns in a reaction time task. Chem Senses 1991;16:183.
4. Buckle J. Clinical Aromatherapy. London, UK: Churchill Livingstone, 2003:127.
5. Culpeper N. Culpeper's Complete Herbal. Ware, UK: Wordsworth Editions, 1995:217.

ROSEMARY

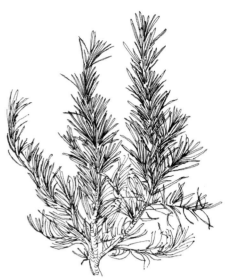

Botanical name: *Rosmarinus officinalis.*

Family: Lamiaceae.

Native to: Mediterranean region. Today it is cultivated worldwide.

Part of plant used: Flowering tops.

Extraction method: Steam distillation

Color of oil: Clear.

Consistency: Thin.

Odor: Strong, camphoraceous, herby smell, with minty overtones.

Chemistry: The three main chemotypes are: (a) Cineole chemotype: mostly grown in Morocco and Tunisia; 1,8 cineole (oxide) 40–44%, α-pinene (monoterpene) 8–14%, camphor (ketone) about 12%. (b) Camphor chemotype: mostly grown in France and Spain; camphor (ketone) 12–28%, α-pinene (monoterpene) 3–27%, 1,8 cineole (oxide) 9–25%. (c) Verbenone chemotype: mostly from Corsica; verbenone (ketone) 15–37%, bornyl acetate (ester). This chemotype is quite rare; it has a totally different aroma, much lighter, rather lemony, and lacking the camphoraceous note of the others.

Precautions: It is probably best to avoid the camphor chemotype during pregnancy and with children, as there have been cases of collapse in infants after a local application of camphor to their nostrils.[1] Many writers advise against using rosemary oil for high blood pressure, but there seems to be no evidence for this precaution.

History and Traditional Uses: Rosemary has been a favorite herb, medicinally and for cooking, since the time of the ancient Egyptians. There are many legends of its rejuvenating and protective powers, such as that of the Queen of Hungary, who transformed herself from an elderly woman into a beautiful young girl courted by the kings of Europe by using rosemary. It has been regarded as a cure-all in folk medicine, burned as a fumigant in hospitals, and carried to ward off sickness.

Main Uses in Massage

The three chemotypes of rosemary all have rather different properties and uses. The cineole and camphor chemotypes are the most similar, both being stimulating[2] and vasodilatory.[3] They are good strengthening tonics for the whole body and are often used in aromatherapy for clients who are tired, run down, lethargic, and perhaps depressed as well. They are helpful for chronic fatigue syndrome and other chronic illnesses that lead to exhaustion.

Valnet[4] and many later aromatherapy writers recommend the topical application of rosemary for muscular and joint pains and stiffness, and this vasodilating property is probably the reason. Stiffness and the related pain are usually relieved if local circulation is improved, and naturopathic doctors often use some kind of local counterirritant to stimulate blood flow to the area. It can also be helpful for headaches, massaged into the neck muscles if they are stiff, and onto the temples to ease the vasoconstriction that often causes pain.

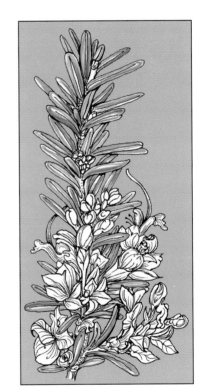

A

B

Therapeutic Effects

Antispasmodic ***
Antiviral ***
Expectorant ****
Stimulant ***
Vasodilator ***

** = mild   **** = extremely powerful

The simulation of blood flow to the brain might also be the cause of rosemary's reputation for improving memory. One study showed that, compared with lavender, "rosemary produced a significant enhancement of performance for overall quality of memory."[5] The same study found that volunteers who smelled the aroma were also more alert than those who smelled lavender, and more content than a control group who were not exposed to the essential oils. Rosemary is definitely useful for clients who would like to be able to concentrate and remember more effectively.

The cineole chemotype seems to be particularly effective for the respiratory system, and many French medical aromatherapists, such as Baudoux, recommend it as a strong expectorant, helpful for infections with a lot of mucus.[6] It can be used for congestion in both the sinuses and the lungs. Various studies also show it to be an antispasmodic,[7] making it an appropriate remedy for asthma and bronchitis.

The verbenone chemotype, because of its high level of mucus-dissolving ketones, is also a good choice for respiratory problems with large amounts of mucus. Blending the cineole and the verbenone chemotypes together for a chest massage or a steam inhalation gives a potent remedy for this particular ailment. It seems to be less stimulating than the other chemotypes, although Mailhebiau considers it to be a powerful immunostimulant.[8]

Notes

1. Tisserand R, Balacs T. Essential Oil Safety. London, UK: Churchill Livingstone, 1999:165.
2. Diego MA, Jones NA, Field T, et al. Aromatherapy positively affects mood, EEG patterns of alertness and math computations. Int J Neurosci 1998;96:217–224.
3. Khatib S, Alkofahi A, Hasan M, et al. The cardiovascular effects of *Rosmarinus officinalis* extract on the isolated intact rabbit heart. Fitoterapia 1998;69(6): 502–506.
4. Valnet J. The Practice of Aromatherapy. Saffron Walden, UK: CW Daniel, 1992:177–179.
5. Moss M, Cook J, Wesnes K, et al. Aromas of rosemary and lavender essential oils differentially affect cognition and mood in healthy adults. Int J Neurosci 2003;113(1):15–38.
6. Baudoux D. L'Aromathérapie. Anglet, France: Éditions atlantica, 2001:192–193.
7. Aqel MB. Relaxant effect of the volatile oil of *Rosmarinus officinalis* on tracheal smooth muscle. J Ethnopharmacol 1991;33(1–2):57–62.
8. Mailhebiau P. Portraits in Oils. Saffron Walden, UK: CW Daniel, 1995:102.

SANDALWOOD

Botanical name: *Santalum album*. An essential oil is also made from the Australian sandalwood (*S. spicatum*).

Family: Santalaceae.

Native to: India and some other parts of Southeast Asia. The best oil is considered to be from Mysore, in south-central India.

Part of plant used: Heartwood and roots.

Extraction method: Water distillation is used, to avoid the powdered wood forming clumps and distilling unevenly, as it does in steam distillation.

Color of oil: Light amber.

Consistency: Very thick.

Odor: Mild, soft, sweet, slightly woody, extremely long lasting.

Chemistry: α-santalol (sesquiterpene alcohol) at least 50%, β-santalol (sesquiterpene alcohol) 19–30%.

Precautions: None known.

History and Traditional Uses: Sandalwood has been used in India for thousands of years, as perfume, medicine, incense, and much more. It was observed in ancient times that termites would not eat the sandalwood trees, so the wood was used to make religious statues, chests to preserve linens, and so on. Sandalwood oil is used in Ayurvedic medicine because it "cools and calms the entire body and mind,"[1] and it is believed to open the third eye. The powdered wood is used in beauty treatments for the skin and in incense; the oil is used in perfumes; and chunks of the wood are burned at Buddhist funerals. Sandalwood oil is also used to make the traditional Indian attars, which are distillations of costly or rare plants into sandalwood oil.[2]

Main Uses in Massage

The calming influence of sandalwood oil, long recognized in Ayurvedic medicine, has been confirmed by numerous laboratory studies. Both α- and β-santalol were found to be sedative and pain relieving;[3] their use increased the length of sleep time and the quality of deep sleep.[4] It is obviously a useful essential oil for those who have insomnia. I also frequently use it with clients who are stressed, are nervous, and tend to worry or obsess, since one of the traditional uses is for meditation, or calming the mind.

One study states that sandalwood has a definite analgesic effect on the central nervous system, which may be caused by santalol binding to opioid receptors in the brain.[5] This may be the origin of its reputation as a gentle antidepressant.

Sandalwood has been used for many centuries in India as an anti-inflammatory, for the skin, respiratory, and urinary systems. Mildly antiseptic, it is one of the most effective essential oils, used in baths, for urinary tract infections; its extreme gentleness on skin and mucous membranes means that it can be used frequently. These qualities also make it an ideal remedy for many skin problems, including acne, dermatitis, itching, and

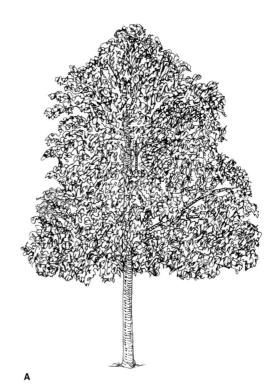

A

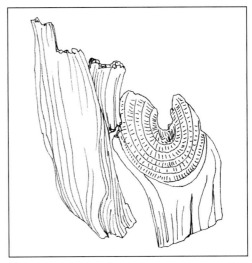

B

Therapeutic Effects

Antidepressant **
Anti-inflammatory for skin
   and mucous membranes ****
CNS relaxant ***
Sedative **

** = mild   **** = extremely powerful

any kind of dermal irritation. It is very soothing for inflamed tissue in the respiratory system, and in a mild dilution can be gargled to ease sore throats. This is not an oil that many people like in steam inhalations—it is too "woody." It is excellent used in a massage on the chest or upper back for chronic bronchitis and dry, persistent coughs.

Notes

1. Frawley D, Lad V. The Yoga of Herbs. Twin Lakes, WI: Lotus Press, 2001:143–144.

2. McMahon C. Attars: Traditional Perfumes of India. Presented at the World of Aromatherapy III Conference Proceedings, Seattle, WA, 2000.

3. Okugawa H, Ueda R, Matsumoto K, et al. Effect of α-santalol and β-santalol from sandalwood on the central nervous system in mice. Phytomedicine 1995;2(2):119–126.

4. Tanak J, Uchimura N, Maeda H, et al. Effects of sandalwood on sleep and biological rhythm. Aroma Res 2002;3(4):355–360.

5. Okukawa H, Kawanishi K, Kato A. Effects of sesquiterpenoids from Oriental incenses on sedative and analgesic action. Aromatherapy Res 2000;1(1):34–48.

SWEET BIRCH

(Compare sweet birch with wintergreen. The two oils are almost identical in chemical composition and therefore uses and precautions.)

Botanical name: *Betula lenta*.

Family: Betulaceae.

Native to: Northern regions, such as North America and Northern Europe.

Part of plant used: Bark.

Extraction method: Steam distillation.

Color of oil: Clear.

Consistency: Thin.

Odor: Minty, green, reminiscent of sports rubs or chewing gum, in which it is often used.

Chemistry: Up to 99.7% methyl salicylate (ester).

Precautions: *Do not take internally under any circumstances.* Sweet birch has been known to cause death when ingested,[1] and as little as 4 mL (less than a teaspoonful) is considered a lethal dose for a child.[2] Cases of hemorrhaging have been observed with people who have used a topical liniment with methyl salicylate, when also taking anticoagulants such as warfarin.[3] (Sweet birch should not be used with any anticoagulants, including warfarin, heparin, or aspirin.) Do not use with children, or during pregnancy or when breast-feeding. It should be used only in dilutions of 3% or less, over a short term, with otherwise healthy adults who are not taking anticoagulants.

History and Traditional Uses: Birch has been much used by Native Americans, as both a tea and as a remedy for any kind of pain.

Main Uses in Massage

Sweet birch is controversial in aromatherapy circles (see box). Most aromatherapy teachers and books strongly advise against using it in any circumstance, yet many aromatherapists use this extremely useful oil with their clients. The reason is that it is unparalleled in its action on painful, overworked muscles and aching joints, and tests show its strong anti-inflammatory and analgesic effects.[4,5] I have never experienced any other essential oil that can relieve musculoskeletal pain so quickly and dramatically. However, any remedy that has such a strong beneficial effect on the body is also likely to have unwanted effects if used unwisely—medicines and poisons historically have been very often one and the same. Used wisely, sweet birch can provide relief for many clients with pain and stiffness in muscles and joints.

  Wise use in this case means that I only use sweet birch with otherwise healthy adults, who are not taking anticoagulant medication. I do not use it in dilutions of greater than 3%, and I often use it in dilutions of only 1% in a blend with other essential oils. I use it for local application only and not for full-body massage. I observe the rule of not using essential oils on broken skin, and I reserve sweet birch for acute situations. This means that I would use a blend with sweet birch for

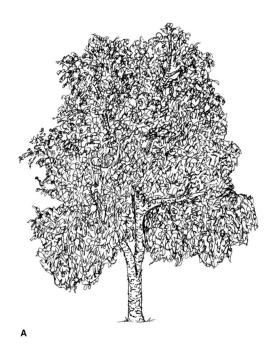

A

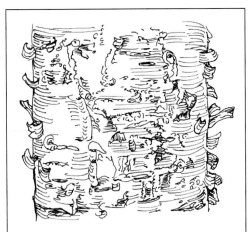

B

Therapeutic Effects

Anti-inflammatory ****
Local analgesic ****

** = mild   **** = extremely powerful

only a few days to help resolve acute or subacute inflammation, and I would not use it with the same client again for at least several weeks. I never sell this undiluted oil to clients who do not have aromatherapy training, and I send blends home with strict advice for proper use.

Notes

1. Hofman M, Diaz JE, Martella C. Oil of wintergreen overdose. Ann Emerg Med 1998;31(6):793–794.
2. Botma M, Colquhoun-Flannery W, Leighton S. Laryngeal oedema caused by accidental ingestion of oil of wintergreen. Int J Ped Otorhinolaryngol 2001;58(3):229–232.
3. Yip AS, Chow WH, Tai YT, et al. Adverse effect of topical methylsalicylate ointment on warfarin anticoagulation: an unrecognized potential hazard. Postgrad Med J 1990;66(775):367–369.
4. Ichiyama RM, Ragan BG, Bell GW, et al. Effects of topical analgesics on the pressor response evoked by muscle afferents. Med Science Sports Exer 2002;34(9):1440–1445.
5. Sur TK, Pandit S, Battacharyya D, et al. Studies on the anti-inflammatory activity of *Betula alnoides* bark. Phytother Res 2002;16(7):669–671.
6. Tisserand RB, Balacs T. Essential Oil Safety. London, UK: Churchill Livingstone, 1999:124.
7. Bell AJ, Duggin G. Acute methyl salicylate toxicity complicating herbal skin treatment for psoriasis. Emer Med (Fremantle) 2002; 14(2):188–190.
8. Chan TY. Ingestion of medicated oils by adults: the risk of severe salicylate poisoning is related to the packaging of these products. Human Exp Toxicol 2002;21(4):171–174.
9. Guba R. Toxicity myths: the actual risks of essential oil use. Int J Aromather 2000;10(1/2):37–49.
10. Baudoux D. L'Aromatherapie. Anglet, France: Editions atlantica, 2001:141.

How Dangerous Are Sweet Birch and Wintergreen?

Most aromatherapy books and teachers seem to agree with Tisserand and Balacs that these oils "should not be used in therapy either internally or externally."[6] Certainly there are enough cases of accidental or suicidal ingestion to demonstrate how dangerous internal use can be. However, the literature reports very few cases of problems with topical use, except when combined with the anticoagulant medication warfarin. The only case I have been able to find of salicylism—poisoning from salicylic acid (including tinnitus, vomiting, and breathing problems)—resulting from dermal application was a 40-year-old man with psoriasis. The report from a hospital in Australia says that "transcutaneous absorption of the methyl salicylate was enhanced in this case due to the abnormal areas of skin and the use of an occlusive dressing."[7] In other words, the preparation was applied on skin that had lost its integrity, probably ensuring a large increase in the levels and rate of absorption.

Methyl salicylate is widely and easily available in over-the-counter topical analgesic ointments from Western and Chinese pharmacies, and few negative side effects have been reported, except when these topical preparations have been ingested, either accidentally or deliberately. Most of the studies on the safety of these medications are focused on changing the packaging to make ingestion more difficult.[8]

The aromatherapist Guba has calculated that even applying 10 mL of a 2.5% dilution of wintergreen oil to the skin (a hefty amount) would result in the same absorption of salicylates as taking one aspirin. He adds that "even with this relatively toxic compound . . . an effective anti-inflammatory preparation can be used with no potential for toxic effects."[9] The respected French aromatherapist Baudoux advises topical use of wintergreen essential oil "up to a maximum dilution of 20%"[10]—far stronger than usually advised. Clearly, aromatherapists should begin to use oils such as wintergreen and sweet birch carefully and judiciously.

TEA TREE

Botanical name: *Melaleuca alternifolia.* Tea tree is a common name in Australia for any of the *Melaleuca* genus, but in aromatherapy and in common use outside of Australia it has come to refer exclusively to *M. alternifolia.*

Family: Myrtaceae.

Native to: Australia.

Part of plant used: Leaves and twigs.

Extraction method: Steam distillation.

Color of oil: Clear to pale yellow.

Consistency: Very thin and watery.

Odor: Penetrating, warm, medicinal.

Chemistry: Terpinen-4-ol (monoterpene alcohol) 30–37%, γ-terpinene (monoterpene) 17–20%, α-terpinene (monoterpene) about 9%, 1,8 cineole (oxide) 3–5%.

Precautions: Possible allergic reaction. The chemistry of the oil and laboratory tests indicate that tea tree is safe when used topically. However, there have been increasing reports of severe allergic reaction to tea tree oil, unusual in such a mild essential oil.[1] One possible explanation is that *M. alternifolia* can now be found in numerous household and bathroom products—everything from toothpaste, to acne lotion, to pet shampoo, to soaps. When someone has prolonged, continual exposure to a substance, no matter how harmless, there is an increased risk of allergic reaction.

Main Uses in Massage

Tea tree is one of the essential oils that has had the most laboratory and clinical testing, primarily because of its possible commercial value. For the massage therapist, its most useful property may be its ability to stimulate the immune system, making it a good element in a blend for those who continually catch colds and the flu, who feel tired and run down, who are recovering from an illness, or who have had chemotherapy or other treatments that depress the immune system.

It has marked antiviral activity, one study noting that the oil "was more effective than that of *Eucalyptus globulus.*"[2] It is useful in a take-home blend for clients who are contraindicated for massage because they are starting a viral infection with a fever; it should be used in a warm bath or in a chest rub. It is also suitable for those who want a home remedy to treat cold sores or warts.

For bacterial infections of the respiratory system, it can be used successfully in a massage on the chest or upper back.[3] Tea tree oil is a powerful antiseptic, and it can be put into blends for clients to use at home to treat any common bacterial infection, such as bladder infections or acne. Studies show that it has fewer side effects than conventional treatment.[4] It seems to be able to kill harmful bacteria without greatly disturbing the normal beneficial bacteria in the body.[5]

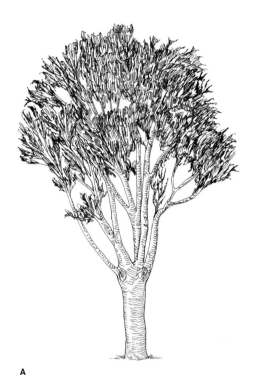

A

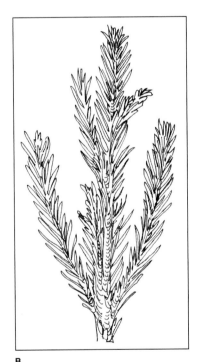

B

Therapeutic Effects

Antibacterial ****
Antifungal **
Antiviral ***
Immunostimulant ***

** = mild   **** = extremely powerful

Tea tree is often recommended as an antifungal, but I do not find it as effective as some other essential oils, such as geranium, palmarosa, or patchouli. It also is sometimes recommended to treat minor burns, but at least one experiment concluded that due to "the reported cytotoxicity of tea tree oil (which could decrease healing and increase scarring), the product was not recommended. . .for the treatment of burns."[6]

Notes

1. Southwell IA, Freeman S, Rubel D. Skin irritancy of tea tree oil. J Essent Oil Res 1997;9:47–52.

2. Schnitzler P, Schon K, Reichling J. Antiviral activity of Australian tea tree oil and eucalyptus oil against *Herpes simplex* virus in cell culture. Pharmazie 2001;56:343–347.

3. Kedzia A, Ostrowski-Meissner H. The effect of selected essential oils on anaerobic bacteria isolated from respiratory tract. Herba Polonica 2003;49(1/2):29–36.

4. Bassett IB, Pannowitz DL, Barnetson R StC. A comparative study of tea-tree oil versus benzoyl peroxide in the treatment of acne. Med J Aust 1990;153(8):455–458.

5. Hammer KA, Carson CF, Riley TV. Susceptibility of transient and commensal skin flora to the essential oil of *Melaleuca alternifolia* (tea tree oil). Aust J Infect Control 1996;24(3):186–189.

6. Faoagali J, George N, Leditschke JF. Does tea tree oil have a place in the topical treatment of burns? Burns 1997;23(4):349–351.

TURMERIC

Botanical name: *Curcuma longa*.

Family: Zingiberaceae.

Native to: India and Southeast Asia.

Part of plant used: Rhizome.

Extraction method: Steam distillation.

Color of oil: Deep yellow.

Consistency: Medium to thick.

Odor: Very warm, soft, deep, slightly spicy.

Chemistry: Ar-turmerone and turmerone (ketones) 30–60%, α-zingiberene (sesquiterpene) about 10%, Ar-curcumene (sesquiterpene) about 8%.

Precautions: None known.

History and Traditional Uses: Turmeric is used extensively in cooking throughout Southeast Asia and especially in India, where it is an ingredient of curry. It is used in both Chinese herbal medicine and Ayurvedic medicine for skin problems, wounds, bruises, joint pain, and digestive issues.[1] I first came across the medicinal use of turmeric when a group of women from Pakistan told me about the application of a paste (made from the spice) to the face as an anti-inflammatory.

Main Uses in Massage

A very new essential oil in the aromatherapy field, turmeric is mostly being used as an antiarthritic agent, its potent anti-inflammatory effects having been explored in laboratory trials.[2] It is reported to have an inhibitory effect on histamine, kinin, and prostaglandins, all of which mediate the body's inflammatory response. As it seems to be rather mild on the skin, it is an ideal oil to add to topical blends in fairly strong dilutions for use locally on painful, arthritic joints, and possibly other inflammatory problems, such as carpal tunnel syndrome.

Research also shows that the essential oil has expectorant properties when inhaled.[3] This effect, along with its anti-inflammatory effects, may make it a good choice for allergic-type respiratory problems, such as hayfever and asthma.

Notes

1. Wuthi-udomlert M, Grisanapan W, Luanratana O, et al. Antifungal activity of Curcuma longa grown in Thailand. Southeast Asian J Trop Med Public Health 2000;31(Suppl. 1):178–182.
2. Ammon HP, Wahl MA. Pharmacology of Curcuma Longa. Planta Medica 1991; 57(1):1–7.
3. Li C, Li L, Luo J, et al. Effect of turmeric volatile oil on the respiratory tract. Zhongguo Zhong Yao Za Zhi 1998;23(10):624–625.

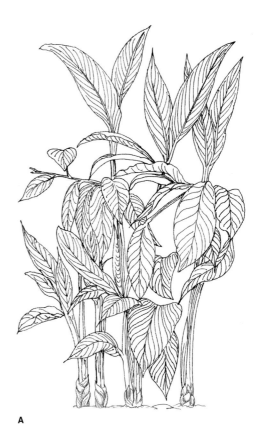

A

B

Therapeutic Effects

Antifungal **
Anti-inflammatory ****
Expectorant **

** = mild   **** = extremely powerful

VETIVER

Botanical name: *Vetiveria zizanioides.*

Family: Gramineae.

Native to: Tropical Asia. Today it is also cultivated in China, Haiti, West Africa, and South America.

Part of plant used: Roots.

Extraction method: Steam distillation.

Color of oil: Olive green to very dark brown.

Consistency: Very thick to molasseslike.

Odor: Earthy, mossy, woody, sweet, lingering; a very powerful aroma.

Chemistry: Vetiverol (various sesquiterpene alcohols) up to 60%, α-vetivone (ketone) 2–7%. Vetiver has a complex chemistry.

Precautions: None known.

History and Traditional Uses: The thin, fibrous roots are traditionally used in Asia to weave mats, baskets, fans, and screens, which give off a cool scent when sprinkled with water, which also helps repel insects. It is grown in many tropical countries to prevent soil erosion during heavy rains. It is used in Ayurvedic medicine to prevent the vomiting that accompanies cholera.[1]

Main Uses in Massage

Vetiver is a powerful and effective sedative. It calms the mind and, appropriate for a root, has a strongly grounding effect, useful for clients who are anxious, hyperactive, insecure, or nervous to the point of being hysterical. In studies it proved to be extremely effective in decreasing both the severity and the frequency of dementia-related behavior.[2] Because it is so useful in calming and bringing people "down to earth," it is also indicated for those who find it difficult to be practical, who are absent-minded, or who neglect to eat or look after themselves.

The essential oil is traditionally used in aromatherapy for its cooling, moisturizing effects on the skin. It is helpful for most inflammatory skin conditions, including acne, dermatitis, psoriasis, and urticaria. The same properties may be useful for other inflammatory conditions, such as arthritis.

Notes

1. Irani F. The Magic of Ayurveda Aromatherapy. West Pennant Hills, Australia: Subtle Energies, 2001:118–120.
2. Bowles EJ, Griffiths DM, Quirk L, et al. Effects of essential oils and touch on resistance to nursing care procedures and other dementia-related behaviours in a residential care facility. Int J Aromather 2002;12(1):22–29.

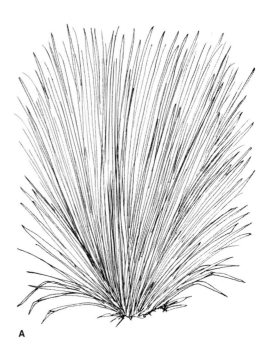

A

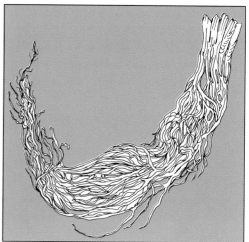

B

Therapeutic Effects

Antibacterial ***
Coolant ***
Moisturizing **
Sedative and calming ****

** = mild   **** = extremely powerful

WINTERGREEN

Botanical name: Two species are used to distill the essential oil, *Gaultheria procumbens* and *G. fragrantissima*.

Family: Ericaceae.

Native to: Many regions, including North America, Asia, and New Zealand.

Part of plant used: Leaves.

Extraction method: Steam distillation.

Color of oil: From clear to deep red, depending on the species.

Consistency: Thin.

Odor: Minty, green, reminiscent of sports rubs or chewing gum, in which it is often used.

Chemistry: Up to 99.7% methyl salicylate (ester).

For precautions, therapeutic effects, and main uses in massage, refer to sweet birch essential oil. Although sweet birch and wintergreen are unrelated species and their oils come from different parts of the plant, the essential oils are almost identical in chemistry, use, and contraindications.

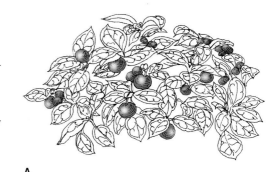

A

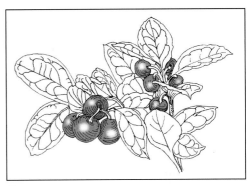

B

YLANG YLANG

Botanical name: *Cananga odorata* var. *genuina*. A closely related species, *C. odorata* var. *macrophylla*, often called cananga oil, is occasionally found in aromatherapy. It is considered to have an inferior aroma and is mostly used in soap making.

Family: Annonaceae.

Native to: Tropical Southeast Asia to Australia. It is also cultivated in Madagascar.

Part of plant used: Flowers, which come in a variety of colors; the yellow is considered to have the finest aroma.

Extraction method: Fractional distillation (see box).

Color of oil: Pale to mid-yellow.

Consistency: Medium.

Odor: Because of the variable quality of the oil, it is difficult to give an accurate description. A fine extra or complete should have an intensely sweet, delicate floral aroma with rich, almost fruit and butterscotch undertones.

Chemistry: Difficult to analyze with any accuracy. Generally, ylang ylang contains ethers (usually *p*-methyl cresol), esters, alcohols (the largest amount usually linalol), and sesquiterpenes (germacrene-D and β-caryophyllene). The extra grades tend to contain more ethers and esters, while the lower grades have increasingly large amounts of sesquiterpenes, giving them their harsher smell.[1]

Precautions: None known. However, I have noticed (and many aromatherapy writers mention) that using large amounts of ylang ylang can lead to headache and nausea.

History and Traditional Uses: In Indonesia, ylang ylang is traditionally spread on the beds of newlywed couples. In the Philippines it is used for hair and skin care and to prevent fevers. The oil was used in Victorian times as part of the well-known hair ointment, macassar oil, because it was thought to encourage hair growth. It is a popular ingredient with perfumers, as it contains both floral top notes and more long-lasting base notes.

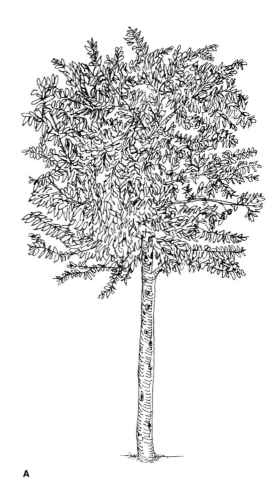

A

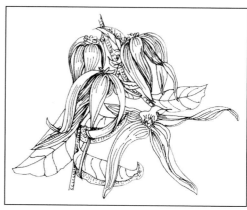

B

Main Uses in Massage

Ylang ylang is one of those oils that people either love or hate. In spite of my admiration for its healing qualities, I have never been able to get over my own dislike of the aroma; it usually reminds me disagreeably of bubblegum. However, most people do like it in blends, even if not on its own. It can be used in relaxation massage for its calming, soothing effects, or given in take-home blends to clients who have insomnia or who find it difficult to relax in the evenings. Ylang ylang is traditionally used in aromatherapy for arrhythmia, tachycardia, and high blood pressure. According to Buckle, midwives in Britain use the essential oil to help reduce hypertension during pregnancy.[2]

Therapeutic Effects

Antidepressant ***
Antispasmodic ***
Hypotensive ****
Sedative ****

** = mild   **** = extremely powerful

Research from the Neuropsychiatry and Seizure Clinic in Birmingham, England, points to its benefits in the treatment of epilepsy: "Aromatherapy was applied to those experiencing particular stress with their epilepsy or where anxiety reinforced their seizures."[3] Ylang ylang was one of the five essential oils used in the study with excellent results. According to the report, "of the first ten patients treated (followed up for over two years) six became seizure free and three withdrew from anticonvulsive medication."[4] Very possibly, ylang ylang's antispasmodic properties, together with its calming quality, may have contributed to this result. The essential oil may be of great benefit in other chronic illnesses in which anxiety or stress trigger the symptoms, such as asthma, irritable bowel syndrome, psoriasis, dermatitis, and digestive problems.

It is also traditionally used in skin care and hair care products and seems to be suitable for all skin types and many dermatological problems.

Notes:

1. Clarke S. Essential Chemistry for Safe Aromatherapy. London, UK: Churchill Livingstone, 2002:154–159.
2. Buckle J. Clinical Aromatherapy. London, UK: Churchill Livingstone, 2003:250.
3. Betts T. Sniffing the breeze. Aromather Quarterly 1994;Spring issue:33.
4. Betts T. Sniffing the breeze. Aromather Quarterly 1994;Spring issue:33.

Fractional Distillation of Ylang Ylang

Fractional distillation is a procedure in which the distillation process is halted after two or more hours and the first part of the distillate is removed. The distillation is continued with the same flowers for about another hour, and another portion of essential oil is obtained and removed. This continues for more than 20 hours, until up to five separate fractions of the oil have been distilled. The first fraction is called extra superior, followed by extra, first, second, and third grades. The extra is most prized by perfumers and aromatherapists because of its fine aroma and therapeutic effects. A complete is sometimes produced by blending the extra, first, and second grades, but in practice this could be a mixture of any of the grades. The quality of the different grades varies considerably from producer to producer because the individual distiller determines the length of distillation of any one grade. As a result, ylang ylang is one of the most difficult oils to compare prices for and to buy successfully, as one essential oil may be totally different in both chemistry and aroma from another, and there are few guarantees that you are actually getting what you are paying for. I have bought the CO_2 extract since it became available because this form gives me more confidence that I am getting what is described on the label.

7

Applications Suitable for the Massage Room

Topical Application
  Relaxation Massage
  Treatment Massage
  Sports Massage
  Manual Lymphatic Drainage
  Polarity and Energy Work
  Hot Stone Massage
  Acupressure and Reflexology
  Facial Massage
Preblended or Custom Formulas
Other Methods of Use
  Compresses
  Foot Baths and Hand Baths
  Diffusers
  Spritzers

Aromatherapy can be incorporated into any form of bodywork, including relaxation massage, treatment work, sports massage, deep tissue work, manual lymphatic drainage, acupressure and reflexology, and forms of "energetic" work such as polarity therapy. The types of essential oils, the strength of dilution, and the application methods used by therapists may vary widely depending on which type of bodywork they are practicing. The applications that are best suited to a professional massage setting are topical application, compresses, foot and hand baths, and diffusers.

Topical Application

Topical application is the form of aromatherapy most favored by massage therapists, for obvious reasons. It is an extremely effective mode of administration because essential oils influence the client by their absorption through the skin into the bloodstream and by the inhalation of aromatic molecules, which have an effect on the brain. Both of these actions occur naturally in an aromatherapy massage, as the warmth from the massage room, the client's body, and the therapist's hands volatilize the essential oils and enable them to be inhaled. In fact, unless strong dilutions or occlusive methods (coverings) are used, inhalation is probably the primary way the client is influenced. The amount of essential oils absorbed may be as low as 4% of a prepared blend during a standard aromatherapy massage and is never higher than 50%, because of the evaporation of the volatile oils in the warm air of the massage room.[1]

For topical application, essential oils can be added directly to any massage oil, lotion, or gel, either in a small bottle, which is shaken thoroughly to disperse the essential oils, or in a blending bowl, which is stirred. Heavy creams are less easy to use, as they need to be stirred for quite some time to completely mix in the essential oils; shaking simply does not work because of the thick consistency of creams.

Relaxation Massage

Relaxation massage typically concentrates on fairly large areas of the body, such as the back, or the whole body. Concentrations tend to be quite low, usually around 1–2%, because the area of skin worked on is large, so absorption rates are higher. The relaxation associated with essential oils is mostly caused by the effects inhalation has on the brain, rather than by absorption into the bloodstream. The dilution also depends to some extent on the odor intensity of the essential oil, as well as the sensitivity of the client's skin. A relaxation massage with rose absolute, for example, may use much less than a 1% dilution because rose has such a powerful fragrance.

The psychological effects of aromatherapy massage are well documented, with clients reporting increased relaxation,[2] ability to cope under stress,[3] and reduced anxiety,[4] among other benefits. These effects work perfectly with the general aims of relaxation massage. Essential oils also can be used to enhance the physiological effects commonly experienced in relaxation massage, such as lowered blood pressure (ylang ylang), increased immune functioning (tea tree and eucalyptus), and deeper breathing (frankincense).

Treatment Massage

Treatment massage includes injury work, bodywork for clients with chronic problems such as digestive issues or asthma, and deeper work on tight muscle groups. In treatment work the therapist rarely does a full-body massage, concentrating instead on particular areas of concern. Dilutions tend to be stronger than for relaxation work because the area of skin that will absorb essential oil is smaller and also because the absorption of a larger amount of essential oil into the bloodstream is desirable to achieve the physiological effects. These effects include increased local circulation, reduced inflammation in connective tissue, and decreased pain in a particular area.

Dilutions for treatment massage usually range from 3% for larger areas of the body to 10% for smaller areas, such as arthritic hands or knees. Dilutions stronger than 10% are used in aromatherapy but are mostly confined to acute situations, such as first aid for a sprain or severe bruising. These higher concentrations can be very effective, and clients often comment that their symptoms seem to diminish quickly. Students who have blending assignments in class sometimes apply these stronger remedies without any soft tissue manipulation at all and still experience significant relief from symptoms within 10 to 20 minutes.

Because treatment massage is often confined to smaller parts of the body, occluding the area that has had essential oils applied is much easier than when larger areas are involved and will ensure a significantly higher and more sustained rate of absorption.[5] An injured knee, for example, can have an essential oil blend applied to it and then be wrapped in plastic wrap and perhaps a towel for warmth and comfort (Figure 7.1). Hands, feet, and limbs can be quickly treated in this way, and even the low back and abdomen can be occluded with a little effort, if necessary.

Including aromatherapy in treatment work is satisfying because the results are often dramatically faster and more effective than massage alone. Moreover, the practitioner has the chance to treat problems for which massage is not appropriate. A good example is varicose veins, for which only light effleurage is possible and a major decrease in symptoms is not expected. By using appropriate essential oils regularly in light effleurage over the area and giving the same blend to the client to use at home, this condition often can be improved over time.

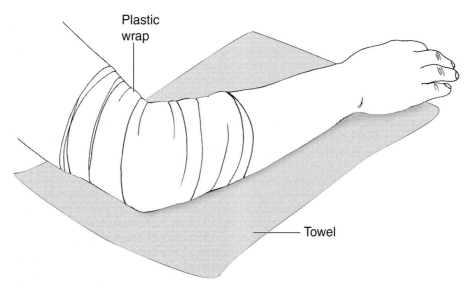

Figure 7.1 Occluding a joint. After an application of essential oils, the elbow is wrapped tightly in plastic wrap and then in a towel to increase absorption.

Deep tissue work could also be loosely classified as treatment massage, using milder or stronger dilutions topically, depending on the size of the area being treated. One particularly useful application with deep tissue work is sending the client home with a blend designed to relieve inflammation, to help alleviate the aching that sometimes follows very deep massage.

Sports Massage

Sports massage can be described in three parts:

1. Pre-event massage consists mostly of jostling movements, compression, friction, and range of motion. This is often performed through the clothes and is not very suited to topical application. Spritzers may be the best option here, to help invigorate and clear the sinuses.

2. Post-event massage is largely first aid and damage control. The therapist applies essential oils to the skin, often in strong dilutions or neat, to treat strains, sprains, and overworked muscles. Anti-inflammatory and analgesic oils, such as wintergreen, sweet birch, German chamomile, and lavender, are the most useful at this point.

3. Massage between sports events can be regarded as treatment work, and uses the same kind of dilution percentages and techniques.

Manual Lymphatic Drainage

The slow pumping movements of manual lymphatic drainage (MLD) do not lend themselves particularly to the application of essential oils. However, oils such as helichrysum, grapefruit, juniper, and cypress, all of which encourage lymph movement, can be applied after the treatment in a light effleurage massage. Dilutions tend to be relatively strong, at around 4%, as these higher concentrations are needed to make the application effective.

Polarity and Energy Work

In energy work, applications tend to be both topical and nontopical, with low concentrations of essential oils, because this form of treatment is intended to affect the energy centers, energy field, and the more subtle layers of awareness. Dilutions may be as mild as 0.5%. In polarity therapy, therapists frequently perform reflex work on the hands and feet, and topical applications of essential oils are appropriate in this part of the treatment. Generally, most other applications in energy work involve some form of diffusion. Essential oils are sometimes chosen to affect particular **chakras**, the energy centers of the body. Rose oil, for example, is traditionally associated with the heart chakra and sandalwood with the base chakra.

Hot Stone Massage

Hot stone massage is becoming increasingly popular with both clients and therapists. It combines extremely well with aromatherapy, as the heat from the stones warms the skin, opens the pores, and increases the absorption of essential oils through the skin into the bloodstream. Most hot stone massages tend to be full-body massages, and the same dilutions apply as for a relaxation massage. Sometimes hot stone therapy is used as part of a treatment session, in which case similar dilutions would apply, with higher concentrations for more acute problems and for smaller areas of skin. Aromatherapists should remember that using heat together with the hotter essential oils, such as ginger or clove, can produce a burning sensation on the skin or skin irritation.

Acupressure and Reflexology

Topical application of essential oils is also used in reflexology and acupressure, even though the area worked on often is extremely small. Gabriel Mojay, an English aromatherapy educator and acupuncturist, has written extensively on aromatherapy from a traditional Chinese medicine perspective. Mojay practices what he calls aromatic acupressure, which involves placing single essential oils, or combinations of oils that would be indicated for the Chinese treatment of the problem, directly onto the appropriate acupuncture or acupressure points. An example from one of his articles is a formula for dysmenorrhea, or painful menstrual cramps, involving what is called in Chinese medicine "stagnation of cold." The oil is composed of ginger (*Zingiber officinale*) as 40% of the essential oil blend, basil (*Ocimum basilicum*) 30%, sweet marjoram (*Origanum majorana*) 20%, and clary sage (*Salvia sclarea*) 10%, to be applied, undiluted, to various appropriate acupressure points.[6]

This same technique can be used in reflexology, in which undiluted essential oils can be applied to reflex areas on the feet or hands. For example, if treating chronic low-back pain, a reflexologist might choose oils such as black pepper (*Piper nigrum*) and sweet marjoram (*Origanum majorana*) and massage them into the reflex area for the low back near the heel of the foot. A respiratory blend of eucalyptus (*Eucalyptus radiata*), spike lavender (*Lavandula latifolia*), and rosemary (*Rosmarinus officinalis*) might be applied neat to the chest reflex area on the ball of the foot. Or the therapist may choose to dilute a combination of essential oils in lotion or oil and massage the whole foot with this blend, as part of the reflexology treatment, usually at the end of the session. Dilutions can be 1–5%, depending on the client's needs and the purpose of the massage.

Facial Massage

Although facial massage is not really a massage specialty, many massage therapists include it as part of a relaxation session in a treatment massage, especially for sinus congestion, stiff neck, and headaches. The skin on the face often is much more sensitive than elsewhere, and if aromatherapy is used as part of the treatment, the therapist may need to dilute the blend further for the face, make a different blend entirely, or use lotion or oil with no essential oils added at all. A 1% blend is generally strong enough for work on the face, although the amount used depends on a client's age and skin sensitivity.

Preblended or Custom Formulas

Some massage therapists use blends formulated for particular problems they frequently encounter in their practice. They make up large batches in oil or lotion to use with many different clients. Others make up an individual blend for each client, taking into account not just the immediate problem but perhaps also the client's constitution, any emotional issues that are presented, and the particular dilution needed for the situation. Neither of these approaches is right or wrong, as massage therapists all have different styles of practice. A busy sports massage therapist may use several ready-made blends because she sees the same problems again and again and works mainly with healthy adults, and her focus is not particularly on emotional work. A massage therapist with a more varied practice doing both treatment and relaxation work, on the other hand, may need to blend for each individual client.

Whether the formulas are preblended or custom made, therapists should have a thorough knowledge of the essential oils in their blends, the reasons they are included in the formulas, and what contraindications exist. I have encountered practitioners in massage clinics, spas, and sports clubs using ready-blended aromatherapy lotions who are uninformed about what they are using, or why, and when they should *not* be using it. This is both unsafe and unethical.

Making large amounts of preblended massage oil also poses the problem of the carrier becoming rancid over time. This can be avoided by refrigerating the blend and decanting small bottles of it to use in the massage room.

Other Methods of Use

Although applications of essential oils other than topical probably will be used less often by massage therapists, other methods are extremely useful in certain situations or for specific problems. Certain types of therapists tend to use some of these applications regularly, such as foot baths for reflexology or compresses in sports massage.

Compresses

Compresses are mostly used in treatment massage and in sports massage for injuries. Compresses can be hot or cold, depending on the client's problem and on the therapist's approach. Because many massage therapists use preheated or prechilled hot or cold packs, the most practical way to use essential oils with compresses is to apply the essential oils to the skin, usually in a strong dilution, or undiluted on very small areas such as a wrist or a sprained thumb, and then to put the thermal pack on top. It is also possible to put the essential oils into very cold or very hot water, dip a small towel in, wring it out, and apply. However, this method tends to be more time-consuming and slightly messier in a massage room setting. This type of compress does not retain heat or cold as long or as well as do the thermal packs.

Dilutions for use under a compress would be similar to straightforward topical application on a small injured area. Dilutions are between 3% and 10%, depending on the problem being treated, whether it is acute or chronic, and the client's age and condition. When using warm or hot compresses it is important to remember that heat will increase the chances of irritation, and this could affect which essential oils are selected. Some of the hotter, more irritating oils should be avoided, especially with hot compresses. For example, the spice oils, such as clove (*Syzygium aromaticum*), may be well tolerated when applied topically but could produce irritation even at the same dilution when heat is added.

Foot Baths and Hand Baths

Foot baths are frequently used as part of a relaxation treatment (Figure 7.2). Some massage therapists routinely offer their clients an aromatic foot bath at the start of a session, especially when they are completing intake forms or chatting before the massage begins. One study showed that adding only 4 drops of lavender (*Lavandula angustifolia*) essential oil to a foot bath led to "small but significant changes in autonomic activity" indicative of greater relaxation.[7] Another study with senior citizens, again using lavender essential oil in an evening foot bath, showed that the subjects not only slept better but also had better moods the following day.[8] Warm baths are a good way to get essential oils into the bloodstream, as warm hydrated skin tends to absorb essential oils more efficiently.

Foot baths and hand baths are also used for treatment work, in much the same way as compresses, and essential oils can be added for the same reasons. They are an ideal way to treat conditions such as athlete's foot, excessively dry cracked skin on the soles of the feet, and dermatitis.[9]

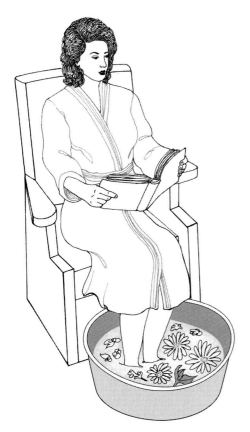

Figure 7.2 A foot bath.

Activity 7.1

Using a Foot Bath or Hand Bath

Using a small plastic tub that is long enough for your feet and can hold water at least 4 inches in depth, try the following exercises over several days:

1. Fill the tub to a depth of at least 4 inches with water that is comfortably warm. Add 3–6 drops of eucalyptus essential oil (*Eucalyptus radiata*). Put your feet in the tub and stay there for 5–10 minutes. Notice the sensations in your feet and also notice if the foot bath has any effect on your sinuses.

2. Fill the tub as before with warm water and add 3–4 drops of peppermint essential oil (*Mentha piperita*). Take your pulse before putting your feet in the tub. Notice any skin sensations, and also notice if you feel warmer or cooler overall after the foot bath. Take your pulse again just before taking your feet out of the tub. Is it faster, slower, or just the same as before?

3. Fill the tub as before with warm water and add 1 drop of rose absolute (*Rosa damascena* or *centifolia*). Can you smell the oil as intensely as those in the other exercises? Note any skin sensations or other feelings.

They also are extremely effective for respiratory problems because the essential oils are absorbed into the skin and also inhaled as they evaporate off the warm water. Foot baths can be useful for headaches (perhaps with peppermint), sore feet, and poor circulation, among many other problems.

Massage therapists may decide to use foot baths for aesthetic reasons as well, because some people arriving at a massage clinic, especially in the summer, have sweaty, odorous feet. A quick aromatic foot bath both refreshes the client and makes the feet more pleasant for the therapist to work on. This is especially true for reflexologists.

Essential oils can simply be added to the water of the foot or hand bath, but it is probably better to dilute them first for a client who has sensitive skin. The essential oils can be dissolved in a commercial emulsifier, honey, full-fat milk, or liquid soap. They can also be dissolved in alcohol, but this method can be somewhat harsh on the skin. As with compresses, heat from the foot bath may increase the effects of essential oils that are skin irritating.

As with topical application, the amount of essential oil added to foot baths or hand baths depends on the type of treatment and on the person involved. For a healthy adult, 3 to 6 drops of essential oil can be added to a foot bath for relaxation; the amount may need to be less if the intense floral oils are used. For a child or an elderly person, 2 to 3 drops would be enough, and dilution in honey, milk, or soap may be necessary. Treatment work may require significantly larger amounts of essential oils, perhaps up to 20 drops for something like a sprained ankle. It would be advisable to dissolve this larger amount before adding it to the foot bath, to avoid skin irritation. The usual hydrotherapy contraindications for heat apply to aromatherapy foot and hand baths.

Diffusers

Using **diffusers** involves vaporizing essential oils into the air to be inhaled. There are several different methods of use, including steam inhalation, putting essential oils into aroma lamps (oil burners) or nebulizers, adding them to a bowl of hot water, and putting a few drops onto a tissue for a client to sniff. Inhaling essential oils increases relaxation and sedation, and reduces anxiety.[10] But studies show that inhalation also produces marked physiological effects, such as boosting immunity,[11] reducing smoking withdrawal symptoms,[12] assisting recovery from exercise,[13] and even reducing the amount of cholesterol in the aorta.[14] Thus, using diffusers is valuable in treatment massage and sports massage, as well as for relaxation.

Direct **steam inhalation** is primarily used for respiratory congestion and coughs. The most convenient device in the massage room is the use of an electric steam inhaler, with a well for heating water (Figure 7.3). Before the water is heated, add 1 to 3 drops of essential oil to the water. Steam inhalation can be used frequently if sinus congestion is acute, for example, but small amounts of essential oil at one time are more effective than large doses, which sometimes can actually worsen congestion. If a client is suffering from sinus or lung congestion, the use of an inhaler at the end of a session may encourage the mucus to flow more easily for a while afterwards, although this is not recommended for a client who will be prone for some time.

Most aromatherapy guidelines advise against using steam inhalation with clients who have asthma. However, several of my clients with asthma have doctors who recommend steam inhalation. Conversely, some people with asthma cannot even sit in a steamroom without precipitating an attack. Always check with an asthmatic client's doctor before attempting to use steam inhalation.

To diffuse essential oils into the air, several devices can be used. Simple **oil burners,** or **aroma lamps** with a tea candle that heats a reservoir, can be effective for inhalation.[15] Always put water in the reservoir before adding the aromatics because essential oils are highly flammable and may catch fire if burned without water. An electrically run **nebulizer,** which shoots out a fine mist of essential oil droplets, may be preferable to an aroma lamp, as it has no open flame, thus making it safer for use in the massage room. The amount of essential oils used in the burner or nebulizer depends on the size of the room and on the preference of the client; as few as 3 or 4 drops can produce a strong aroma in a small room. Cool-air **fan diffusers** that use a battery or electrically run fan to waft essential oils into the air are also an option for smaller rooms.

With any kind of diffusion it is necessary to air the space before the next client arrives. This can be difficult in a professional setting in which other therapists use the same room, or in a clinic. Even in a room used exclusively by one therapist, the smell can become so intense that it is difficult to remove quickly and effectively. For this reason, therapists who most often use diffusion tend to be those who work at home and do not book clients back to back. However, using the diffuser for just 10 or 15 minutes may not be overwhelming for most clients. In my massage practice, if I decide to diffuse essential oils, I often do it for a short time at the beginning of a session, to give the smell some time to dissipate, or when I don't have another client scheduled immediately afterward.

Scheduling can be important for client comfort because every person who comes into the massage room will not necessarily welcome fragrances. However, inhalation is a very safe way to introduce essential oils into a massage session, when there may be reasons to avoid topical application, such as highly sensitive skin.

When an aroma is being used mainly for psychological reasons, or to help avoid congestion when a client is prone, you can place a couple of drops of essential oil on a tissue

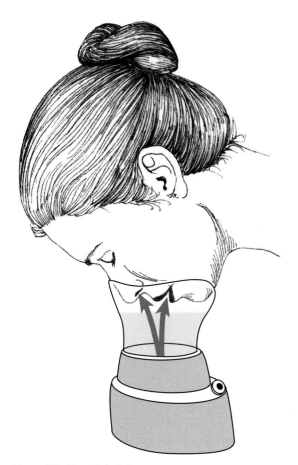

Figure 7.3 Steam inhalation.

and tuck it into the face cradle cover. This technique avoids the complication of diffusing essential oil throughout the entire massage room.

Spritzers

A **spritzer** is one of the simplest and most effective ways to diffuse essential oils, and consists of a light dilution, usually 1–2%, in a spray bottle filled with water. The bottle is shaken before each spraying so that the water-insoluble essential oils hang in suspension for a few seconds, giving a better mix of water and oils.

The solution can be sprayed into the air in the massage room for a brief diffusion, avoiding the situation with burners and nebulizers wherein rooms have to be aired thoroughly afterward. It is also nice to mist over clients in extremely hot weather to refresh each body section after massaging it. In this case, the spritzer bottle should be held high above the client—at least 2 feet or more above—as it should fall as a light mist and not a spray, which may startle the client.

Because of its ease and convenience for people with busy lives, who may work in open areas where they do not want the after-effects of diffusers, using a spritzer is a good take-home method for clients. They should be warned, however, not to spray directly onto the skin because that would constitute a neat application (due to the fact that the essential oils do not dissolve in the water), which may not be appropriate. I knew someone who made a spritzer containing bergamot oil and sprayed it directly onto her face; she ended up with little red spots where the tiny undiluted droplets of bergamot had photosensitized the skin. It is better to hold the spritzer above the head, to let the mist fall gently over the body, or to spray into the air.

SUMMARY

- The most appropriate methods of application within a professional massage setting are topical application, compresses, foot and hand baths, and diffusion.

- For topical application, the different massage styles often use varying dilution percentages. Dilutions tend to be mild for relaxation massage and stronger for treatment massage, including sports massage and MLD.

- For energy work, including polarity work, dilutions are generally mild (as low as 1%).

- Hot stone massage increases the absorption of essential oils. Dilutions are similar to regular massage.

- Small amounts of undiluted essential oils can be used on acupressure points or reflexology points.

- Dilutions should be mild for facial massage (around 1%) because the skin on the face is sensitive.

- Essential oils can be preblended in large amounts for a particular problem, or custom blended for individual clients. In both cases, therapists should have a thorough knowledge of the essential oils used.

- For compresses, the most convenient method is a strong dilution (or neat application) to the local area, covered with a hot or cold thermal pack.

- Foot baths and hand baths are useful for relaxation and to relieve sprains, strains, headaches, and respiratory problems. Although 3 to 6 drops is common, the amount may be higher, especially for acute injury work.

- Direct steam inhalation is used for respiratory congestion and coughs. Lower amounts (1–3 drops) used more frequently tend to have a better effect than larger amounts. Caution is advised with asthmatic clients, and a doctor's release might be necessary.

- Diffusion can have psychological and physiological effects. Methods commonly used are oil burners (aroma lamps), electric nebulizers, and spritzers. Diffusion for 10 or 15 minutes during a session is sufficient. The massage space should be aired out after each session.

Review Questions

1. Relaxation massage generally uses milder dilutions, as full-body massage is common in this treatment modality. (T/F)
2. Spritzers can safely be sprayed directly onto the face. (T/F)
3. Dilutions for treatment massage are often between _____ and _____%, although they may be even stronger for work with acute injuries.
4. Why would an aromatherapist occlude an area of the body that has just had essential oils applied to it?
5. Topical application is probably *least* appropriate during which part of sports massage: pre-event, post-event, or between events?

6. How could a reflexologist or acupressure practitioner include aromatherapy in his or her treatment session? (List two possible methods mentioned in the chapter.)

7. The most convenient (and least messy) method of using compresses with aromatherapy is to use a towel that is wrung out in hot or cold water that contains essential oils. (T/F)

8. Foot baths can be used to treat headaches and sinus congestion. (T/F)

9. An average amount of drops of essential oil added to a foot bath is _____ to _____.

10. It may not be appropriate to use a steam inhaler with a client who suffers from _____.

11. Blends for the face should be stronger, as the skin is tougher in this area. (T/F)

12. Aroma lamps (oil burners) are not effective for diffusing essential oils in massage rooms. (T/F)

13. What challenge is associated with diffusing essential oils in the air in a professional massage setting?

14. Essential oils do not dissolve in water; therefore, when using a spritzer, it should be _____ just before it is used.

15. Direct steam inhalation is most often used for _____ problems.

Notes

1. Guba R. Toxicity myths—the actual risks of essential oil use. Int J Aromather 2002;10(1/2):37–49.

2. Hadfield N. The role of aromatherapy massage in reducing anxiety in patients with malignant brain tumors. Int J Palliat Nurs 2001;7(6):279–285.

3. Waldman CS, Tseng P, Meulman P, et al. Aromatherapy in the intensive care unit. Care Crit Ill 1993;9(4):170–174.

4. Corner J, Cawley N, Hildebrand S. An evaluation of the use of essential oils on the well-being of cancer patients. Int J Palliat Nurs 1995;1(2): 67–73.

5. Fuchs N, Jager W, Lenhardt A, et al. Systemic absorption of topically applied carvone: influence of massage technique. J Society Cosmet Chem 1997;48(6):277–282.

6. Mojay G. Healing the jade pool—the phyto-aromatic and acupressure treatment of dysmenorrhoea and menopausal syndrome: an East-West approach. Int J Aromather 2002; 12(3):131–141.

7. Saeki Y. The effect of foot-bath with or without the essential oil of lavender on the autonomic nervous system: a randomized trial. Complement Ther Med 2000;8:2–7.

8. Moriya K. The effect of foot bathing with lavender oil on the nocturnal sleep. Aroma Res 2000;1(4):62–69.

9. Iwase N, Sato H, et al. Effect of bath additive containing eucalyptus extracts for skin care. Aroma Res 2000;1(4):70–76.

10. Buchbauer G, Jirovetz L, Jager W, et al. Aromatherapy: evidence for sedative effects of the essential oil of lavender after inhalation. Zeitschrift fur Naturforschung Teil C 1991;46(11–12):1067–1072.

11. Fujiwara R, Komori T, et al. Effects of a long-term inhalation of fragrances on the stress-induced immunosuppression in mice. Neuroimmunomodulation 1998;5:318–322.

12. Rose JE, Behm FM. Inhalation of vapor from black pepper extract reduces smoking withdrawal symptoms. Drug Alcohol Depend 1994;34(3):225–229.

13. Romine IJ, Bush AM, Geist CR. Lavender aromatherapy in recovery from exercise. Percept Motor Skills 1999;88:756–758.

14. Nikolaevskii VV, Kononova NS, Pertsovskii AI, et al. Effect of essential oils on the course of experimental atherosclerosis. Patologicheskaia Fiziologiia I Eksperimentalnaia Terepiia (Moskva) 1990;5:52–53.

15. Overhofer B, Nikiforov A, Buchbauer G, et al. Investigation of the alteration of the composition of various essential oils used in aroma lamp applications. Flavor Fragr J 1999;14:293–299.

8

Measurements and Dilutions

Measuring essential oils and deciding how much of them to put in your massage oil or lotion can be confusing. It is extremely important to understand dilution methods because different clients and different massage modalities will require varying concentrations of essential oils. In pricing your treatments or remedies, it is also helpful to be able to calculate the cost of the essential oils that have been used, by the drop.

Measurements

Part of the confusion for most therapists in America is that essential oils usually are not measured in the conventional fluid ounces, unless you are buying them in bulk. They usually are sold in much smaller quantities. In this book, therefore, essential oil measurements are given in milliliters (one thousandth of a liter). In 1 fl. oz. there are about 30 mL. At the retail level, essential oils generally are sold in amounts of 5–15 mL (roughly 0.15–0.5 oz.) (Figure 8.1).

Precious essential oils or absolutes are frequently retailed in much smaller quantities. For example, the flower oils are generally sold in 2 mL sizes, or even as small as 1 mL sizes, the reason being the high cost of these oils. The flowers yield only small amounts of essential oil and the plants require high amounts of labor, such as caring for and hand-picking the flowers. Suppliers, however, often will put these small amounts of oil into larger bottles, not for deceptive purposes but because the larger bottles (conventionally 5 mL) are easier to handle and easier to pack later and display. This bottling practice can lead to confusion because a bottle may appear to be only half full.

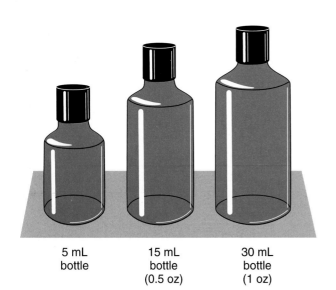

5 mL	15 mL	30 mL
bottle	bottle	bottle
	(0.5 oz)	(1 oz)

Figure 8.1 Bottle sizes.

Calculating Costs

When buying an essential oil or absolute, it is always a good idea to calculate how much it will cost you per drop. While this might seem overly precise, knowing the exact cost of each drop is necessary for determining the cost to you of any massage blends or other products you create. You may think twice about including a particular blend of jasmine, sandalwood, and chamomile in the set price of an aromatherapy massage session when you calculate that it has cost you $12.00 to make! And the realization that your rose essential oil retails for $1.50 per drop might prompt you to reserve it for those occasions when it is absolutely necessary.

The calculation for determining the cost per drop is straightforward: Simply divide the price you paid for your essential oil by the number of drops in the bottle. However, the size of a drop can vary considerably, depending on whether the essential oil is thick or thin. Just imagine trying to measure equal amounts of lemon juice and molasses by counting the number of drops of each you use and you can begin to see the problem. What's more, bottle dropper inserts tend to vary in size among manufacturers, producing varying sizes of drops. One nursing study found significant differences between different manufacturers' drop size of the same essential oil (bergamot).[1]

As a general guideline, we can say that most aromatic oils contain *between 20 and 35 drops per milliliter*. If you want to be more precise about your calculations, you can look at the thickness of the oil and decide if it is closer to 20 drops per mL (very thick oils, such as vetiver and vanilla absolute) or closer to 35 drops per mL (very thin oils, such as lemon and peppermint).

A quick calculation for the cost of peppermint oil would be as follows:

Price of bottle of essential oil: $6.50.

Size of bottle: 5 mL.

Number of drops per mL: about 30.

Number of drops in the bottle: 30 per mL × 5 mL = 150 drops.

Divide price by number of drops: $6.50 divided by 150 = about 4 cents per drop.

It's a good idea to keep a price list from a reputable supplier at hand and to consult it when studying essential oils or making blends. You will quickly build up a basic knowledge of which essential oils are expensive, which are midrange in price, and which are inexpensive.

Dilutions

For use in massage work and most other methods of application, essential oils are diluted in massage oil or lotion, which are called **carriers** or **base oils** in aromatherapy. The consensus among aromatherapy teachers, and in aromatherapy books, is that you should use a 1–3% dilution for massage. But what does a "percent dilution" mean, how can you calculate it, and is that figure always correct in all situations and for all clients?

Calculating Dilutions

A **percent dilution** simply means that for every 100 drops of carrier oil or lotion you use, you will need to add 1 drop of essential oil to make each 1%. Therefore, a 3% dilution means 3 drops of essential oil in 100 drops of massage oil or lotion. Counting out 100 drops of your massage oil is obviously going to be a waste of time, so some common measurements are needed. It is useful to know that there are about 6 *teaspoons in a fluid ounce*, so that 1 *teaspoon = 5 mL*.

If we say that a massage oil has 20 drops per mL (for simplicity's sake only, as many commonly used essential oils have more than 20 drops per mL), this means a teaspoon contains roughly 100 drops (20 drops × 5 mL per teaspoon). Therefore, you can add 1 drop of essential oil to 1 teaspoon of massage oil (1 drop per 100 drops) to get a 1% dilution. A rough estimate of how many teaspoons of oil or lotion you are using for a massage will let you know how many drops of essential oil you need to use. For example, if you want to make a 3% dilution in about 4 teaspoons of lotion:

4 teaspoons = 400 drops of lotion.

1% dilution in 400 drops = 4 drops of essential oil in 400 drops of lotion.

3% dilution in 400 drops = 3 × 4 = 12 drops of essential oil in 4 teaspoons of lotion.

It is important to remember that these 12 drops are a *total* of all of the essential oils used, not 12 drops of *each* essential oil in your blend. For example, if you used lavender, geranium, and bergamot in this particular blend, you might have 4 drops of each essential oil, to make up the 12 drops needed for the 3% dilution.

As another example, if you have 2 oz. of massage lotion and you want to make a 3% dilution:

1 oz. of lotion = 6 teaspoons = 600 drops.

2 oz. of lotion = 1200 drops.

1% dilution in 2 oz. (or 1200 drops) = 12 drops of essential oil.

3% dilution in 2 oz. = 3 × 12 = 36 drops of essential oil in 2 oz. of lotion.

It should be obvious that these kinds of measurements are imprecise; they give an approximation of the dilution because drop sizes vary so much. However, this kind of calculation is usually accurate enough for our purposes, if we remember that we are dealing with absorption through the skin rather than oral ingestion as used in medical aromatherapy, wherein measurements are required to be much more precise. As we will see in Chapter 10 on safety, the amount of essential oil absorbed through the skin into the bloodstream varies, depending on the client's amount of body fat, the warmth of the room, the temperature of the client's skin, whether the part of the body just massaged is covered immediately afterward, and so on. Because this method of absorption is fairly safe on the whole, approximate calculations give us enough information to know if what we are doing is sensible and appropriate. As the herbalist Mills says, "the exact dosage is less important than the correct choice of approach."[2]

Table 8.1   Dilutions for Essential Oils in Teaspoons of Carrier

Amount of Carrier	1 Teaspoon = 100 Drops = 5 mL	2 Teaspoons = 200 Drops = 10 mL	3 Teaspoons (1 Tablespoon)	4 Teaspoons
Essential oil 1%	1 drop – *2 drops*	2 drops – *3 drops*	3 drops – *5 drops*	4 drops – *7 drops*
Essential oil 2%	2 drops – *3 drops*	4 drops – *7 drops*	6 drops – *10 drops*	8 drops – *14 drops*
Essential oil 3%	3 drops – *5 drops*	6 drops – *10 drops*	9 drops – *16 drops*	12 drops – *20 drops*
Essential oil 4%	4 drops – *7 drops*	8 drops – *14 drops*	12 drops – *20 drops*	16 drops – *28 drops*

Table 8.2   Dilutions for Essential Oils in Ounces of Carrier

Amount of Carrier	$^1/_2$ oz. = 3 teaspoons = 15 mL	1 oz. = 6 teaspoons = 30 mL	2 oz.	3 oz.	4 oz.
Essential oil 1%	3 drops – *5 drops*	6 drops – *10 drops*	12 drops – *20 drops*	18 drops – *30 drops*	24 drops – *40 drops*
Essential oil 2%	6 drops – *10 drops*	12 drops – *20 drops*	24 drops – *40 drops*	36 drops – *60 drops*	48 drops (about $^1/_2$ tsp) – *80 drops*
Essential oil 3%	9 drops – *16 drops*	18 drops – *32 drops*	36 drops – *64 drops*	54 drops – *96 drops*	72 drops – *128 drops*
Essential oil 4%	12 drops – *20 drops*	24 drops – *40 drops*	48 drops (about $^1/_2$ tsp) – *80 drops*	72 drops – *120 drops*	96 drops (about 1 tsp) – *160 drops*

Refer to Table 8.1 for a reference guide for dilutions in teaspoons of carrier and Table 8.2 for a reference guide for dilutions in ounces of carrier. Drop amounts are given for thicker oils with about 20 drops per mL. Amounts listed in italics are for thinner oils with about 35 drops per mL. Most essential oils will fall somewhere in the middle.

Choosing a Dilution

Having established how to calculate dilutions, the next step is choosing what dilution you need. The 1–3% dilution recommended in many aromatherapy books does not take into account the varying needs of the professional massage practitioner, who may be doing full-body relaxation massage, injury work, or sports massage and who may be working with clients with chronic health problems, such as arthritic joints, whiplash, irritable bowel syndrome, or chronic respiratory problems. Massage therapists tend to treat most of these problems more locally, perhaps spending a large part, or even all, of the session time working intensively on the smaller area involved. Using a 2–3% dilution of an essential oil on an ankle that has just been sprained may not give the rapid healing results that a 20–30% dilution would provide.

It is important to make wise dilution decisions. A thorough knowledge of the properties, chemistry, and contraindications of the essential oils you work with will enable you to balance considerations of safety with those of effectiveness. The chapters on methods of application (Chapter 7) and safety (Chapter 10) provide more detailed guidelines on dilution percentages used in holistic aromatherapy.

Strong Dilutions. In medical aromatherapy, French practitioners often use topical formulas with dilutions greater than 10%, and the use of neat, or undiluted, oils is quite common. The French aromatherapist Baudoux suggests diluting certain essential oils to a 50% dilution "for those with sensitive skin,"[3] not the type of dilution that would normally be advised in the holistic tradition for sensitive skin. As a result of my own work, I believe that there is a place in the massage practice for the use of essential oils at a significantly higher concentration than the standard 1–3%.

Considerations for Dilutions. How does the massage therapist decide when it is beneficial to use stronger dilutions and what safety precautions should be taken? Here are some general points to consider:

1. *Your own experience.* Unless you have very delicate and reactive skin, you can get a good idea of the character of an essential oil at different dilutions by experimenting with it on your own skin. Try it first over a large area with fairly sensitive skin—the abdomen, perhaps—in a 2–3% dilution. Wait for 5 or 6 hours and see if there is any reaction, and then increase the dilution, perhaps to 10%, and wait for a similar length of time to judge if this oil is especially irritating. A few days later, if you have no reaction, you might use it in a 50% dilution on a smaller area of skin, and even later use it neat, or in a 100% dilution on a small patch of skin. This experimenting with increasing doses should give you a good idea of the nature of the essential oil. How did your skin react? Was there any kind of rash or redness? Was there any feeling of irritation or itching? Did it simply feel warm, or cold, or tingly?

2. *The client.* When deciding on a dilution, you must keep the client in mind. Use milder dilutions, often much milder, with babies and small children, the elderly, people with any kind of allergy, and people with extremely sensitive skin. These people all have a higher risk of adverse skin reactions to essential oils. Because essential oils vary widely in their effects, there is no substitute for a knowledge of the specific strengths and properties of each one when deciding on dilutions.

3. *The size and area of the body.* The rule of thumb is that if you are doing a full-body massage, a dilution of 1–3% is appropriate. If you are working specifically on a smaller area, you are probably doing so because of a particular problem in that region, such as low-back pain or tight hamstrings, and a stronger dilution may give you better results. The overall number of drops of essential oil absorbed into the bloodstream will be similar if you use a mild dilution over a large area or a strong dilution on a small area of skin. The smaller the area is on which you work, the stronger the dilution you can use. A client with irritable bowel syndrome may be suited to an abdominal massage with essential oils at a 5–6% dilution. Someone with severe low-back pain, as a result of strained muscles, for example, often will benefit from a blend of the appropriate essential oils applied locally in a dilution of 10% or even more. A recently sprained ankle, or acute carpal tunnel syndrome, may warrant the use of oils in an extremely strong dilution in the range of 30–100% for these very small areas of the body.

4. *The essential oils being used.* Some essential oils are more irritating to the skin than others, even commonly used oils such as peppermint. Chapter 10 on safety lists all the essential oils that are commonly known as potential skin irritants. However, your in-depth study of the properties of the essential oils you are using, together with your experience of how the essential oils react on your own skin, will give you a clear indication of which essential oils are appropriate, and in what proportion. If a potentially irritating essential oil is to be used—perhaps thyme CT thymol (*Thymus vulgaris* CT thymol)—because of its highly antiseptic nature, it should make up only a small part of the whole blend, the other oils ideally being nonirritant in nature and thus acting as buffers for the thyme. Oils that will likely cause skin reactions should not make up more than 25% of the entire essential oil blend. Also, formulas that include such oils are more safely used diluted than undiluted.

5. *The goal of your treatment session.* Massage therapists work on many different levels with their clients, usually concentrating on the particular approach that will be most beneficial for the client overall, or for that session in particular. Is the treatment primarily physical, or is it more psychological, emotional, or energetic in nature? This goal of the session will affect the percentage dilution of the essential oils you use. Generally, the more grossly physical the work is, the stronger the appropriate dilution is likely to be. As the treatment works on increasingly subtle levels, the concentration level is likely to decrease. While this is a personal choice for each massage practitioner, most therapists working on an energetic level seem to agree that "less is more," and some rarely use more than a 0.5 % dilution for this kind of work. For purely physical massage work, the dilution is often decided by whether the problem is acute or chronic. Acute problems mostly respond best to stronger dilutions, while in chronic situations milder dilutions tend to work better. The exceptions are chronic problems that affect very small areas of the body, such as plantar warts or acne.

Activity 8.3

Deciding on Appropriate Dilutions

You have three clients below. Decide on appropriate dilutions for each client.

1. Mrs. S. sprained her wrist within the last 5 hours. You decide to use an ice pack on the area, with essential oils below the compress.

2. Mr. B. would like a full-body relaxation massage. He does not have any particular physical issues, but feels stressed, anxious, and overwhelmed. He is age 35 with no chronic illnesses.

3. Ms. F. is an 85-year-old woman with cancer, in hospice care, who has developed a bad chest cough. She has asked you to make up a blend to rub on her chest to help with the cough.

SUMMARY

- Undiluted essential oils and very strong dilutions (greater than 30%) should be used only on adults, on a small area of skin that is not highly sensitive, and generally in acute situations so that the application is short term.

- Medium to strong dilutions (4–30%) are best on adults and children older than age 8 for physical conditions, acute or chronic, involving small to medium areas of the body. The stronger dilutions tend to be best for short-term use.

- Mild dilutions (1–3%) may be used on adults or children older than age 5 for full-body massage, or on medium-sized areas of the body, for relaxation massage, and for psychological and emotional work. The milder dilutions are more suitable for young children, the elderly, pregnant women, and people with sensitive skin or allergies.

- Very mild dilutions (0.5–1%) are best on the very young or the very old, on the very sensitive, and for more subtle work on emotional, psychological, and energetic levels.

Review Questions

1. Small amounts of essential oils usually are not sold in fluid ounces but in _____.
2. To calculate the cost of an essential oil per drop, you need to divide the price of the bottle by _____.
3. How many drops of essential oil are there usually in 1 mL?
4. How many drops of essential oil do you need to add to 1 teaspoonful of carrier to make a 1% dilution?
5. If you want to make a 3% dilution in 2 oz. of carrier, how many drops of essential oil would you need (assuming that there are 20 drops of this essential oil in 1 mL)?
6. If you want to make a 2% dilution in 5 oz. of carrier, how many drops of essential oil would you need (assuming that there are 35 drops of this essential oil in 1 mL)?

Notes

1. Oleveant NA, Humphris G, Roe B. How big is a drop? A volumetric assay of essential oils. J Clin Nurs 1999;8(3):299–304.
2. Mills S. The Essential Book of Herbal Medicine. London, UK: Penguin, 1991.
3. Baudoux D. L'Aromathérapie. Anglet, France: Éditions atlantica, 2000.

Although animal fats, such as goose grease, traditionally have been used in both healing work and beauty care, today this is rare, and oils from plants are primarily the ones used in massage and aromatherapy. In aromatherapy, these are interchangeably called **carrier oils, vegetable oils, base oils, or fixed oils** (the latter to distinguish them from the volatile oils, or essential oils, of aromatherapy). The word "carrier" is somewhat misleading when it comes to good-quality vegetable oils, as they do not simply "carry" the essential oils but have distinct healing properties of their own, which have been known to nutritionists for a long time. Just as essential oils can be blended for a synergistic effect and a beautiful aroma, fixed oils can be combined to create particular textures and healing applications.

Vegetable oils are my preferred carriers for many reasons. I appreciate their intrinsic therapeutic properties, and I enjoy sourcing new and exotic oils from around the world. I also find it easier to assess the quality and properties of an oil from a single botanical source rather than a commercially produced cream or gel with many different ingredients, some of which I am familiar with, many of which I am not. When I buy an organic sunflower oil from a reputable supplier, I can be fairly sure of what I am getting.

Characteristics of Oils

Aromatherapists have to make choices about which oils to use and in which situations to use them. Oils and fats are the same thing: Both are known as **lipids.** We tend to use the word "oil" for substances that are liquid and "fat" for those that are solid, but the difference is simply a matter of temperature. If you heat any fat to a high enough temperature, it will melt, and many oils will become solid if you put them in the refrigerator or the freezer.

Lipids consist of one molecule of glycerol attached to three fatty acid molecules. **Fatty acids** are the main component of all the fats in the body, including triglycerides in the bloodstream, adipose tissue, and the membranes enclosing the cells and the organelles within cells. Fatty acids play important roles in the construction and maintenance of cells in any part of the body.

Plant oils may be found in any part of the plant, but the highest concentrations are in the seeds (Figure 9.1). This is because the **seed** (sometimes called the **nut**) is the part that grows into a new plant. Before the tiny seedling can produce leaves and synthesize its own food, it has to be given an adequate supply of nutrition from its parent. Since lipids are the most concentrated form of energy in the plant or animal world (more concentrated even than sugars), the parent plant packs the seed with oil to sustain the growing plant. This is why most of the oils that we use for food and for our skin are made by crushing seeds and nuts and some fruits.

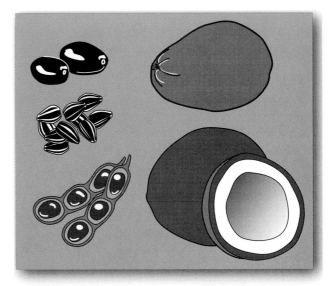

Figure 9.1 Various seeds, nuts, and fruits used to make oil. Sunflower seeds, soybeans, olives, avocado, and coconut.

Oils from plants are saturated, monounsaturated, and polyunsaturated. These terms derive from their chemical structures. **Saturated fatty acids** consist of carbon chains, with the maximum possible number of hydrogens attached to them. **Unsaturated fatty acids** have one (monounsaturates) or more (polyunsaturates) double bonds between the carbon atoms, with fewer hydrogen atoms attached as a result. This means that unsaturated molecules end up with a kink in their molecular chain, unlike the straight chains of the saturated molecules. Because the straight chains stack together more easily, saturated fats have a denser, heavier structure, making them more likely to be solid at room temperature, which is easily seen in saturated animal fats such as butter and vegetable fats such as coconut and palm oils. Unsaturated fats tend to be liquid at room temperature, as are most vegetable oils.

Double bonds tend to be weaker than single bonds and more easily broken, so that unsaturated fatty acids react more rapidly with oxygen. As a result, unsaturated oils have a tendency to break down and turn rancid more quickly than the stable saturated fats. This is especially true with a particular group of unsaturated fatty acids, linoleic acid and alpha-linolenic acid, known as **essential fatty acids (EFAs).** They are called "essential" because they are necessary nutrients the body cannot manufacture, so they must be provided in the diet. Oils that are particularly high in EFAs, such as flax, hemp, and pumpkin seed, are extremely healing and are used by the body to synthesize important hormonelike compounds called prostaglandins and to maintain the most active tissues, such as the brain, adrenal glands, and testes. However, these oils are also the most reactive with oxygen, so their shelf life is very short.

Other Components of Oils. Oils and fats contain components such as lecithin, which helps the body break down fats and oils by emulsifying them or joining them with water. This process helps reduce the amount of cholesterol in the blood, for example. Lecithin is also a skin softener, and vegetable oils such as soybean oil are extremely beneficial for sensitive skin. Other components are essential for maintaining the myelin sheath that covers certain nerves and for building cell membranes.

Natural, unrefined oils contain vitamins, such as A, D, E, and K, necessary for good eyesight, clear skin, strong bones, and blood clotting. They are also good anti-aging compounds, antioxidants, and anti-inflammatories. Unrefined oils also contain compounds that help reduce low-density lipoprotein ("bad" cholesterol) in the blood; various trace minerals such as copper, calcium, and magnesium; and chlorophyll.

Extracting Oils

We have a perception of vegetable oil as being very close to natural—after all, we just need to crush the seed and collect the oil, right? That is the way our ancestors did it, in batch presses that simply applied pressure on the seeds from the top (Figure 9.2). A lot of pressure is required, so oil pressing was a cottage industry, rather than something done in every household. Oil was produced in small amounts and consumed quickly, as it would spoil much more easily than the seed itself.

Industrialization took over the oil-producing market, and presses became larger, oil-bearing crops became big business, and pesticides were introduced. Manufacturers

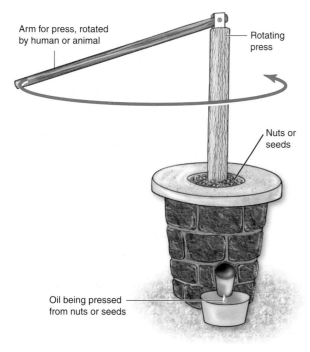

Arm for press, rotated
by human or animal

Rotating press

Nuts or seeds

Oil being pressed
from nuts or seeds

Figure 9.2 An old-fashioned oil press.

suddenly had a problem with spoilage because oil was being produced in much larger quantities, much farther away from the consumer. So they turned to different crops, whose oils have a much longer shelf life (though lower nutritional value) and started to produce **refined oil,** extracting the constituents of vegetable oil that are most likely to cause it to degrade. This process resulted in the pale yellow vegetable oils, with little odor, that fill supermarket shelves today. As Udo Erasmus, one of the world's experts in edible oils, remarks: "Over the years, natural, unrefined oils were replaced by bland, refined oils without taste, and we have come to believe that oil *should* be tasteless. But fresh, natural seed oils have the delicate aromas and flavors of the seeds from which they are pressed."[2]

Industrial Processing of Oils. Seeds or nuts are usually cleaned and then cooked at about 248°F (120°C) to release the oil and make it easier to extract. It is then **expeller-pressed.** A large spiral-shaped auger squeezes the seeds against a metal plate, which has holes in the sides for the oil to run out. Although the pressure and friction are extremely high, leading to temperatures of up to 200°F (95°C), this method is described as **cold-pressed** because no extra heat is applied. At this point the oil may be filtered and sold as crude or unrefined oil. Some oils are routinely extracted using industrial solvents, such as hexane, which are then evaporated off, often leaving solvent traces in the oil.

The refining process consists of many different steps, including **degumming, refining** (in which a kind of soap is produced and skimmed off), **bleaching** to remove pigments, steam distilling to deodorize the oil, and **winterizing** (in which the oil is cooled and any solid particles filtered off). These processes may use toxic chemicals and high temperatures (up to 518°F or 270°C), which damage any EFAs in the oils; remove nutrients such as lecithin, chlorophyll, vitamins, and minerals; and form new and toxic compounds such as peroxides and trans-fats (fat molecules with arrangements of molecules not found in nature). Oils may *still* be sold as cold pressed as long as no external heat was used in the actual pressing stage.

In aromatherapy, a profession that sees itself as a more "natural" alternative, the use of oils refined in this way poses a problem. But using unrefined, crude oils has its own issues. These closer-to-nature products may have quite a strong smell, be highly colored, and have a tendency to go rancid much more quickly. They need to be bought in small amounts, preferably refrigerated, and used quickly. The advantages of the crude oils are their health benefits and their lack of toxic by-products.

Topical Application of Oils

There is a certain amount of controversy about how effectively our body absorbs fixed oils when they are applied to the skin. One study reported that safflower oil did not correct EFA deficiency in surgical patients when applied topically.[3] Another case report on a 19-year-old man receiving fat-free intravenous fluids states that "the EFA deficiency was reversed after 21 days by daily, topical application of linoleic acid to the patient's skin."[4] Clinical studies on animals showed that vitamin E was absorbed from one patch on the skin and found in other skin areas, and in the liver and heart.[5]

According to Erasmus, "the kinds of oil that work best are those that our skin absorbs—oils containing EFAs that it can use for nourishment. To a smaller extent, skin also absorbs monounsaturated oleic acid. Saturated fats are poorly absorbed. Non-natural, artificial mineral oil and petroleum jelly are not absorbed at all, providing only a protective coat."[6] For aromatherapists, who generally want carriers with the best absorption rates for the essential oils they use, vegetable oils high in EFAs, such as hemp and flax, would seem to be ideal—except for their strong odor and short shelf life. However, there are other oils containing moderate amounts of EFAs that do not have these drawbacks, such as almond, rice bran, sunflower, soybean, safflower, and walnut. Mineral oil ("baby oil") and lotions containing mineral oil are not used for aromatherapy at all, because of their lack of absorption. Topically applied EFAs have been shown in clinical trials to improve atopic dermatitis,[7] prevent pressure sores, maintain skin elasticity, and hydrate the skin.[8]

Safety in Topical Application.
A common concern among aromatherapy clients and practitioners is whether fixed oils, particularly the nut oils, can cause allergic reactions in people with sensitivities to those foods when the oils are applied to the skin. Certainly allergic reactions are possible when *any* substance is placed on the skin, and vegetable oils are no exception. One study on 27 people with food allergies stated that the choice of a topical ointment is important because of the possibility of topical sensitivity to the same substances.[9] Another study found that "refined peanut oil-containing dermatologic preparation is safe to use, even in persons who are sensitive to peanuts."[10]

In my experience, I have found people who have reactions to seed or nut products, no matter whether they eat them or apply them topically. As a result, I strongly advise against the use of an oil on the skin of a client who is allergic to the food from which the oil is prepared.

Base Oils

The base oils are listed below in two categories, according to how they are generally used: oils for full-body massage and specialty oils. I have included information about the color and odor of the unrefined oil, as well as how long it is likely to keep in cool, dark conditions. "Very stable" means that it should not go rancid within a year, "fairly stable" means it will last for 6 months to a year, "less stable" means it should keep for up to 6 months, and "unstable" means it should be used as soon as possible, probably within 2 or 3 months.

Oils for Full-Body Massage.   These oils are light to medium in texture, have a low odor, and are reasonably priced. For these reasons they are suitable for use for a full-body massage.

Almond (*Prunus amygdalis*): Pale yellow, light odor, fairly stable, high in oleic acid with some linoleic acid (EFA). It also contains vitamin E. This is a medium-weight oil that absorbs fairly slowly. It is often recommended as soothing for dry or inflamed skin.

Apricot (*Prunus armeniaca*): Medium yellow with quite a strong odor (the refined, odorless oil is more often sold), fairly stable, high in oleic acid with some linoleic acid (EFA). It is a light, easily absorbed oil, often used for delicate skin, such as the neck, face, and around the eyes.[11]

Canola (*Brassica napus*): Pale yellow, light odor, fairly stable, high in oleic acid, with both EFAs (about 30% combined). On the surface this is an ideal oil, but in practice most canola oil is highly processed and often used for inexpensive body products. Organic, cold-pressed, unrefined canola oil is an excellent massage oil, and one study reported its effectiveness in helping to heal damaged, irritated skin.[12]

Coconut (*Cocos nucifera*): Pale yellow, distinct coconut odor, solid at room temperature, very stable, high in saturated fats. What is usually sold in stores is a highly refined coconut oil, white and odorless, or a "fractionated" or "light" liquid coconut oil, which is also very processed. Because of the saturated fats, it does not absorb well beyond the top layers of skin but is very emollient and moisturizing and is a good addition to thick ointments or skin care items. It is used in Indonesia to treat wounds and injuries.[13]

Corn (*Zea mays*): Pale yellow, low odor, fairly stable, high in linoleic acid. Unfortunately, most corn oil is solvent-extracted[14] and very refined, the EFA linoleic acid and its vitamin E content having been processed out. Unrefined corn oil keeps well and absorbs well.

Grapeseed (*Vitis vinifera*): Dark green, medium odor, less stable, high in linoleic acid (EFA). This oil is usually solvent-extracted and highly refined, yielding the familiar colorless, odorless store-bought product. It is frequently used by massage therapists who are uninformed about the processing this oil usually undergoes.

Hazelnut (*Corylus avellana*): Medium yellow, light nutty odor, fairly stable, high in oleic acid. Avoid the refined oil; the unrefined oil is a wonderful, inexpensive massage oil. It is light and absorbs quickly, leaving no greasy residue, but is rich and nourishing for dry skin.

Jojoba (*Simmondsia chinensis*): Golden yellow, light odor, very stable, high in eicosanoic acid. Not actually an oil, but a wax, its chemical structure makes it liquid at room temperature and extremely stable, so it does not oxidize or go rancid, even in very warm temperatures. It has been used by Native Americans for hundreds of years to treat sores, cuts, bruises, and burns. When the use of sperm whale oil was banned in the United States in 1974, jojoba oil was used as a substitute.[15] It is well tolerated by the skin, as it has a similar structure to human sebum, the skin's moisturizer. It is ideal for balancing sebum and can be used for either greasy or dry skin, acne, cold sores, psoriasis, and damaged hair. This is a wonderful oil to keep in a warm massage room, due to its stability.

Peanut (*Arachis hypogaea*): Yellow, strong peanut aroma, fairly stable, high in oleic acid. The unrefined oil absorbs well but has a strong smell, which is probably not desirable in most full-body aromatherapy massages. Be sure to ask clients about allergic reactions before using this oil, as most nut allergies are to peanuts.

Rice bran (*Oryza sativa*): Dark brown color, medium odor, fairly stable, high in oleic acid. The refined oil is most often used in aromatherapy massage, due to the dark color and stronger odor of the unrefined oil. Even refined, it is moisturizing and soothing, and seems to have an anti-inflammatory effect on the skin.

Safflower (*Carthamus tinctorius*): Pale yellow, light odor, less stable, very high in linoleic acid (EFA). The unrefined oil makes a beautifully light, easily absorbed oil that is low in cost. A high-oleic oil is also available, with fewer nutritional benefits but a much longer shelf life.

Sesame (*Sesamum indicum*): Medium yellow, pleasant nutty aroma, very stable, high in linoleic acid (EFA) and oleic acid. According to Erasmus, it "contains natural preservatives (sesamol, sesamin) that stabilize this relatively LA-rich oil, so it keeps longer than expected."[16] It is applied topically in Ayurvedic medicine to treat burns, boils, and ulcers and is used in shirodhara treatments, in which the oil is poured steadily over the forehead for 30 minutes, to calm and balance the mind.[17] It is regarded in India as warming.

Soybean (*Glycine max*): Very pale yellow, low odor, less stable, high in linoleic acid (EFA) and lecithins. This oil is almost always solvent-extracted, and as a result it has little use in topical applications.

Sunflower (*Helianthus annuus*): Deep yellow, nutty odor, less stable, high in linoleic acid (EFA), contains vitamins A and E. The difference between the common refined oil and a good, organic crude oil is startling, in color, odor,

and texture. Sunflower is frequently used to make infused oils (e.g., calendula or St. John's wort). It is a little heavy but makes a fairly inexpensive, good general massage oil, and clinical trials show that "a single application of sunflower seed oil significantly accelerated skin barrier recovery within 1 hour."[18]

Walnut (*Juglans regia*): Golden yellow, light odor, unstable, high in both EFAs. It is difficult to find the unrefined oil, but well worth it, given its smooth, rich texture and exceptional emollient properties. It is extremely nourishing for dry skin, without being heavy or greasy. Because of the high oil content in the nut, it is surprisingly reasonable in price.

Specialty Oils. These are heavier or more expensive oils, used for their particular healing properties on smaller areas of skin, or blended with the oils mentioned in the first section to increase their effects. There are an increasing number of exotic vegetable oils on the market; I have concentrated on those that are quite well known and documented and that are relatively easy to find.

Avocado (*Persea Americana Miller*): Very dark green, strong "green" odor, unstable, high in oleic acid. The refined oil is pale yellow and odorless. The unrefined oil turns brown and goes rancid quickly, and should be bought in small amounts to be used within a few weeks. It is a heavy, exceptionally emollient oil. Kusmirek remarks that "repeated massage applications reveal an increase in hydration of the upper layers of the skin, and an improvement in the skin's elastic properties."[19] I frequently use it in oil blends to prevent stretch marks, and one study remarks on its effectiveness for psoriasis.[20]

Camellia (*Camellia japonica*): Pale yellow, light odor, less stable, high in oleic acid. This is an oil traditionally used in Japan for skin and hair care. It is highly moisturizing and skin repairing, making it a good ingredient in blends for mature or damaged skin.

Calophyllum (*Calophyllum inophyllum*): (Also called foraha or tamanu) Dark green, strong smoky, nutty odor, less stable, high in saturated fats. Calophyllum will turn solid at cooler temperatures. It is traditionally used in the South Sea Islands as an anti-inflammatory and cicatrizant, for serious external problems such as leprosy and severe ulcerations. It is an excellent remedy for scar healing, psoriasis, burns, and shingles. Kusmirek suggests its use for cracks and lesions, painful joints and muscles, and neuralgia.[21]

Cocoa butter (*Cacao theobroma*): Pale yellow, strong, pleasant "chocolate" odor, very stable, high in saturated fats. Although cocoa butter smells and feels wonderful on the skin, it does not absorb well into the body because of its high levels of saturated fats. It has protective and moisture-conserving properties, however, and may be melted (it is solid at room temperature) and mixed with lighter oils to treat dry skin.

Evening primrose (*Oenothera biennis*): Yellow, light odor, unstable, high in linoleic acid (EFA) and gamma-linolenic acid (GLA). Evening primrose has been extensively researched because of its high GLA content. GLA is converted by the body into prostaglandins, hormonelike substances that regulate cellular functions. Evening primrose oil has been extensively studied for the treatment of PMS, menopausal problems, multiple sclerosis, eczema, high blood pressure, arthritis, and much more. (Borage oil has about twice the amount of GLA as evening primrose and is probably beneficial for all the same conditions, but it has a strong, almost fishy odor that makes it difficult to use in topical work.)

Hemp (*Cannabis sativa*): Greenish, pleasant nutty odor, less stable, high in both EFAs. Hemp is a rich, heavy oil, very nurturing for dry skin. It reduces roughness and irritation and is useful for cracked hands and feet.

Kukui (*Aleurites moluccana*): Pale yellow, light odor, less stable, high in both EFAs. This Hawaiian oil is light and easily absorbed—a perfect massage oil, except for the high cost. It is used traditionally in Hawaii for eczema, dry chapped skin, psoriasis, and burns.

Macadamia (*Macadamia tenuifolia*): Colorless, light odor, fairly stable, high in oleic acid. It is extremely light and easily absorbed, but very nourishing and moisturizing to the skin. It is sometimes used in expensive skin care products.

Rose hip seed (*Rosa rubiginosa*): Orangish-red, strong odor, less stable, high in both EFAs. Rose hip seed oil usually is extracted with solvents, but a CO_2 extraction exists, which is preferable. This is an amazing remedy for reducing scars, even keloid (abnormally raised) scar tissue. Its regenerating properties also make it excellent as a skin oil to reduce or avoid wrinkles or stretch marks and to improve skin texture. Its heavy, almost sticky texture makes it suitable for only small areas. It also gives good results when blended with lighter fixed oils.

Shea (*Butyospermum parkii*) (also called karite): Pale yellow, quite strong odor, very stable, high in oleic acid and saturated fats. Shea butter is solid at room temperature and has to be warmed gently to be used on the skin. It is both solvent-extracted and cold-pressed; the latter form is more expensive. In western and central Africa, it is used as an emollient for cracked or damaged skin. It is extremely rich and has a luxurious creamy texture that seems to absorb very well, leaving the skin smooth and soft. It often is used in expensive skin creams.

Wheatgerm (*Triticum sativum*): Orange, pleasant bready smell if fresh, very stable, high in linoleic acid (EFA), and one of the richest sources of vitamin E. It is an extremely emollient oil, with a thick, sticky texture. It is best blended with other carriers. Although aromatherapists often add it to blends to delay rancidity, it does not seem to extend the shelf life significantly.

Lotions

Lotions, creams, and massage **gels** are essentially an emulsion of oil and water. Oil and water, which usually do not mix, are made to combine by the use of another substance that does not allow them to separate again. In commercial products, these substances include stearic acid (a saturated fatty acid from animal fats, coconut, palm oil, etc.), sterols (e.g., cholesterol), and sulfated alcohols, such as sodium lauryl sulfate. These emulsions generally do not feel as greasy on the skin as a plain vegetable oil, and the water content also benefits dry skin, which may lack water in the stratum corneum. Creams and lotions are also the carriers that penetrate the stratum corneum most quickly.

Ingredients of Lotions

Many massage therapists prefer creams, lotions, or gels to oils because clients often request these less "greasy" alternatives and because they leave less residue. However, it is important to read the ingredient lists on massage lotions carefully. Although some may be extremely high in quality, others may have questionable constituents. Remember that all lotions and creams are based on oil, and they are only as good as the oil they contain.

While browsing in a local massage supply store, I came across a range of massage lotions made of a blend of various expeller-pressed vegetable oils, including sunflower, avocado, wheat germ and jojoba, Shea butter, herbal extracts, and vegetable-derived emulsifiers—a nice combination of high-quality ingredients. A different lotion listed mineral oil as the only lipid—not an ideal carrier for essential oils because of its large molecular size, which makes it nonabsorbent. Mineral oil will prevent the skin from losing more moisture, but it is a petroleum product, which I would rather not use on my clients.

Commercial lotions, creams, and gels labeled "unscented" actually often contain what is called a **masking fragrance,** used to disguise any unpleasant odors in the product. Manufacturers can add this and still legally call the product "unscented." However, masking fragrances are not ideal for aromatherapy work because they can be quite strong, clashing with the essential oils. It is better to look for products labeled "fragrance-free."

Other ingredients of lotions are also important because they may irritate the skin or cause other health problems. **Triethanolamine (TEA)** is a common constituent of many massage lotions, body lotions, shaving creams, and shampoos. According to Winter, TEA is "the most frequent sensitizer among the common emulsifiers used in cosmetics" and "in products intended for prolonged contact with the skin, the concentration should not exceed 5 percent and be used only in 'rinse-off' products."[22] Manufacturers do not state the percentages of their ingredients in massage lotions. As well, an amount that might be safe for a client who has a massage once a week may not be safe for a massage therapist who uses the same lotion on up to 30 clients (or more) per week.

Safety of Lotions

There seems to be an increasing incidence of massage therapists developing allergic reactions to the lotions and creams they are using professionally. A person may become sensitized to *any* substance, no matter how pure and natural, if it is used on the skin day after day. It is good practice for massage therapists to regularly change the type and brand of carrier they use with clients, to keep themselves healthy. I use several different carrier oils, which I may or may not mix with each other, as well as two different lotions of varying weight and a hypoallergenic gel.

Making Your Own Lotions

I prefer using vegetable oil as a carrier because it has no extra chemical ingredients, no masking fragrance, no added color, and no known skin irritants or sensitizers—all of which appear frequently in commercial lotions. Vegetable oil is also a completely natural product the human body has been absorbing in various ways for millions of years with few problems. You might like to make your own lotions and creams for use in massage. This will take some experimentation, since everyone has different preferences about weight, absorbency, and "slippage." The following recipes are ones I have used with consistent success. The more unusual ingredients, such as stearic acid, can be easily found in soap-making stores or from online suppliers.

Ointments

Ointments, heavier products than lotions and creams, traditionally are a mixture of oil and some kind of wax. They do not contain water, and this is the main difference between ointments and lotions or creams. Commercial ointments may contain as many chemical ingredients as lotions or creams, and making your own is a good option. The easiest to make are combinations of oil, beeswax, and/or cocoa butter (or

---

Recipe 1

1 cup distilled or filtered water

2 cups light oil, such as apricot kernel or rice bran oil

4 tablespoons beeswax

$\frac{1}{2}$ teaspoon borax powder

Dissolve the borax in the water. Separately heat the oil and beeswax in a double boiler (or in a heat-resistant bowl over a saucepan of water) until the wax has melted. Heat the water mixture until it is almost boiling and slowly stir it into the oil mixture. Either beat well or mix it in a blender briefly. Pour into jars. This lotion thickens as it cools.

Recipe 2

1 cup light oil, such as apricot or rice bran

1 cup stearic acid powder (available from craft stores or soap-making stores)

2 teaspoons baking soda

8 tablespoons glycerin

4 cups distilled or filtered water

Combine the oil and stearic acid, and heat until it is a clear liquid. Separately, combine the baking soda, glycerin, and distilled water, and heat until the mixture begins to boil. Slowly add the water mixture to the oil mixture. It will foam up as CO_2 is released. Blend on high for 1 or 2 minutes. Pour into jars.

---

any other vegetable fat that is solid at room temperature, such as Shea butter). It can be fun to play around with these ingredients; they can be combined to make something solid, like a lip balm, or much softer products.

Because the constituents do not absorb well, or absorb only slowly, ointments are used in aromatherapy to nourish the skin or as a vehicle for the slow release of essential oils. The first use is appropriate in pregnancy massage, for example, when a heavier, richer product may be desirable to help prevent stretch marks. The second use may be appropriate for a stiff, painful, arthritic knee, in which anti-inflammatory and analgesic essential oils may provide the most relief if they are absorbed over a longer period of time.

SUMMARY

- A carrier is a substance used to dilute essential oils. The term usually refers to oils and lotions used in aromatherapy massage.

- Factors to consider when choosing which carrier to use are the type of bodywork, the preferences or needs of the massage therapist or client, the skin type of the client, the condition being treated, the size of the area of skin being treated, and the smell of the carrier.

- Emulsions (lotions and creams) absorb the fastest, followed by solutions such as essential oils in vegetable oils or alcohol, then gels, and then ointments. Varying absorption rates will be appropriate for different treatments.

- Vegetable oils (also called fixed oils) may be saturated (usually solid at room temperature) or unsaturated (usually liquid at room temperature). Saturated fats are more stable and turn rancid less easily. The shelf life of vegetable oils ranges from only a few months to about a year or possibly longer, depending on their chemical structure.

- Cold-pressed, unrefined vegetable oils have more healing properties and fewer toxic by-products, but also a shorter shelf life and possibly a stronger odor.

- It is best to avoid using a vegetable oil on the skin with clients who are allergic to the food from which the oil is extracted. (Peanut allergies are common.)

- Vegetable oils vary from light and easily absorbed, suitable for full-body massage, to rich and heavy, for use on smaller areas or mixed with lighter oils. They have many different healing properties.

- Lotions, creams, and gels are based on oils. Ingredients that include high-quality vegetable oils (not mineral oil or petroleum products) are recommended, and they can be made at home.

- The lotions or gels used in massage should be rotated to avoid sensitization from prolonged regular use of one particular product.

- Heavier ointments are a mixture of oil and wax. They do not absorb well but are useful for skin treatments or for the slow release of essential oils.

Review Questions

1. Rich and heavy carrier oils are more suitable for full-body massage. (T/F)
2. Put the following carriers into order, from fastest to slowest, according to their absorption rates: (a) gels, (b) creams or lotions, (c) wax–based ointments, (d) vegetable oils.
3. Creams and lotions are based on _____ and _____.
4. Fats and oils are both known as _____, and are most often found in the _____ of plants.
5. _____ fats are usually solid at room temperature, and _____ fats are usually liquid at room temperature.
6. Oils that are high in essential fatty acids (EFAs) tend to turn rancid more easily and should be kept in dark bottles in the refrigerator. (T/F)
7. Almond, safflower, and rice bran oils would all be good choices for full-body massage, since they are light and easily absorbed. (T/F)
8. Clients may experience allergic reactions to vegetable oils if they have food allergies to that nut or seed in the oil. (T/F)
9. What is an emulsion?
10. Two excellent carriers to treat scar tissue are _____ and _____.
11. What steps can a massage therapist take to avoid developing an allergy to his or her massage lotion?
12. Commercial lotions always contain oils that are suitable for aromatherapy work. (T/F)
13. Ointments are basically a mixture of _____ and _____.
14. Given their slow absorption rate, what type of treatment or bodywork would ointments be good for?
15. What is the advantage of making your own lotions or creams?

Notes

1. Essential Oil Resource Consultants. Advanced Clinical Aromatherapy Part 1, Course notes.
2. Erasmus U. Fats That Heal, Fats That Kill. Burnaby, Canada: Alive Books, 1993:87.
3. O'Neill JA, Caldwell MD, Meng HC. Essential fatty acid deficiency in surgical patients. Ann Surg 1977;185(5):535–542.
4. Skolnik P, Eaglstein WH, Ziboh VA. Human essential fatty acid deficiency: treatment by topical application of linoleic acid. Arch Dermatol 1977;113(7):939–941.

5. Trevithick JR, Mitton KP. Uptake of vitamin E succinate by the skin, conversion to free vitamin E, and transport to internal organs. Biochem Mol Biol Int 1999;47(3):509–518.

6. Erasmus U. Fats That Heal, Fats That Kill. Burnaby, Canada: Alive Books, 1993:294.

7. Mayser P, Mayer K, Mahloudjian M, et al. A double-blind, randomized, placebo-controlled trial of n-3 versus n-6 fatty acid-based lipid infusion in atopic dermatitis. J Parenteral Enteral Nutr 2002;26(3):151–158.

8. Declair V. The usefulness of topical application of essential fatty acids (EFAs) to prevent pressure ulcers. Ostomy/Wound Manage 1997;43(5):48–52.

9. Guillet G, Guillet MH. Percutaneous sensitization to almond oil in infancy and study of ointments in 27 children with food allergy. Allergie et Immunologie (Paris) 2000;32(8):309–311.

10. Yunginger JW, Calobrisi SD. Investigation of the allergenicity of a refined peanut oil-containing dermatologic agent in persons who are sensitive to peanuts. Cutis 2001;68(2):153–155.

11. Kusmirek J. Liquid Sunshine, Vegetable Oils for Aromatherapy. Somerset, England: Floramicus, 2002:92–93.

12. Loden M, Andersson AC. Effect of topically applied lipids on surfactant-irritated skin. Br J Dermatol 1996;134(2):215–220.

13. Sachs M, Eichel J von, Asskali F. Wound treatment with coconut oil in Indonesian natives. Der Chirurg 2002;73(4):387–392.

14. Erasmus U. Fats That Heal, Fats That Kill. Burnaby, Canada: Alive Books, 1993:239.

15. Sims J. Jojoba oil. Gale Encyclopedia of Alternative Medicine. Available at: www.findarticles.com. Accessed May 1, 2005.

16. Erasmus U. Fats That Heal, Fats That Kill. Burnaby, Canada: Alive Books, 1993:245.

17. Irani F. The Magic of Ayurveda Aromatherapy. West Pennant Hills, Australia: Subtle Energies, 2001:83–85.

18. Darmstadt GL, Mao-Qiang M, Chi E, et al. Impact of topical oils on the skin barrier: possible implications for neonatal health in developing countries. Acta Paediatrica 2002;91(5):546–545.

19. Kusmirek J. Liquid Sunshine, Vegetable Oils for Aromatherapy. Somerset, England: Floramicus, 2002:98.

20. Stucker M, Memmel U. Vitamin B(12) cream containing avocado oil in the therapy of plaque psoriasis. Dermatology 2001;203(2):141–147.

21. Kusmirek J. Liquid Sunshine, Vegetable Oils for Aromatherapy. Somerset, England: Floramicus, 2002:166–167.

22. Winter R. A Consumer's Dictionary of Cosmetic Ingredients. New York: Three Rivers Press, 1999:442.

10

Essential Oil Safety

There is a huge amount of debate in aromatherapy circles about the possible hazards of essential oils and how to use them safely. Opinions range widely. Some therapists state that essential oils are on the whole very safe, especially when compared with conventional medical drugs, also known as **allopathic medications.** Others point out that little scientific testing has been done to determine the specific effects of essential oils. Both of these viewpoints have merit. It is true that some aromatic extracts have a long history of use, generally by untrained members of the public, with relatively few recorded side effects of any seriousness. It is also true that aromatherapy in its present form is not very old—dating back to the 1930s at the earliest—and that we now use many aromatic plants that have no traditional history of use, at least in the very concentrated form of essential oils that we now regularly employ.

The Importance of Studying Essential Oil Safety

As we saw in Chapter 4, essential oils can have marked pharmacological and psychological effects, and any substance that affects the body chemically is bound to have unwelcome effects in certain situations, or with certain people. It would be misleading and therefore irresponsible to try to claim that essential oils are both powerful in their beneficial effects and totally harmless otherwise. In most countries, however, essential oils are easily bought over the counter without any restrictions on their use and are often purchased by the general public, with no particular training or instruction. Given this freedom of use, their safety record up to now has actually been very good, and the majority of serious ill effects have been caused by the accidental ingestion of essential oils by children and, occasionally, adults. However, because the use of essential oils in the home has risen exponentially in the past few years, as a result of the increasing popularity of aromatherapy, this type of accident has become more common. Essential oils have the potential to be of great help, but as with many other substances we use daily, such as coffee or aspirin, they can also be abused, either accidentally or through ignorance.

The need for greater public awareness of the possible effects of essential oils is clearly shown in an article from 1999 that reports on two people who developed facial dermatitis after putting essential oil of lavender on their pillows to help with insomnia. Even though one of the people involved knew that she was sensitive to perfume products, "in both cases, the patients had not considered that a natural product such as lavender essential oil could be responsible for acute allergy."[1] Obviously, education on how to utilize essential oils in a safe manner is necessary—both for the aromatherapy supplier or therapist and for the purchaser. These highly concentrated substances are used for therapeutic and even medicinal purposes; thus, as with any remedies or treatments, safety must be considered.

Individual Reactions to Essential Oils

Individual reactions to essential oils, both positive and negative, are extremely unpredictable and vary greatly. One study on childhood poisoning with eucalyptus essential oil in Australia reported that 80% of the children involved were entirely asymptomatic, even though one child had ingested around 45 mL of essential oil, while other children who had swallowed much less had serious symptoms. The authors stated that "there was no correlation between the amount of oil ingested and the presence or severity of symptoms."[2]

These differences in reaction to a substance are not restricted to essential oil use. For example, one of my clients takes a prescribed one quarter of the usual dose of an allopathic drug because her doctor recognized that the usual dose is actually an overdose for her. By contrast, a friend has to have at least three times the average amount of local anesthetic for dental work, as any less is completely ineffective. This range of tolerance for drugs, herbs, essential oils, and any other therapeutic substance is quite normal, but makes it difficult to predict with any accuracy what dosage will be both safe and effective from one person to the next. The herbalist Mills remarks: "Even after taking all such predictable variables into account it is likely that most individuals may vary by as much as 50 per cent from expected levels in their reactions to any remedy, and that about 5 per cent of the population may react dramatically differently."[3]

Scientific Testing and Medical Case Histories

Scientific testing can establish how much of a particular substance can be used without the risk of **toxicity** (poisoning) or other harmful effects. However, since humans are not often willing to be test subjects, many of these experiments are performed on animals. Leaving aside the question of whether animal testing is ethical, these studies present other problems. The toxicity of essential oils and other substances is most often tested by oral ingestion or intraperitoneal injection, not topical application, which is the most common method of use in aromatherapy massage. The amounts involved usually are much larger than would be used in any form of holistic aromatherapy treatment, and they give us little idea whether these substances would be dangerous if applied topically or inhaled. When the tests involve topical applications, they become much more relevant to aromatherapy massage work, but again, human skin is very different from animal skin, which is generally much more sensitive, and comparisons are still difficult (though by no means impossible) to make.

More useful are the case histories written by doctors and nurses of accidental and deliberate overdosing, by ingestion, topical application, or inhalation. These cases provide a clearer picture of what effects a precise amount of essential oil can have. The most serious problems in essential oil use occur because of:

- Accidental or deliberate ingestion.
- Topical application of huge or inappropriate amounts of essential oils.
- Repeated use of *undiluted* essential oils.
- Repeated use over time of the same essential oil, whether used topically or inhaled.

Factors That Affect Safety

Medical case histories, scientific testing, observations by practitioners using essential oils, and medical knowledge of skin sensitivity and allergic reactions provide a basis on which massage therapists can formulate some guidelines for the safe practice of aromatherapy. The primary variables to consider are:

1. The method of application.
2. How much of the essential oil is used overall in the treatment.
3. The person being treated.
4. The potential toxicity of the essential oil used and any drug interactions.
5. The purity and freshness of the essential oil.

Methods of Application

There are various ways to treat the body using essential oils. Internal use, including ingestion, suppositories, and pessaries, is outside the scope of practice of massage practitioners in most countries. The three aromatherapy modalities most often used in massage work are topical application, some form of hydrotherapy, and occasionally inhalation.

The route of absorption is very important when assessing toxicity. Some essential oils may have undesired effects by one route and be perfectly safe by another. A good example is pennyroyal (*Mentha pulegium*), which is now almost unused in aromatherapy because of its safety record. According to Tisserand and Balacs, it has high oral toxicity, and they recommend that it not be used at all in aromatherapy, either internally or externally.[4] However, it is an excellent and harmless remedy for respiratory infections when inhaled—the safest method of application.

Topical Application

Topical application of an essential oil is usually an integral part of the massage. The essential oil is typically dissolved in the massage oil or lotion, which is then used to lubricate the skin. As we read in Chapter 4, many factors influence the absorption of essential oils, including the age and quality of the skin, whether skin is occluded, and skin temperature and hydration. Massage therapists must bear in mind that absorption may be faster and more effective in certain situations and adjust the dosage accordingly. A percentage dilution may need to be slightly lower if a client had just taken a sauna and was having an aromatherapy massage prior to having a spa wrap—both the heat from the sauna and the occlusion from the spa wrap would encourage greater absorption.

It is possible to poison someone with topical application, although the dose would have to be extraordinarily high. An extreme example of topical use is the case of a 6-year-old girl whose parents treated her for itching hives with a topical blend of vinegar, olive oil, methylated spirits, and eucalyptus essential oil. A dose of 25 mL of the essential oil was applied every 2–4 hours under occlusion, and when this did not resolve the problem, the dose was doubled. The child eventually lost consciousness. Fortunately, she improved rapidly within 6 hours after removing the wrap and was discharged from the hospital.[5] The fact that this young child did not present long-term symptoms after this huge dose seems to show that on the whole, topical application is remarkably safe.

Irritation and Sensitization. The most common hazard associated with topical use of aromatic extracts is the possibility of skin irritation or sensitization. It is important to understand the distinction between them; the latter is much more serious. **Skin irritation,** a straightforward problem, results when a strong chemical substance causes redness, rash, and occasionally skin damage. The reaction is almost immediate, but subsides quickly once the irritant is removed.

Skin sensitization is an allergic response. A reaction might not occur the first time an allergenic substance is used, but subsequent exposure causes inflammation, an immune system response, and even tiny amounts of the allergenic substance can produce a significant reaction. If an essential oil is suspected of causing an allergic reaction, this substance should *never* be used on the client again. Other essential oils in the same genus, or with a similar chemistry, should be used cautiously or avoided, as studies show that there may be cross-sensitization in such cases.[6]

Skin Irritants. Any volatile oil may be irritating to the body, depending on how it is used. *Essential oils should never be used in or near the eyes.* Therapists must be very careful when applying oils to mucous membranes or to delicate skin, such as the axillary region.

Several essential oils have been identified as usually irritating to the skin—that is, they tend to consistently cause irritation in many people, if used in a strong enough concentration or on delicate areas of skin. The aromatherapy industry does not have the resources to monitor these kinds of reactions worldwide, but the fragrance organizations, such

Table 10.1	Skin Irritants
Essential Oil	**Botanical Name**
Cade*	*Juniperus oxycedrus*
Cassia	*Cinnamomum cassia*
Cinnamon bark and leaf	*Cinnamomum zeylanicum*
Clove bud, leaf, and stem	*Syzygium aromaticum*
Fennel	*Foeniculum vulgare*
Fig leaf absolute*	*Ficus carica*
Oregano*	*Origanum vulgare*
Parsley seed and leaf	*Petroselinum sativum*
Savory, summer	*Satureia hortensis*
Savory, winter	*Satureia montana*
Terebinth*	*Pinus palustris*
Thyme	*Thymus vulgaris CT thymol*
Verbena	*Lippia citriodora*

*Strong irritant

Table 10.2	Skin Sensitizers
Essential Oil	**Botanical Name**
Benzoin	*Styrax benzoin*
Cassia	*Cinnamomum cassia*
Cinnamon bark	*Cinnamomum zeylanicum*
Costus	*Saussurea costus*
Elecampane	*Inula helenium*
Fig leaf absolute	*Ficus carica*
Oakmoss absolute	*Evernia prunastri*
Tea absolute	*Camellia sinensis*
Treemoss	*Evernia furfuracea*
Verbena essential oil and absolute	*Lippia citriodora*

as the International Fragrance Research Association (IFRA) and the Research Institute for Fragrance Materials (RIFM), gather information on adverse reactions from member companies and scientific studies and commission research on fragrance raw materials.[7]

Essential oils that are occasionally sold by aromatherapy suppliers but are generally regarded as skin irritating are listed in Table 10.1. These oils can be irritating when used neat or in strong dilutions, but many can be used topically in lower concentrations. There are other essential oils, such as horseradish, mustard, onion, and garlic, that are never used in holistic aromatherapy because they are extremely strong skin irritants, but they can be found in food flavorings in tiny amounts.

Essential oils that are high in monoterpenes, such as the citrus oils or the needle oils (spruce, fir, pine, etc.), have been shown to be skin irritating when oxidized. It is important that these oils are fresh when used in skin applications. One study stated: "In animal models, *d*-limonene of high purity gave no significant allergic reaction, but limonene exposed to the air for two months sensitized the animals."[8] (Limonene is the main chemical component in all expressed oils from citrus rinds.)

Skin Sensitizers. It is difficult to make a list of essential oils that cause allergic skin reactions because almost any substance may have this effect on someone, somewhere. However, some essential oils and absolutes seem to be more consistently sensitizing than others (Table 10.2). Most people will not have allergic reactions even to the oils considered strongly sensitizing, or they may develop a sensitivity after a period of time. Practitioners using aromatherapy must be careful with clients who have already noticed allergic reactions to other substances. Aromatherapists should also be very careful about using essential oils that are new to the field and have not yet undergone any testing for irritation and sensitization; they are essentially using their clients as test subjects.

Undiluted Essential Oils. The use of undiluted essential oils on the skin is discouraged, except for acute care (first aid), which involves short-term use, on small areas of skin, in otherwise healthy adults. Typical situations in which neat, or undiluted, essential oils are appropriate are, for example, a very recent sprain, bug bites, and minor burns. The repeated use of an undiluted essential oil seems to increase the likelihood of an allergic response, as in the case of applying neat essential oil to acne or athlete's foot for several weeks or longer. Several case studies demonstrate the development of an allergy to tea tree (*Melaleuca alternifolia*) from repeated use over a long period of time of the neat essential oil.[9]

Undiluted oils can also be dangerous when used on mucous membranes or more sensitive areas, such as the face or axillary region. One case was reported of a woman who spilled neat clove oil (*Syzygium aromaticum*) onto her face while trying to relieve a toothache. Eleven months later she had a patch of dry, irritated skin from just below the eye to the upper lip, and sensation within this area was reduced to that of deep pressure only.[10]

Skin Quality. The integrity of the skin is also important to consider. Skin acts as both a physical and chemical barrier to many toxins and slows down the absorption of other substances into the bloodstream. If the skin is broken or abraded, the rate and level of absorption become unpredictable and may, in fact, be very high. Also, some essential oils, even those generally considered mild, may have adverse effects on damaged skin.

In one study, the authors mentioned the **cytotoxicity** (possible harmful effect on cells of the body) of tea tree essential oil (*Melaleuca alternifolia*) and stated that it "could decrease healing and increase scarring," and as a result they recommend against its use for the treatment of burns.[11] Another study on tea tree oil noted that seven patients who had been applying the undiluted essential oil over a period of 3 years for fungal infections, pimples, and rashes developed allergic dermatitis. The authors commented that "the application of diluted oil to healthy skin may cause no sensitivity reaction."[12] For this reason, essential oils should not be used undiluted, or for long periods of time, on skin that has been broken or has lost its integrity.

Repeated Use of Essential Oils. There are many medical case histories showing that the repeated use of the same essential oils tends to result in the development of an allergic response to those substances. This occurs most often in therapists who apply the oils to their clients' skin with their hands. It is a strong reminder to massage therapists using aromatherapy that they need to be careful—not only for their clients but also, more urgently, for themselves. One case study reports that a holistic beauty therapist who had worked for 12 years giving aromatherapy massages and facials tested positive for allergies to lemongrass, Cananga, rose, ylang ylang, clary sage, and patchouli essential oils and lavender absolute.[13] These oils are listed by Tisserand and Balacs as posing only a slight risk of allergic reaction, or they "almost certainly will not cause skin sensitization."[14] The authors of the report also noted that the therapist was sensitive to her own blended foot and facial lotions.

Anyone using the same single essential oil or blend for a long time runs a greatly increased risk. A study in Japan between 1990 and 1998 demonstrated a sudden increase in allergies to lavender essential oil from 1997. The writers concluded that "the incidence of lavender oil allergy had risen in Japan due to increased exposure to lavender flowers and essential oil."[15] The authors of a case study of contact dermatitis in a young girl who had used a children's perfume observed that "commercial fragrance products aimed at the child and teenage markets are already commonplace. The prevalence of fragrance intolerance among the young population is subsequently increasing."[16]

The message is clear: We need to be careful that we use all types of aromatic oils wisely, and avoid overusing them either for pleasure or for therapeutic work. The practice of changing the topical blends clients use at regular intervals is a good idea. This is particularly advisable for take-home blends, which may be used up to two to three times a day on the skin. I generally change the essential oils in these blends about every 4 to 6 weeks, if a client is treating something intensively.

Hydrotherapy

Although hydrotherapy as an aromatherapy modality in massage mainly involves hand baths and foot baths of varying temperatures, some of the information here also applies to compresses and heating pads. Evidence shows that heat increases the irritating or damaging effects of certain essential oils. The essential oils listed in Tables 10.1 and 10.2 as skin irritants or skin sensitizers should be avoided or used in small amounts when applied with heat. One case study also states that substances high in menthol, such as peppermint essential oil (*Mentha piperita*), or methyl salicylate, such as wintergreen, (*Gaultheria procumbens*) or sweet birch (*Betula lenta*), may have a damaging effect on skin and underlying tissue if used topically with heat.[17]

Baths of any kind are actually topical applications because the essential oils in the water touch the skin directly. Many people simply add several drops of essential oil to the water to create an aromatic bath. In effect, this is an undiluted application, since essential oils and water do not mix and the oils will float on top of the water, coming directly in contact with the skin. As mentioned above, heat increases the irritating effects of the oils, and neat application tends to encourage both skin irritation and allergic reaction. For both of these reasons, it is advisable to dilute the essential oils before they are added to the bath water, in small amounts of liquid soap, honey, full-fat milk, or a commercial emulsifier. Valnet, who frequently mentions the benefits of aromatic baths, writes of using "various mixtures of whole natural essences *in emulsion form* for use in ordinary bathing and washing."[18] Most people will find that they can easily tolerate undiluted essential oils in a foot bath, but it is definitely safer to dissolve them beforehand.

Guba states that higher amounts of essential oils can be safely used in baths when they are emulsified; 10–60 drops (about 25 mg per drop) can be used without causing skin irritation.[19] This amount probably refers to a full bath, and drop amounts for the hand baths and foot baths used in a massage practice would be much smaller, even for treatment work. Of course, any discussion of a safe or appropriate amount of essential oils in a bath must depend on the specific essential oils used.

Inhalation

Inhalation of essential oils is generally regarded as the safest route of absorption. Problems associated with inhaling tend to be fewer and less severe than with topical application. Burfield, an aromatherapy educator who often writes on safety issues, estimates that the actual doses inhaled from a room nebulizer would be extremely small,[20] and most cases of acute effects from inhalation are in industrial accidents involving extraordinarily large amounts of aromatics. Milder side effects, such as headache and nausea, almost always disappear quickly once the offending aroma has been removed.

With steam inhalation it is important to protect the eyes by avoiding the use of essential oils high in phenols or aldehydes, such as thyme CT thymol (*Thymus vulgaris* CT thymol) or lemongrass (*Cymbopogon citratus*), which can irritate the eyes. Some aromatherapists advise not using steam inhalation with clients who have asthma, for fear of provoking an asthmatic attack. People seem to have a range of different reactions; I have encountered asthma sufferers whose doctors recommended steam inhalations to help with symptoms, while I know other people with asthma who cannot even go into a steam room without having a severe reaction.

More disturbing are reports of allergic reaction involving inhalation. One case study involved a 53-year-old man who developed persistent eczema on his scalp, neck, and hands and was found to have sensitization to lavender, jasmine, rosewood, laurel, eucalyptus, and pomerance oils. The authors noted that "due to the persistence of the volatile essential oils in the patient's home after a year-long use of aroma lamps, complete renewal of the interior of the flat was considered vital."[21] There are other case studies of allergic airborne contact dermatitis, with less exposure, but obviously the greatest risk in this situation is to aromatherapists since inhalation exposure is always greater for them than for a client. It is extremely important to air out the massage room between clients and to launder sheets and pillow cases thoroughly to minimize risks to the therapist.

I have encountered several people who experienced mild allergic symptoms (slight sinus congestion, wheezing, itchy or inflamed eyes) for a short time after simply smelling a particular essential oil from the bottle. One student remembered a childhood allergic reaction to scented geranium plants after having the same response to the essential oil. Some people may have a sensitivity only to the aroma and may be able to use the essential oil topically with no apparent symptoms, and vice versa. I have also seen people who have become so sensitized to an essential oil because of frequent undiluted topical use that even inhaling the oil from a bottle produces an allergic response. As with sensitization to topical applications, individuals should always avoid essential oils that cause an inhalation allergic reaction.

The Client

So far we have been discussing safety aspects that relate to adults with no chronic health problems or other special needs, but there are several groups of clients who require particular care. These include children, the elderly, people with especially sensitive skin or skin problems, pregnant women, people with epilepsy, and those with high blood pressure.

Children, the Elderly, and Clients With Sensitive Skin

Children younger than age 7 or 8 have thinner skin than adults and therefore have a higher absorption rate for essential oils. Combined with their smaller body weight and size, this means that the doses of essential oil they receive should be proportionately smaller, as we saw in Chapter 8. Also, the skin of infants and children is much more sensitive, becoming gradually more tolerant as they grow older, so essential oils used topically with the youngest children need to be the mildest possible on the skin. It is probably advisable not to use essential oils at all on premature or newborn babies, unless the benefits outweigh the risks, and the use of hydrosols would certainly be preferable here if treatment is needed.

The same guidelines apply to older people, whose skin becomes gradually thinner as they age, and for people who have naturally sensitive skin that tends to be irritated easily by detergents or cosmetics. Clients with nonallergic dermatitis, psoriasis, and other skin problems tend to do better with milder oils in lower concentrations. Some of the essential oils that are easily tolerated topically by clients with sensitive skin are listed in Table 10.3.

Particularly relevant to young children are case studies that demonstrate the dangers of certain essential oil constituents, such as a case of acute poisoning of an infant by the topical application of oils containing camphor, menthol, and thymol.[22] Another study examined the effects of the inhalation of menthol fumes by premature infants, which caused a rise in heart rate and a drop in respiratory rate.[23] Essential oils such as peppermint (*Mentha piperita*), thyme (*Thymus vulgaris* CT thymol), camphor (*Cinnamomum camphora*), sage (*Salvia officinalis*), and *Lavandula stoechas*, which have medium or high amounts of these chemicals, should be avoided completely with young children (younger than age 8).

Table 10.3	Mild Essential Oils for Sensitive Skin
Essential Oil	**Botanical Name**
Cardamon	*Elettaria cardamomum*
Chamomile, German	*Matricaria recutita*
Chamomile, Roman	*Chamaemelum nobile*
Clary sage	*Salvia sclarea*
Geranium	*Pelargonium graveolens*
Lavender	*Lavandula angustifolia*
Neroli	*Citrus aurantium* var. *amara*
Palmarosa	*Cymbopogon martinii*
Rose	*Rosa damascena* or *R. centifolia*
Rosewood	*Aniba roseadora*

Pregnant Women

There are many case studies of women who have attempted—usually unsuccessfully—to abort a fetus by ingesting large amounts of essential oils. The most commonly used oil is pennyroyal (*Mentha pulegium*). However, there is not a single reported case of any problem, including miscarriage, being caused by the topical use or inhalation of any essential oil during pregnancy.

The term **emmenagogue**, a substance that stimulates menstrual discharge, is often misinterpreted to mean **abortifacient**, a substance that causes miscarriage. As a result, many mild and harmless essential oils, such as rose (*Rosa damascena*) and lavender (*Lavandula angustifolia*), have been contraindicated for pregnancy in some aromatherapy books. There are other safe essential oils, such as juniper (*Juniperus communis*) and Virginian cedar (*Juniperus virginiana*), that have been contraindicated, presumably because they were in the same genus as the more hazardous savin oil (*Juniperus sabina*). Also, some essential oils have been shown in studies to be harmful when taken internally during pregnancy, but they are perfectly safe when used topically or inhaled.

There is also no evidence indicating that most women have increased skin sensitivity during pregnancy and therefore need milder dilutions. I sometimes use smaller amounts both topically and inhaled for pregnant clients, but only because a woman's sense of smell seems to be particularly acute during pregnancy, not because of any safety concerns.

In addition to the obviously toxic oils such as mustard or rue, a few essential oils should be avoided because animal tests have shown them to have some effects that are abortifacient and **fetotoxic**, or harmful to the fetus; in addition, toxicity is suspected due to their chemistry.[24] These oils are high in apiol, sabinyl acetate, camphor, and pinocamphone and are listed in Table 10.4.

Epilepsy

Several commonly used essential oils, including rosemary (*Rosmarinus officinalis*), are routinely contraindicated for use in treating people with epilepsy. However, Tisserand and Balacs remark that "in the only recorded cases where seizures have been induced by essential oils, most of them apparently in non-epileptics, the oils were taken orally."[25] Used externally and in inhalation, essential oils appear to be perfectly safe for people with epilepsy, unless they have an oversensitivity to odor stimuli. In fact, one study suggests that strong aromas may even suppress seizures and recommends the use of olfactory stimulation in anticonvulsant therapy.[26]

High Blood Pressure

Several fairly common oils, such as rosemary, are routinely contraindicated for use with clients who have hypertension,

Table 10.4	Essential Oils to be Avoided During Pregnancy*	
Essential Oil	**Botanical Name**
Camphor or Ho leaf	*Cinnamomum camphora*
Cotton lavender	*Santolina chamaecyparissus*
Hyssop	*Hyssopus officinalis*
Indian dill	*Anethum sowa* *Lavandula stoechas*
Oakmoss absolute	*Evernia prunastri*
Parsley leaf and seed	*Petroselinum sativum*
Perilla	*Perilla frutescens*
Rue	*Ruta graveolens*
Spanish sage	*Salvia lavandulifolia*
Savin	*Juniperus sabina*
Treemoss absolute	*Evernia furfuraceae*

*List is not complete because of space limitations. Any essential oils not mentioned in this book should be checked for safety or avoided.

with no evidence established against them. Tisserand and Balacs conclude that "there is no need for contraindication of essential oils in either hypertension or hypotension in any route of administration."[27]

Potential Toxicity

Aside from the essential oils that should be avoided with particular groups of clients, several other essential oils probably should not be used in aromatherapy at all or should be used with great care, as a result of their proven or suspected toxicity (Table 10.5). Table 10.5 does not include oils that are safe topically but toxic internally

Table 10.5	Essential Oils With Potential Toxicity	
Essential Oil	**Botanical Name**
Artemesia arborescens	
Camphor, brown and yellow	*Cinnamomum camphora*
Ho leaf	*Cinnamomum camphora*
Lanyana	*Artemisia afra*
Melaleuca bracteata	
Sassafras	*Sassafras albidum*
Savin	*Juniperus sabina*
Tansy	*Tanacetum vulgare*
Tarragon	*Artemisia dracunculus*
Thuja	*Thuja occidentalis*

because internal use is outside the massage therapist's scope of practice. For reasons of space, the table includes only essential oils or absolutes that are in common use in aromatherapy and can be easily obtained from an aromatherapy supplier. *If an essential oil is not included, it does not mean that it is safe for use, and its toxicity should be researched.* Most of the oils listed in Table 10.5 are high in chemicals such as thujone, methyl eugenol, safrole, camphor, estragole, or other constituents that have been shown in studies to be **carcinogenic** (cancer-causing), neurotoxic, or hepatotoxic or that are **systemic toxins** (substances that are harmful to the whole body).

Photosensitization

The oils listed in Table 10.6 have been shown, both by reported cases and studies, to be **photosensitizing**, or **phototoxic**. This means that they increase the potential of the skin to burn in ultraviolet (UV) light and should not be used for at least 12 hours before sunbathing, using a tanning bed, or simply spending more than a short amount of time in direct sunlight.

Essential Oil and Drug Interactions

There are few known interactions between topically applied or inhaled essential oils and medically prescribed drugs. Most contraindications are for oral ingestion of essential oils with prescription drugs. However, one clear contraindication is the use of wintergreen (*Gaultheria procumbens*) or sweet birch (*Betula lenta*) with a client who is taking an anticoagulant medication. Case studies report hemorrhaging in patients who have used large topical applications of commercial methyl salicylate (found in sweet birch and wintergreen at about 97% concentration) while taking warfarin, a prescription anticoagulant.[28]

Table 10.6	Photosensitizing Essential Oils
Essential Oil	**Botanical Name**
Angelica root*	*Angelica archangelica*
Bergamot*	*Citrus x bergamia*
Bitter orange	*Citrus aurantium* var. *amara*
Grapefruit	*Citrus x paradisii*
Lemon	*Citrus limon*
Lime*	*Citrus aurantifolia*
Mandarin petitgrain	*Citrus reticulata*
Rue*	*Ruta graveolens*
Tagetes*	*Tagetes minuta*
Verbena essential oil and absolute	*Lippia citriodora*

*Strong sensitizer

Chemotypes

As we saw in Chapter 5, some essential oils have various chemotypes. Every chemotype has different chemical constituents and therefore possibly different contraindications. One of the most important oils from the point of view of safety is thyme (*Thymus vulgaris*), which has several chemotypes commonly used in aromatherapy: thymol, linalool, and carvacrol. Other chemotypes are also sold by suppliers, such as geraniol and thujanol, so it is important to ask your supplier which one is being offered, if this information is not already provided. The thymol chemotype is the one most traditionally used in aromatherapy and the most skin irritating, because of its relatively high phenol content (32–63%). The carvacrol chemotype is also supposed to be irritating because it is also high in phenols. The linalool, geraniol, and thujanol chemotypes, on the other hand, are extremely mild on the skin and mucous membranes, as they have mainly an alcohol–ester combination, with none of the contraindications of the phenol chemotypes. However, thyme essential oil is often contraindicated in aromatherapy books, without regard as to which chemotype is used.

Purity and Freshness

Essential oils are not always what they pretend to be, in either the fragrance world or the aromatherapy world. One study on sensitization from volatile oils states that the "concentration of essential oils used in patch tests appeared to be of minor importance, provided that they were pure" and concludes that "good quality and lack of aging" seemed to be the most important factors in avoiding skin sensitization.[29] The purity of essential oils often is in question.

In another case report, a middle-aged man developed dermatitis and photosensitivity of the face after using a new aftershave containing sandalwood oil. The "sandalwood" was found to be composed of synthetic geranium, geranium bourbon, synthetic and natural sandalwood oil, cedarwood oil, and patchouli oil, and the client in fact tested positive for the synthetic and natural geranium, not for the sandalwood.[30]

Managing Skin Irritation and Sensitization With Clients

In general, minor skin irritation is not a difficult problem to deal with, and the symptoms—mostly redness, occasionally small red bumps, burning, or itching sensations—are usually mild with the types of dilution commonly used in aromatherapy massage. One study on cases of accidental eucalyptus exposure states that "irritation of the skin subsided one hour after the removal of the oil."[31] In my experience, irritation often resolves itself even more quickly than that, and the client frequently does not notice any symptoms herself. If irritation is more severe, the practitioner can gently wipe the affected area with mild soapy water to remove the irritant, or apply aloe vera gel or a similar soothing substance to calm the skin.

Sensitization is a more difficult problem, and in many cases the symptoms are similar to skin irritation, so it can be difficult to know whether it is an allergic reaction. Typically, the client has no noticeable reaction the first time an essential oil is used and then has increasingly strong responses to later doses. If in doubt, the situation must be regarded as sensitization and the substance avoided in all use. In my experience, the clients most likely to develop sensitivities to essential oils are those who already have had some kind of allergic reaction to other substances, such as detergents and fragrances.

Patch Testing

Patch testing can be done by a massage therapist to determine whether a client is likely to have skin irritation or a sensitivity to a particular essential oil or absolute. To test for irritation, the essential oil is applied to the skin, usually on the inside of the forearm, at double the concentration normally used (perhaps 5–10%) and covered for 24 hours. This test should be repeated to identify a skin sensitization, which might not be noticeable on first use.

Patch testing might not be convenient for massage therapists who tend to meet their clients for the first time just before the massage session starts, or who may see a particular client only once. The most practical course of action when using essential oils with a first-time client is to conduct a thorough intake interview to establish whether the client has sensitive skin or allergies. Essential oils that are known skin irritants and sensitizers should be avoided in this first session, and moderate to mild dilutions should be used. However, patch testing is prudent if a client has already shown allergies to other substances. Also, if an aromatherapist is sending a blend home with this type of client for long-term use for a chronic issue, then patch testing of the essential oils in the blend is definitely appropriate.

SUMMARY

- Most severe ill effects of essential oils are caused by accidental or deliberate ingestion.

- Individual reactions to essential oils vary widely. Laboratory and clinical tests may be helpful in establishing toxic limits, but the results from animal testing do not always transfer well to humans.

- Internal use is the most hazardous method of application and is outside the scope of practice for massage therapists.

- The main risks in topical application are skin irritation, skin sensitization, and photosensitization.

- Any essential oil that causes an allergic reaction should not be used with that client again.

- The citrus and needle essential oils may be more skin irritating when oxidized; these oils should be used very fresh.

- Undiluted essential oils should not be used on the skin, except for acute care, with adults or older children, for short periods of time. Undiluted oils should never be used on sensitive areas of skin (axillary region, face, mucous membranes), on diseased skin, or for long periods on broken skin.

- Therapists should vary the essential oils they use. Repeated use of the same oils may make the therapist or client more susceptible to allergic reactions.

- Heat with oils high in menthol (peppermint) or methyl salicylate (wintergreen and sweet birch) should be avoided.

- Inhalation is the safest method of application. Steam inhalation may need to be avoided with asthmatics.

- Milder dilutions should be used with children, the elderly, and those with sensitive skin and chronic skin problems. Essential oils containing high amounts of camphor, menthol, and thymol should be avoided with young children.

- Aromatic oils high in apiol, sabinyl acetate, camphor, and pinocamphone should be avoided during pregnancy.

- Sweet birch and wintergreen should be avoided with clients on anticoagulant medications.

- Skin irritation can be soothed by washing the area with a mild soap and/or applying aloe vera.

- Patch testing, in which a strong dilution of an essential oil is applied to the forearm and covered, can be used to test for skin sensitivity or irritation.

Review Questions

1. Massage therapists may use essential oils with clients topically, internally, and in inhalation, within their scope of practice. (T/F)
2. The most hazardous method of application is: (a) ingestion, (b) inhalation, (c) topical application, (d) foot bath.
3. The biggest risks in topical application are of _____ and _____.
4. Mild essential oils such as lavender should never irritate the skin. (T/F)

5. Essential oils that are more irritating when older include essential oils extracted from: (a) spices, (b) resins and woods, (c) needles and citruses, (d) flowers and roots.

6. If a client has an allergic reaction to an essential oil, the oil can be used again after a few days have passed to allow the skin to calm down. (T/F)

7. Essential oils should be diluted in _____, _____, _____, or _____, if they are added to a foot bath for someone with sensitive skin.

8. Young children, the elderly, and people with sensitive skin need: (a) stronger dilutions than adults, (b) milder dilutions than adults, (c) the same dilutions as adults.

9. It is possible to have an allergic reaction to an essential oil just from smelling it. (T/F)

10. Pregnant women sometimes require milder dilutions because they frequently have an increased sensitivity to _____.

11. Sweet birch and wintergreen are contraindicated when a client is taking: (a) antidepressants, (b) anticoagulants, (c) anti-inflammatories, (d) antispasmodics.

12. Why should bergamot oil be avoided in topical applications before going out in sunlight?

13. All chemotypes of thyme essential oil (*Thymus vulgaris*) have the same properties and safety indications. (T/F)

14. Patch testing should be done with: (a) undiluted essential oils, (b) an extremely mild dilution (0.5%), (c) essential oils at the same dilution as the therapist plans to use them, (d) essential oils at double the dilution as the therapist plans to use them.

Notes

1. Coulson IH, Khan SA. Facial 'pillow' dermatitis due to lavender oil allergy. Contact Dermatitis 1999;41:111.

2. Webb NJA, Pitt WR. Eucalyptus poisoning in childhood: 41 cases in south-east Queensland. J Paediatr Child Health 1993;29:368–371.

3. Mills S. The Essential Book of Herbal Medicine. London, UK: Penguin, 1991:346.

4. Tisserand R, Balacs T. Essential Oil Safety. London, UK: Churchill Livingstone, 1999:159.

5. Darben T, Cominos B, Lee CT. Topical eucalyptus oil poisoning. Australas J Dermatol 1998;39:265–267.

6. Selvaag E, Erikson B, Thune P. Contact allergy due to tea tree oil and cross-sensitisation to colophony. Contact Dermatitis 1994;31:124–125.

7. www.ifraorg.org/GuideLines.asp

8. Chang Y-C, Karlberg AT, Maibach HI. Allergic contact dermatitis from oxidized *d*-limonene. Contact Dermatitis 1997;37:308–309.

9. Knight TE, Hausen BM. Melaleuca oil (tea tree oil) dermatitis. J Am Acad Dermatol 1994;30(3):423–427.

10. Isaacs G. Permanent local anaesthesia and anhidrosis after clove oil spillage. Lancet 1983;16:882.

11. Faoagali J, George N, Leditschke JF. Does tea tree oil have a place in the topical treatment of burns? Burns 1997;23(4):349–351.

12. Knight TE, Hausen BM, ibid.

13. Cockayne SE, Gawkrodger DJ. Occupational contact dermatitis in an aromatherapist. Contact Dermatitis 1997;36:306.

14. Tisserand R, Balacs T. Essential Oil Safety. London, UK: Churchill Livingstone, 1999:203–211.

15. Sugiura M, Hayakawa R, Kato Y, et al. Results of patch testing with lavender oil in Japan. Contact Dermatitis 2000;43:157–160.

16. Vilaplana J, Romaguera C. Contact dermatitis from the essential oil of tangerine in fragrance. Contact Dermatitis 2002;46:108.

17. Heng MC. Local necrosis and interstitial nephritis due to topical methyl salicylate and menthol. Cutis 1987;39(5):442–444.

18. Valnet J. The Practice of Aromatherapy. Essex, UK: CW Daniel, 1992:74.

19. Guba R. Aromatherapy from your keyboard. Aromather Today 2000;16:6.

20. Burfield T. Safety of Essential Oils. Int J Aromather 2000;10(1/2):16–29.

21. Schaller M, Korting HC. Allergic airborne contact dermatitis from essential oils used in aromatherapy. Clin Exp Dermatol 1995;20(2):143–145.

22. Dupreyon JP, Quattrocchi F, Castaing H, et al. Acute poisoning of an infant by cutaneous application of a local counterirritant and pulmonary antiseptic salve. Eur J Toxicol Environ Hyg 1976;9(5):313–320.

23. Javorka K, Tomori Z, Zavarska L. Protective and defensive airway reflexes in premature infants. Physiol Bohemoslov 1980;29(1):29–35.

24. Tisserand R, Balacs T. Essential Oil Safety. London, UK: Churchill Livingstone, 1999:105–112.

25. Tisserand R, Balacs T. Essential Oil Safety. London, UK: Churchill Livingstone, 1999(68):105–112.

26. Ebert U, Loscher W. Strong olfactory stimulation reduces seizure susceptibility in amygdala-kindled rats. Neurosci Lett 2000;287(3):199–202.

27. Tisserand R, Balacs T. Essential Oil Safety. London, UK: Churchill Livingstone, 1999:65.

28. Chan TY. Potential dangers from topical preparations containing methyl salicylate. Hum Exp Toxicol 1996;15(9):747–750.

29. Woeber K, Krombach M. Sensitisation from volatile oils (preliminary report). Berufsdermatosen 1969;17(6):320–326.

30. Starke JC. Photoallergy to sandalwood oil. Arch Dermatol 1967;96:62–63.

31. Spoerke DG, Vandenburg SA, Smolinske SC, et al. Eucalyptus oil: 14 cases of exposure. Vet Hum Toxicol (Manhattan) 1989;31(2):166–168.

11 Blending

"I make my perfumes by trial and error,"
admits Quraysh somewhat forlornly.

"That's how they all do it," Turin yells. The
Indian looks at him sharply, wonderingly.
Turin raises both eyebrows, grins, nods.
"Those guys in their big gleaming expensive
labs in Switzerland and France, they
gas-chromatograph everything, and then in
the end they just try sticking everything
with everything else and smell it all.
And that's it."[1]

Perfume blending is both extremely easy and unbelievably complex. It is easy in that an absolute beginner with a good nose can produce a pleasant mixture given good materials, yet the process is so complex that the large perfume houses employ hundreds of people and spend millions of dollars each year attempting to come up with something new and appealing. The basic problem, outlined in Chandler Burr's fascinating book *The Emperor of Scent*, is that no one thoroughly understands smell, and it is difficult to predict how different combinations of molecules will end up smelling.[1] In most cases, perfumers make blends by trial and error.

Therapeutic blending is a different matter. Instead of a purely cosmetic fragrance, the aromatherapist is attempting to create a blend that produces a particular effect on the body or on the emotions. However, even for holistic aromatherapists, who concentrate on topical application and inhalation, it is desirable to produce something that is pleasant to the client, especially for take-home blends, simply to ensure that the client will enjoy the experience and be more inclined to use the remedy.

Blending for Fragrance

Most aromatherapists, whether they specialize in purely treatment work or in more pampering methods in a spa setting, enjoy creating beautiful combinations of essential oils. The most important guideline in fragrance blending is to please your own nose or that of your client. Blending for fragrance is subjective; what pleases one person may not appeal to another. For this reason, there are no strict rules about which essential oils should or should not be mixed together. Some general guidelines can help the beginner gain experience, without being overwhelmed by the complexity of the choices.

Learning About Your Essential Oils

The initial concern in aesthetic blending is developing an accurate sense of what each of your essential oils smells like, not what you *think* they smell like. Most people in our culture assume they know the smell of ginger (*Zingiber officinale*), but if you hand them a ginger essential oil on a tester strip and ask them what it is, many will not be able to identify it. It is interesting to watch people sniff tobacco absolute (*Nicotiana tabacum*). Most people like the smell very much, until I tell them what it is, and then they screw their faces up in disgust. Also, most people think they know what lavender smells like, but there are many different species and varieties of lavender, each with remarkably varied aromas.

Developing an accurate sense of an essential oil's smell requires that you become familiar with the aroma's character, volatility, and intensity.

Character. The **character** of an oil's aroma is defined as how you would describe it. Place a drop of one essential oil on a professional tester strip (or pH-neutral card from an art supply store). It is even better to ask someone else to do this for you, so you don't know which essential oil it is and therefore have fewer preconceptions about it. It is preferable to put the oil on a tester strip than to smell it from the bottle, as you will get a fuller sense of the smell when the larger heavier molecules warm up, evaporate, and travel to your nose. (Placing a drop on your skin will heat it up even faster.)

Spend some time smelling it and writing your impressions of the fragrance. Is it cool, warm, hot, dry, powdery, mossy, sweet, bitter, deep, light? If it was a color, what color would it be? Does it remind you of a place or an activity? All of these questions help to establish the character of the aroma.

Volatility. An essential oil's **volatility** is its rate of evaporation. Does the smell disappear quickly or linger for a long time? Does it change with time? (Perfumers refer to this change as "drydown.") You can even put it away and come back to it several days or even weeks later, and see how much it has changed.

Many essential oils have a mixture of molecules with different volatilities. As a result, the aroma of the oil changes considerably when exposed to air. The lighter, more volatile molecules evaporate quickly and are smelled first, leaving the heavier, less volatile molecules to be inhaled later. The larger, less volatile molecules seem to smell sweeter, so blends often become sweeter over time. Professional perfumers always allow their blends to stand for at least several weeks, until they stop changing in character before selling them. You may be surprised by how much your blends continue to develop and change for weeks after a blending session.

Some oils change very little over time because they are made up primarily of less volatile components. For instance, you could place a drop of sandalwood (*Santalum album*) on a tester strip and leave it for 3 months; it will still smell strongly of sandalwood at the end of that time. Table 11.1 lists volatility rates of the most commonly used essential oils.

Intensity. An aroma's **intensity** can be defined as how easily it can be smelled even in small amounts. Equal amounts of jasmine absolute and lavender essential oil, for example, would not make a balanced blend because the jasmine has a much stronger scent than the lavender and would completely overpower it. It is not possible to recommend exactly how many drops of jasmine would balance a certain number of drops of lavender, as different aromatherapists will own jasmine and lavender from different parts of the world and the oils will not match in intensity.

Table 11.2 presents the odor intensities of the most commonly used essential oils. Intensity in this context relates to smell only. Some of the intensely smelling oils have a mild effect when applied to the skin, while others may be strong in both odor and effect. You should use less of the

Table 11.1	Volatility Rates of Some Commonly Used Essential Oils		
Extreme Volatility	**Strong Volatility**	**Moderate Volatility**	**Slow Volatility**
Grapefruit (*Citrus x paradisii*)	Basil (*Ocimum basilicum*)	Bay laurel (*Laurus nobilis*)	Blue cypress (*Callitris intratropica*)
Lemon (*Citrus limon*)	Cardamon (*Elettaria cardamomum*)	Black pepper (*Piper nigrum*)	Carrot (*Daucus carota*)
Mandarin (*Citrus reticulata*)	Clary sage (*Salvia sclarea*)	Roman chamomile (*Chamaemelum nobile*)	Cedar (*Cedrus atlantica* or *C. deodara*)
Melissa (*Melissa officinalis*)	Eucalyptus (*Eucalyptus radiata* or *E. globulus*)	Cinnamon (*Cinnamomum zeylanicum*)	German chamomile (*Matricaria recutita*)
Peppermint (*Mentha piperita*)	Hyssop (*Hyssopus officinalis*)	Cypress (*Cupressus sempervirens*)	Cumin (*Cuminum cyminum*)
	Juniper (*Juniperus communis*)	Fennel (*Foeniculum vulgare*)	Frankincense (*Boswellia carteri*)
	Spike lavender (*Lavandula latifolia*)	Fir (*Abies alba*)	Ginger CO_2 (*Zingiber officinale*)
	Palmarosa (*Cymbopogon martinii*)	Geranium (*Pelargonium graveolens*)	Jasmine (*Jasminum grandiflorum*)
	Rosemary (*Rosmarinus officinalis*)	Ginger ess. oil (*Zingiber officinale*)	Sandalwood (*Santalum album*)
	Sweet birch (*Betula lenta*)	Helichrysum (*Helichrysum italicum*)	Turmeric (*Curcuma longa*)
	Tea tree (*Melaleuca alternifolia*)	Inula (*Inula graveolens*)	Vetiver (*Vetiveria zizanioides*)
		Lavender (*Lavandula angustifolia*)	
		Marjoram (*Origanum majorana*)	
		Neroli (*Citrus aurantium* var. *amara*)	
		Nutmeg (*Myristica fragrans*)	
		Ylang ylang (*Cananga odorata*)	

Table 11.2	Odor Intensities of Some Commonly Used Essential Oils		
Extremely Intense	**Strongly Intense**	**Moderately Intense**	**Mildly Intense**
Cumin (*Cuminum cyminum*)	Basil (*Ocimum basilicum*)	Bergamot (*Citrus x bergamia*)	Cedarwood (*Cedrus atlantica* or *C. deodara*)
Cinnamon (*Cinnamomum zeylanicum*)	Carrot (*Daucus carota*)	Bay laurel (*Laurus nobilis*)	Cypress (*Cupressus sempervirens*)
Clove (*Syzygium aromaticum*)	*Eucalyptus globulus* and *E. radiata*	Black pepper (*Piper nigrum*)	Fir (*Abies alba*)
German chamomile (*Matricaria recutita*)	Fennel (*Foeniculum vulgare*)	Blue cypress (*Callitris intratropica*)	Grapefruit (*Citrus x paradisii*)
Roman chamomile (*Chamaemelum nobile*)	Ginger (*Zingiber officinale*)	Cardamon (*Elettaria cardamomum*)	Rosalina (*Melaleuca ericifolia*)
Peppermint (*Mentha piperita*)	Helichrysum (*Helichrysum italicum*)	Clary sage (*Salvia sclarea*)	Sandalwood (*Santalum album*)
	Jasmine (*Jasminum grandiflorum*)	Frankincense (*Boswellia carteri*)	
	Neroli (*Citrus aurantium* var. *amara*)	Juniper (*Juniperus communis*)	
	Nutmeg (*Myristica fragrans*)	Lavender (*Lavandula angustifolia*)	
	Patchouli (*Pogostemon cablin*)	Lemon (*Citrus limon*)	
	Rose absolute (*Rosa damascena*)	Marjoram (*Origanum majorana*)	
	Vetiver (*Vetiveria zizanioides*)	Melissa (*Melissa officinalis*)	
	Ylang ylang (*Cananga odorata*)	Myrrh (*Commiphora myrrha*)	
		Palmarosa (*Cymbopogon martinii*)	
		Petitgrain (*Citrus aurantium* var. *amara*)	
		Pine (*Pinus sylvestris*)	
		Tea tree (*Melaleuca alternifolia*)	

Activity 11.1

Blending by Nose Alone

Choose a few essential oils you like and think might combine well. Open the bottles, hold them in your hands, and wave them under your nose. Alternatively, place a drop of each onto a tester strip. Is there one that dominates the others? Are there any that seem to clash? You may want to put aside the oil that does not really fit with the others, or use less of the oils that dominate. Take an empty glass blending bottle and add one drop of each essential oil that you have chosen. Roll the bottle between your hands briefly to help the oils mix, and then smell the result. If it is not exactly how you want it, add another drop of one of your group of oils, and keep doing this until the blend smells balanced to you. Remember that the smell of your blend will change, sometimes quite significantly, over the next few days or weeks. Keep a record of the number of drops of each oil you use, so that you can reproduce the recipe if you want to.

Activity 11.2

Blending the Notes

Choose at least two essential oils you consider to be bases (long volatility, often deeper, heavier smell), at least two mid notes (medium volatility, warm character), and two or more top notes (high volatility, sharp character). Starting with the base notes, put 1 drop of each into an empty glass blending bottle, and then add 1 or 2 drops of each mid note. Smell your blend before adding 1 drop of each top note. Recheck the result and decide if you need more base, mid, or top notes. Keep adding 1 drop at a time until you have reached a balanced fragrance. You may find you need a different essential oil to fill in any spaces if your top, mid, or base notes are too far apart.

essential oils from the very intense list when blending with oils from the other lists. For example, if you are making a blend with Roman chamomile, lemon, and sandalwood, you might use 1 drop of chamomile, 4 drops of lemon, and 7 drops of sandalwood to produce a balanced aroma.

Getting Started

Once you have an idea of the character, volatility, and intensity of the different essential oils you own, it is much easier to imagine how they will combine with each other. There are some blending techniques and styles that are enjoyable to ex-

periment with, but basically anyone can make aromatherapy blends. Start by blending with only three or four different essential oils or absolutes, and then progress to using more as you get more comfortable with combining scents. Some people naturally start by blending a lot of different aromatic oils, whereas others may make the most exquisite perfumes with three or four constituents and never want to use more.

Top-Mid-Base Note Blending

Top-mid-base note blending, invented by a French perfumer named Piesse, is a process intended to create a balanced fragrance that will last for some time when worn. It combines **base notes,** essential oils that are very stable and have a long volatility, with **top notes,** oils that are very volatile for immediate interest, to showcase the **mid notes,** the medium volatility essential oils that make up the main character of the blend. A good example is the long-lasting sandalwood as a base note, with lavender as a mid note, and lemon as a lively top note.

Therapeutic Blending

Most massage therapists are concerned more with therapeutic blending than with fragrance blending. The therapist combines several essential oils that have been chosen to help with any problems the client is experiencing. Therapeutic blending may concentrate on physical issues such as muscular tension or pain, or emotional issues such as anxiety or depression.

Synergy

A perfumer blends many different fragrances because people find beauty in complexity. An aromatherapist blends several different essential oils to create a **synergy,** a blend of two or more essential oils that together may be much more effective therapeutically than one single oil. One study showed, for example, that the antifungal effects of tea tree (*Melaleuca alternifolia*) and lavender (*Lavandula angustifolia*) essential oils were increased by using them together, even though "there was no chemical interaction resulting in a new compound."[2]

Mixing essential oils that all focus on the same therapeutic treatment can increase the benefits to the client, especially if the oils chosen all have slightly different modes of action. A blend for sunburn, for example, might include peppermint oil to provide relief to the burned area by stimulating the cold receptors in the skin and lavender essential oil as an anti-inflammatory and skin-healing agent.

It is important in any kind of healing work not to dilute the focus of a treatment by trying to work on too many problems at one time. Of course, physical problems often lead to emotional and mental difficulties (and vice versa), and it is possible and desirable to create a remedy that helps the client on these different levels. However, trying to make

Activity 11.3

Blending by Chemistry

Referring back to Chapter 5 (Essential Oil Chemistry), decide on an appropriate formula for:

1. An inflammatory flare-up of rheumatoid arthritis in the knees

2. A long-term treatment for lowered immune response

Bear in mind the precautions for skin irritation or other possible problems. Decide first which chemical groups would be most effective in these situations, and then see if they have any potential hazards that could be balanced by other groups. Look for essential oils that are high in these chemical constituents, and decide on a blend.

a blend that addresses every physical and emotional difficulty occurring at once in the client's life is both unrealistic and much less effective, since you may be combining oils having contradictory properties. One study on the effects of combinations of essential oils on smooth muscle showed that "in some cases there was no activity at all as opposite activities cancelled each other out."[3] The authors gave as an example a blend of nutmeg, geranium, and bergamot, in which presumably the stimulant effects of nutmeg on smooth muscle cancelled out the relaxing, antispasmodic effects of the geranium and bergamot. A mixture of several essential oils does not necessarily create a synergy.

The optimal number of essential oils to use in a therapeutic massage blend is a matter of personal choice. Some aromatherapists prefer using a single essential oil for one treatment, and others combine up to 15 oils in one blend. My preference is to use between three and seven oils.

Blending by Chemistry

A good working knowledge of essential oil chemistry can be useful in making a choice of oils for a blend. Essential oils with a high level of chemical constituents that tend to have particular properties can be combined to make an effective treatment formula, while keeping safety in mind. For example, phenols are compounds that are generally good broad-spectrum antifungals, seemingly an ideal choice for athlete's foot, until we realize that they can also be skin irritating. Primary alcohols, such as geraniol, citronellol, and nerol, also are antifungal but are rarely irritants. A formula such as thyme (*Thymus vulgaris* CT thymol), geranium (*Pelargonium graveolens*), and lavandin (*Lavandula* x *intermedia*), which uses both phenol-rich and alcohol-rich essential oils, would be an ideal remedy for this problem.

Avoiding skin irritation can be a major factor in deciding on an essential oil formula. For instance, Guba recommends the use of phenol-rich essential oils as 10% of a formula, with the remaining 90% composed of nonirritant essential oils, such as lavender, tea tree, or *Eucalyptus radiata*.[4] The decision to include a potentially skin-irritating oil in the formula may dictate the character of the other ingredients.

Blending by Plant Part

Blending by plant part, sometimes called **morphological blending,** is an interesting method that owes something to the Doctrine of Signatures of the medieval herbalists. The underlying premise is that different plant parts have different functions, and that as a result, the essential oils from those parts have certain properties in common. For example, the leaves or needles of trees are used by the plant to take in oxygen and carbon dioxide, and to release more oxygen. According to this theory, a blend of tree leaves and needles would benefit the respiratory system. In fact this is the case, with essential oils such as pine, fir, tea tree, and eucalyptus being included in the recommended formula. I find the idea too generalized because there is little opportunity to fine-tune for different types of respiratory problems. However, you may like it as an easy way to remember some of the properties of a broad range of oils.

To continue the morphological theory, roots and rhizomes such as vetiver and ginger would be good for grounding and for digestion. Woods transport liquids and therefore benefit the urinary and lymphatic systems, while resins such as myrrh are antiseptic and wound healing—identical to their function in the tree. Flowers, as the reproductive part of the plant, work well on the reproductive system, while fruits and seeds tend to influence the digestive system (most are foods) and the endocrine system because of their potential for growth and development. Morphological blending can also be used as an interesting and novel way to approach aesthetic blending. Putting together some or all of the essential oils in one group can lead to some lovely and unusual results.

Including the Client in the Blending Process

Having picked several essential oils you think are most appropriate for your client's needs, you might like to invite her to become part of the blending process by asking her to smell them and choose those to which she is most drawn. Including your client in this way has several benefits. She takes an active part in her own treatment, and as a result the mixture becomes "her" blend, one that she is more likely to use because she has chosen and likes the individual components. In addition, if you have faith in the intuitive ability of the human body, you will find that what your clients choose (from a selection of essential oils that you know are appropriate to the problem) works better for them than what you might have chosen.

SUMMARY

- Blending for fragrance has no set rules, just guidelines for creating a balanced or interesting blend.

- Learning about the odor character, volatility, and intensity of your essential oils will help with fragrance blending.

- Top-mid-base note blending is a process that mixes essential oils of different volatilities to create a balanced blend.

- In therapeutic blending it is desirable to create an attractive fragrance so that clients will have a pleasant experience and will want to reuse the remedy.

- In therapeutic blending, several essential oils may produce a synergy. However, oils that cancel out each other's effects should be avoided.

- The number of essential oils to use in one blend is at the therapist's discretion.

- Understanding the chemistry of essential oils can help a therapist create a synergistic blend, while avoiding possible skin irritation or other complications.

- Blending by plant part is called morphological blending and can be used for its therapeutic effects or for fragrance blending.

- Including the client in the blending process means that she is likely to enjoy the blend and use it more frequently.

Review Questions

1. It is difficult to predict what a blend of several essential oils will smell like. (T/F)
2. You will get a better idea of the full scent of an essential oil if you: (a) smell it out of the bottle, (b) put it on a professional tester strip, (c) dilute it in water and spray it in the air, (d) dilute it in oil and then smell it.
3. If an essential oil is of good quality, it should smell exactly the same after a few hours on a tester strip. (T/F)
4. Which of the following oils is most volatile (evaporates fastest at room temperature)? (a) sandalwood, (b) patchouli, (c) lavender, (d) lemon.
5. Explain how to do top–mid–base note blending.
6. What is a synergistic blend, in therapeutic blending?
7. If you use an essential oil that is very stimulating together with an essential oil that is very sedative, they will not cancel each other out therapeutically. (T/F)
8. Phenols (which are often skin irritating) can be mixed with alcohols (which are usually mild on the skin) to minimize the irritating effects. (T/F)
9. In blending by plant part, a respiratory blend would be made from the following essential oils: (a) spruce, cypress, and petitgrain, (b) jasmine, chamomile, and rose, (c) nutmeg, cinnamon, and clove, (d) spikenard, ginger, and vetiver.
10. The following number of essential oils should be combined for a satisfactory blend: (a) 2–4, (b) 3–7, (c) more than 7, (d) the number is up to the therapist.

Notes

1. Burr C. The Emperor of Scent. New York: Random House, 2002:292.
2. Cassella S, Cassella JP, Smith I. Synergetic antifungal activity of tea tree (*Melaleuca alternifolia*) and lavender (*Lavandula angustifolia*) essential oils against dermatophyte infection. Int J Aromather 2002;12(1):2–15.
3. Lis-Balchin M, Deans S, Hart S. A study of the changes on the bioactivity of essential oils used singly and as mixture in aromatherapy. J Altern Complement Med 1997;3(3):249–256.
4. Guba R. Toxicity myths—the actual risks of essential oil use. Int J Aromather 2002;10(1/2):37–49.

12

Supplies and Equipment for Aromatherapy Massage

Setting up to practice aromatherapy massage may seem as simple as purchasing a few essential oils and getting to work. Many of us have started this way and then learned more efficient ways of organizing our equipment and our space by trial and error. Some supplies are essential for the massage therapist who wishes to practice aromatherapy, while other items are useful but not essential. Along with equipment and supplies, the therapist must consider his or her workspace as a whole and determine whether the room, or even the building, is suited to an aromatherapy practice.

The main things to consider when preparing to practice aromatherapy are the following:

- The suitability of the massage room and building for aromatherapy, and how to work with any potential difficulties.
- Extra supplies and equipment you may need.
- The essential oils to start with, bearing in mind the type of massage you practice.
- How to organize the physical space in the room.

Your Workplace

Your workplace consists of many elements, including the massage room itself, the suite or building it is in, your immediate colleagues and clients, and other people who use the building.

Your Colleagues and Clients

Many massage therapists reading this book will have already set up their practice—as an employee, as an independent contractor renting a room in a massage clinic or chiropractor's office, or as a business proprietor sharing a workspace with colleagues. Incorporating aromatherapy into this kind of practice may present issues because of shared space or other features of the building. The first thing to consider is how your aromatherapy work may impact other people using the same area. I often forget when I am teaching a class or doing a massage with aromatherapy how quickly my own nose adapts to the scents, and how overpowering they may be for someone else walking into that space. It is important to inform colleagues, and other people sharing the area, of how you intend to work and to negotiate how this can happen without making them uncomfortable or creating problems for them.

Colleagues will almost certainly have questions and concerns about how strong the aromas will be and how the scents in the room might affect their own clients. You may decide to suggest using aromatherapy for a trial period of a few weeks to let them judge how it will fit in and then revisit the issue at the end of that time. I have practiced aromatherapy in many different shared workplaces and have never had serious problems, even when another practitioner would use my room immediately after I had finished working there. Some points to consider are the following:

1. If you are an employee, your employer needs to agree to your use of essential oils in your work. Not only is it good work etiquette to ask, but your employer may have specific concerns about how the business is presented and about possible safety issues regarding clients.

2. If you are sharing a space, make sure the room is well ventilated to the outside of the building, so that aromas can be dispersed quickly and effectively and not waft into waiting areas, other practice rooms, or changing rooms. A fan to increase air flow toward a window can be useful.

3. In shared massage spaces, you may decide not to use equipment such as aroma lamps or steam inhalers, which diffuse essential oils into the air much more rapidly, making it more difficult to clear the scents away afterward.

4. If you are sharing linen, reassure colleagues that essential oils are easily removed by laundering and that their crisp professional sheets will not necessarily smell of jasmine or patchouli. The smell of massage oil is actually more difficult to remove than that of essential oils.

5. If another person is using the same room after you, try to schedule your clients so that you have 10 or 15 minutes at the end of your work time to air the room out thoroughly for the next practitioner.

The Massage Room

Even if you are practicing completely by yourself, with no one else to object to what you use in your work, there are some aspects of your physical space you need to consider. The most important of these is room size. A few bottles of essential oils may not take up much physical space, but your room must be large enough to accommodate a work surface where you can have your essential oils, carriers, and blending bowls or bottles, at the very least (Figure 12.1). A massage room should not be so small that it can hold only a massage table, with barely enough room to maneuver around it. Although a small space may be suitable for a therapist who

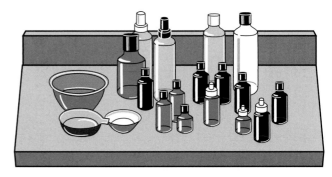

Figure 12.1 A typical work surface with essential oils, blending bowls, carriers, and bottles.

simply works with a bottle of massage lotion in a holster, it is a practical impossibility for aromatherapy work and the extra supplies needed.

Even if you are not sharing a room with another practitioner, the room's ventilation must be adequate because some of your clients will not appreciate aromas or want aromatherapy. It is also healthier for the practitioner not to have a buildup of essential oil aromas in her system. A good flow of air via a window in one wall and a door in the opposite wall is ideal. If your massage space is an inside room with no windows, use a fan to clear the air.

Supplies and Equipment

Some supplies are absolutely necessary to an aromatherapy practice, if you wish to present a professional image. Apart from your essential oils, these supplies generally are quite inexpensive and easy to find, but they will make your sessions run much more smoothly if you have them within easy reach. Which essential oils are appropriate for your particular practice are discussed later in the chapter.

Carriers

Chapter 9 discussed carrier oils, lotions, and ointments, in some depth, and it is important to bear in mind a couple of basic principles. First, different clients will prefer different carrier types. Even though you may prefer using oil for a massage, you should also have lotion and gel in your massage room, in case clients ask for them. Second, it is healthier for practitioners to have a variety of carriers because they will also be absorbing them through their hands. Research suggests that regularly repeated doses of any substance on a long-term basis has a tendency to lead to allergic sensitization. I recommend that massage therapists have on hand at least two or three different massage oils, a good unscented lotion, and a gel.

If you are using unrefined vegetable oils, remember that they tend to turn rancid rather rapidly, especially in a massage room, which is often considerably warmer than a living space. It is probably a good idea to have smaller bottles of oil in the massage room and keep any larger amounts in a refrigerator. One of the oils I use frequently is jojoba, partly because I like its consistency and qualities but also because it is a liquid wax and does not turn rancid, even when kept in warm temperatures for some time. Sesame oil also seems to have a long shelf life.

Carriers should be kept on a surface that will not stain if they are spilled and that can be wiped off easily. No matter how careful I try to be with oil or lotion, I always end up with greasy rings on all the surfaces in my massage room. Bottles with pump tops spill less easily, but they still ooze and get sticky. Essential oils can damage surfaces if spilled on paint or varnish.

Bottles and Jars

To mix the essential oils with a carrier, you need some kind of container. Small plastic bottles are the most convenient, and I usually use a 1 oz. or 2 oz. size. A 1 oz. bottle holds enough for a full-body massage, and a 2 oz. bottle holds enough to give a treatment and send a reasonable amount home with the client. You can buy bottles with a flip top, and you can purchase them in bulk, which makes the price reasonable. It is hard to find pump tops for these small bottles, and many massage therapists who are used to using a lotion bottle with a pump in a holster may have some difficulty at first transitioning to the smaller, pumpless bottles that are more convenient for aromatherapy massage. Larger bottles can be used, but as many aromatherapists blend for individual clients and for individual sessions, they tend to be less appropriate.

If you often use lotion, especially a heavier one, you may find that blending in a bottle requires some practice. To experience how the thicker essential oils can refuse to dissolve completely, put some German chamomile, vetiver, or some other very colorful, heavy essential oil in a bottle of lotion and watch the streaks form as you shake it. I usually find that the oils mix easily into the lotion if I layer the blend, putting about half the lotion in first, then the essential oils, and then more lotion. Leave some space in the top of the bottle, so that everything will blend together when you shake it. If the oils still have not dissolved completely into the lotion, you can use a small stick to stir it quickly. The best are the wooden stirring sticks found in coffee shops, and you can buy them from a catering retailer cheaply.

If you send very heavy lotions or ointments home with clients—the most common one I use is a heavy beeswax and oil ointment for cracked heels—it is best to use a small plastic jar. Jars are available in stores or through suppliers that sell bottles.

Some aromatherapists prefer to put all their blends in colored glass bottles. Although colored glass is ideal for preserving the quality of the essential oil and carrier, plastic is less expensive, and it is lighter and less likely to break if clients want to carry their blends in purses or pockets. You can use colored glass if a client wants you to make up a larger amount of an aromatherapy blend or a spritzer as a gift for someone else.

The 1 oz. and 2 oz. plastic bottles with spray tops are useful to have on hand to make spritzers for clients to take with them. I occasionally make neat (undiluted) blends of essential oils for a client to use at home, in a steam inhaler or dropped onto a tissue to inhale; for these mixtures small glass bottles are necessary because undiluted essential oils can dissolve plastic. These bottles are available in many sizes, from about 1 mL and up; I find the 5 mL size to be the most convenient. They can be purchased with lids that have dropper tops and tamper-proof seals; you simply screw the lid on firmly and the dropper top will be inserted into the bottle, ready for use.

Reusing bottles that have contained aromatherapy blends is possible, but the aroma of the essential oils tends to cling to any bottle, whether it is glass or plastic. Rinse the bottles with rubbing alcohol to remove any residue, and then wash them on the hottest cycle in a dishwasher. This often works, although it may not be successful with bottles that have contained the more intense oils such as patchouli or jasmine. I prefer to recycle the used bottles and put my next blends into fresh containers. Doing so prevents bacterial contamination.

Bowls

Bowls are useful when you need to make only a small amount of a blend. Sessions in which the aromatherapist makes a strong blend to apply to a painful low back and a milder blend with different oils entirely to use on the shoulders, neck, and face for relaxation are common. The same session may involve a homework blend for the client to take away and apply to his persistent athlete's foot. Using three bottles for one client soon starts to add up financially, so a better option is to make the blends used during the session in a couple of small bowls, which can be cleaned thoroughly after the massage and reused. For therapists who are not used to handling a bowl full of oil or lotion in a massage, this may take some practice, but it is well worth doing.

Bowls can be made of glass, glazed ceramic, or even stone. They should not be made of wood, plastic, or unglazed pottery because they will absorb the blend to some extent and will be more difficult to wash out. It is a good idea to have several small bowls, as you may need at least two per client, and you will want to have enough for several clients to save time between sessions. Bowls with beautiful colors or patterns will add to the aesthetic quality of your massage setting.

Other Useful Items

There are many pieces of equipment that are not necessary for practicing aromatherapy massage, but you may decide to buy them at some point to enhance the treatments you give your clients. All the items listed below are reasonable in price and small enough to be stored easily.

- *Diffuser or nebulizer.* Either a diffuser or a nebulizer can be used for inhalation during sessions, to affect mood, improve breathing, or relieve stress.
- *Steam inhaler.* A steam inhaler is useful for clients with respiratory problems; it is more professional, quicker, and less messy than using a bowl of steaming water and a towel over the head.
- *Foot bath.* A foot bath with essential oils is such an inexpensive and useful way to treat so many different problems that it is almost indispensable. A small plastic tub is

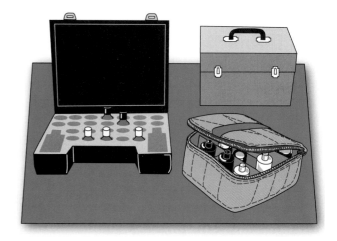

Figure 12.2 Different types of carrying cases for essential oils.

sufficient, though there are numerous ways to make a foot bath more interesting, such as placing small round pebbles or sand in the bottom of the tub to create a "natural" texture. Foot baths should always be sanitized between clients.

- *Aromatherapy charts.* Wall charts are handy references for therapists who are a little unsure of the subject. These charts can help educate clients and stimulate interest in those who otherwise may not have thought of an aromatherapy treatment. Charts can be bought from aromatherapy suppliers or they can be home-made.
- *Carrying cases.* Carrying cases for oils are useful for aromatherapists who may need to take their essential oils to a talk or demonstration, and they are indispensable for therapists who do outcall work. Many types of custom cases are available from aromatherapy suppliers, ranging from beautiful wooden boxes, to plastic briefcases, to padded cases sewn from soft materials (Figure 12.2). Anything that is easy to carry and prevents your bottles from breaking is suitable. I prefer a case with some kind of foam interior or soft padding, and with individual holes for each bottle, because it is safer and does not rattle when carried. Fishing tackle boxes can also be used, as they have enough space for essential oils, bottles of carrier, and other small items.

Establishing a Basic Set of Essential Oils

Which essential oils are the most useful? Which 10 oils would you not want to do without? Which essential oils should you buy first? The answers depend on the style of massage therapy or bodywork you practice, because different essential oils are appropriate for each one. Your choices will also be based on personal preference. I asked several experienced massage therapists who have practiced aromatherapy for years to name the 10 oils they use the most often. Every list differed greatly, reflecting not just the various massage styles but also the personalities of the therapists involved.

Here are some ideas for building a working supply of oils:

1. *Invest in essential oils that you yourself like.* Although this may seem unprofessional, essential oils work on the senses as much as they work pharmaceutically, and the person who will smell them most often is you! I ignored the fact that I dislike ylang ylang (*Cananga odorata*) and bought a large, fairly expensive bottle of this useful oil early in my career. The bottle remained practically untouched until I discovered that I could tolerate the scent only when I blended the ylang ylang with certain other essential oils.

2. *Consider the needs of your massage practice.* If you are doing primarily relaxation work with elderly people, or if you practice only pregnancy massage, then using essential oil of sweet birch (*Betula lenta*) would not be at all appropriate for your particular clients. If you work mostly with athletes, you will probably want to invest in essential oils that have particularly good effects on skeletal muscle, such as rosemary (*Rosmarinus officinalis*) and ginger (*Zingiber officinale*).

3. *Choose essential oils with a broad range of uses.* You do not need to start out with a large number of oils if the ones you choose have several potential uses. It is a good idea to restrict yourself to somewhere between 10 and 20 oils for the first year or so, because it is hard otherwise to remember their properties and get a real sense of their strengths and weaknesses. You can begin practicing aromatherapy with only four or five essential oils, if you choose them wisely. You may decide to concentrate on the therapeutic effects of the oils, selecting one or two stimulants, sedatives, warming oils, and anti-inflammatories, plus a strong immune booster and a respiratory decongestant, for example. Or you could choose one flower oil, a citrus, a root oil, a wood, a leaf oil, and an herb, a selection that would also represent a wide range of aromas and properties.

4. *Begin with the standard essential oils.* Essential oils in regular use, such as lavender and lemon, rather than the exotics like tuberose and *Ammi visnaga* tend to have a broader range of action, have more documented safety testing, and are usually much less expensive.

5. *Choose moderately priced essential oils.* If your budget is limited, there are many essential oils that are inexpensively to moderately priced. It makes more sense to have several high-quality oils, such as lavender, rosemary, and mandarin, than lower-quality grades of some more expensive oils, such as jasmine.

Essential Oils to Suit Your Practice

Some massage styles or techniques combine particularly well with certain essential oils.

- *Relaxation massage.* Relaxation massage often, though not exclusively, utilizes a lot of the sedative, calming oils, such as lavender, Roman chamomile, clary sage, cedarwood, marjoram, frankincense, rosalina, the citruses, and many of the flowers, such as ylang ylang, rose, jasmine, and neroli.

- *Treatment massage and sports massage.* Therapists who specialize in treatment work and sports massage derive much benefit from essential oils that are painkilling, anti-inflammatory, and antispasmodic, such as sweet birch and wintergreen, lavender, German chamomile, helichrysum, rosemary, and peppermint. The hot essential oils, such as black pepper, ginger, and nutmeg, which help warm tissue prior to stretching, are also useful.

- *Manual lymphatic drainage.* Essential oils that promote lymph flow are obviously useful in manual lymphatic drainage. These include juniper, cypress, grapefruit, fennel, helichrysum, rosemary, and peppermint.

Organizing Your Space and Your Oils

A work surface for making your blends, setting up a diffuser, or simply storing your oils and lotions is essential (see Figure 12.1). If you have a lot of storage space in the massage room, your surface area can be quite small. I prefer to keep all my essential oils in drawers so the space looks less cluttered and to keep them away from clients with allergies who need to be in a scent-free environment. Make sure, however, that you keep your essential oils close enough to the area where you interview clients so that you can include them when you select oils, if desired.

If you use blending bowls, you will need more level surfaces that stay available for blending. You can use a small side table or chair, strategically placed, or a low shelf or wide window ledge.

Organizing your essential oils will probably present no problem when you first start practicing, as most aromatherapists begin with a relatively small collection of oils. However, as you will discover, aromatherapy tends to be somewhat addictive, and most aromatherapists I know accumulate large collections of many different essential oils once they have been in business for some time. Labeling the bottles on the tops of the lids makes it much easier to find the ones you need, and arranging the oils alphabetically also helps. Color-coding the labels makes identification even quicker, and you can use different colors for stimulating and sedating oils, or for essential oils from different plant parts (e.g., green for leaf oils, pink for flower oils). Another idea is to keep different types of essential oils in separate small boxes. Whatever system enables you to locate the appropriate essential oil quickly and easily is the right one for you.

It can be difficult for beginning aromatherapists to remember the effects of the essential oils. Give yourself some reminders of the properties of each of your oils, perhaps in the form of a brightly colored chart on the wall, a small laminated list on your work top, or labels on the bottles themselves. Anything that helps you remember the qualities of your remedies will help you and ultimately your clients.

SUMMARY

- Plans to use aromatherapy should be discussed with colleagues and other people who share the work area.
- Good ventilation in the massage room avoids problems for colleagues, nonaromatherapy clients, and the aromatherapist.
- The massage room should be large enough to have a workspace for blending and for supplies and equipment.
- Plastic bottles with flip tops and spritzer tops, small glass bottles, and jars may all be necessary for making blends.
- Blending bowls are useful for mixing smaller amounts of carrier and essential oils, and should be made of glass, glazed ceramic, or stone.

- Other useful items include a diffuser or nebulizer, a steam inhaler, a foot bath, aromatherapy charts, and carrying cases.
- Essential oils should be selected for personal preference, appropriateness for a specific massage practice, broad range of use, and quality.
- Essential oils can be organized by labeling the tops and separating the bottles into categories, or arranging them alphabetically.

Review Questions

1. Name three methods you can use to ensure your use of aromatherapy will not have a negative impact on your colleagues or other people in your workplace.
2. Why are work surfaces essential in a massage room when doing aromatherapy work?
3. The most useful sizes of bottles for individual sessions are _____ oz. and _____ oz.
4. Why are bottles that have already been used for aromatherapy blending difficult to reuse?
5. Why are bowls sometimes used for blending?
6. What materials should blending bowls be made of?
7. Why are standard essential oils generally more useful than exotic ones?
8. Relaxation massage frequently uses the following type of essential oils: (a) sedative, (b) anti-inflammatory, (c) analgesic.

13 The Aromatherapy Consultation and Treatment

The consultation and treatment draws on all the skills of the aromatherapy massage therapist. The therapist must be a good listener to obtain the information he or she needs during the intake part of the session. Knowledge of the essential oils, application methods for aromatherapy, and massage techniques are all essential in making appropriate choices for the best treatment for the client.

The Consultation

The consultation is arguably the most important part of the aromatherapy session. If good communication is established between the therapist and client, the selection of appropriate essential oils to use in the treatment becomes much easier, and the entire session has a more significant impact. Most massage therapists are already experienced and skilled in the techniques of interviewing and obtaining information from their clients. Doing an intake for an aromatherapy session is not dramatically different from that of a regular massage, but it is somewhat longer, as questions for both massage and aromatherapy need to be asked. Areas to cover in an aromatherapy interview that are not always explored in a standard massage intake include the following:

- Skin sensitivity.
- Allergies.
- Medications.
- Stress levels and emotional issues.
- Scent preferences.

Skin Sensitivity

Since most aromatherapy massage sessions involve applying diluted essential oils to the skin, information about a client's tolerance for various substances and general sensitivity is vital. The most common adverse reactions to aromatherapy are skin irritation and allergic reaction. When asked if they have sensitive skin, many clients will be unsure how to answer. Asking specific questions will yield answers about the delicacy of the skin and possible contact allergies:

"Has your skin ever reacted badly to detergent or perfumes?"

"Have you ever developed a rash just from touching something?"

"Do you ever break out after you've used household cleaners?"

"Have you ever had an aromatherapy session before; if so, how did you react to it?"

Allergies

It is important to be aware if your client has any known allergies. A sensitivity to aspirin will eliminate the possibility of using wintergreen and sweet birch oils, as their main component, methyl salicylate, is related to the active substance in aspirin. You should also avoid using essential oils from plants to which clients are allergic. Although this additional precaution is not essential because most allergies are to the pollen the plant produces, which is not present in the essential oil, if the body has an adverse reaction to one part of the plant, it might be better for the whole system to avoid the essential oil from that plant.

Allergies of any kind—whether dermal, digestive, or respiratory—indicate a hypersensitive immune system. It is best to start with smaller doses of essential oils until you can assess how the client responds to aromatherapy. For example, if a client tells me she has an allergy to strawberries or suffers from hay fever in the spring, I will use the same dilutions topically with her as I would for someone with very sensitive skin.

Medications

It is useful to know what medications your clients are taking because it gives you a sense of their general state of health. For instance, if a client tells you he has type II diabetes but his doctor thinks that diet and lifestyle changes are sufficient to control it, you have a very different picture of his overall well-being than if he tells you that he takes insulin. If someone with diagnosed high blood pressure does not take medication but keeps her blood pressure down by going to yoga and relaxation classes, you have a good idea that stress might be a major factor in any other ailments she may have.

Some essential oils are clearly contraindicated for clients taking particular medications. Wintergreen (*Gaultheria procumbens*) and sweet birch (*Betula lenta*) essential oils must not be applied topically to clients who are taking anticoagulants, as there have been cases of older patients hemorrhaging when synthetic methyl salicylate has been used with certain anticoagulant medications.

Stress Levels and Emotional Issues

Many massage therapists are told during their training that they should not inquire about their clients' emotional lives, and that a massage practitioner is not a counselor or a trained psychotherapist. However, aromatherapy has a strong effect on mood and emotions. It seems natural to ask clients something about their emotional life to work more effectively with them on all levels of their health, both physical and psychological. Clients generally are only too eager to talk about what is affecting them emotionally, and you might find it more of a challenge to get some people to stop talking than to open up!

If either the therapist or the client is uncomfortable with what is essentially a very private part of someone's life, you can simply say you don't need to know any specifics but that it will be easier for you to decide which essential oils to use if you have a general idea about what the client is experiencing—whether it is depression, grief, anger or irritation, frustration, anxiety, and so on. A nonthreatening way to ask about emotional issues is to inquire about how much stress they are experiencing in their life at the moment. For some reason, stress seems to be a perfectly acceptable topic of conversation, even for people who shy away from talking about emotions.

Scent Preferences

With new clients it is a good idea to ask what type of scents they like or if there are any they dislike. This is not strictly a therapeutic question; you want the client to enjoy her session as much as possible and also to use any blends you send home with her. Therefore, you want to stay away from aromas she would normally avoid or that have unpleasant memories for her. A surprising amount of people have very strong opinions about what scents they do (and do not) want to be applied to them, ranging from the very general—"no floral smells please!"—to the very specific—"I really love lavender."

You may wish to include certain clients in the process of selecting the essential oils to use in the massage. During the consultation, pick six or seven oils you consider appropriate for the issues you will be working with, and ask the client if there are any within this range that she is particularly attracted to or that she dislikes. This step is particularly relevant for relaxation massage or when a client wants to work with emotional issues, as the main mode of action in these cases is via the olfactory system to the limbic brain. The blend is primarily designed to be smelled and should therefore appeal to the client. It is not as important in blends that are meant to treat physical problems, such as an aching low back or a sprained wrist. If the remedy has the desired effect, the client will probably continue using it, no matter how it smells.

Taking A Case History

As a massage therapist, you are accustomed to charting your clients' physical problems, health history, progress, and so on, on some kind of intake form, whether a Subjective, Objective, Assessment, Plan (SOAP) chart or something simpler. It is equally important to record the aromatherapy part of your sessions, not only the extra information described above but also details of the essential oils you used, the dilution percentage, the method of application, and any results observed. This information is necessary and desirable for many reasons. The primary reason is that your client may love the smell or may obtain excellent results from the blend you made and want to have more of it. If you have not recorded the exact essential oils and amounts used, you probably will not be able to duplicate the blend by smell alone, as blends tend to change in aroma significantly, even within a few days.

Case histories should also be taken for safety reasons. If your client has an allergic reaction, either during the session or when using a take-home blend, you need to know which essential oils you used so you can avoid them in the future. Information about irritation and allergic reactions is extremely valuable because the record of published case histories on this subject is minimal. A central database wherein massage therapists and other practitioners using aromatherapy could exchange experiences of safety issues would be useful.

Good record-keeping will also remind you of how long a client has been using a particular combination of oils and when that blend should be changed, to minimize the client's risk of building up a tolerance or of having an allergic reaction. Through good record-keeping, over time you will construct an excellent database of the results obtained from specific essential oils, directly from your own experience.

Figures 13.1 and 13.2 are examples of intake forms used in aromatherapy massage treatments. Forms can be extremely simple, as in Figure 13.1, or much more comprehensive, as in Figure 13.2.

Selecting Essential Oils for Treatment

Whether or not you decide to include your client in choosing which essential oils to use in treatment, you are responsible for determining which oils are most appropriate for an individual and his or her issues. This can be challenging for a new aromatherapist. The best way to learn about the properties and effects of essential oils is to use them and observe how effective they are in various situations. Until you have a certain amount of experience doing so, selecting the best oils for your clients can be difficult.

Guidelines for Selection

Three main factors should be considered when selecting essential oils:

1. *The problem to be treated.* Massage therapists who are starting to use aromatherapy sometimes try to treat too many problems at once. While it is natural for us as healers to try to make our clients feel better, treatments are most effective if the therapist focuses on one or two main issues. Try to understand from the consultation what the most important, or most urgent, problems are, or perhaps which issues the client would most like to focus on in this particular session.

2. *The therapeutic effects of the oils.* From your basic supply, determine which essential oils would be most appropriate for this particular problem. Remember to consider not only which oils will resolve the problem quickly but also other

Confidential Client Intake Form

Name _____   Date _____

Address _____   Phone _____

E-mail address _____

Occupation _____   Date of Birth _____

Please check any of the following that apply to you:

___   High blood pressure or heart problems

___   Pregnant (if so, how many months:_____)

___   Taking medications (please list _____)

___   Currently consulting a physician (please describe health issue _____)

___   Allergies

___   Sensitive skin

___   Varicose veins

___   Digestive problems

___   Asthma or other respiratory problem

___   Eczema, dermatitis, etc.

___   Muscle or joint pain (please describe _____)

___   Any other long-term health issue (please describe _____)

How would you rate your stress level?   Low   Medium   High

Figure 13.1 A simple client intake form.

Confidential Client Intake Form

Name _____   Date _____

Address _____   Phone _____

E-mail address _____

Occupation _____   Date of Birth _____

Primary Healthcare Provider (PCP) _____   PCP phone _____

Permission to consult with healthcare provider Yes / No

Health History

Have you ever received a professional massage treatment? If yes, give frequency

_____.

Have you ever received a professional aromatherapy treatment? If yes, give frequency

_____.

Are you currently seeing a medical practitioner? (MD, chiropractor, physical therapist,

psychotherapist, etc.) Yes / No   If yes, please explain_____ .

List current medications _____.

Surgeries (year and treatment received)_____

Accidents (year and treatment received)_____

Stress level (please circle)   High   Medium   Low

Figure 13.2 A comprehensive client intake form.

Check all conditions that apply and explain.

Never   Past   Current

General

Headaches

Sleep problems

Fatigue

Infections

Fever

Depression/anxiety

Skin

Skin conditions (rash, athlete's foot, warts, other)

Allergies (scents, lotions, detergents, other)

Sensitivity (reacts easily to strong substances)

Muscles and Joints

Arthritis

Joint problems or pain

Weak or sore muscles or cramps or spasms

Spinal or disk problems

Temporomandibular joint dysfunction, jaw pain

Sprains or strains

Sciatica, nerve pain, shooting pain

Figure 13.2 (*Continued*)

Cardiovascular

Heart disease

Stroke

High or low blood pressure

Poor circulation

Blood clots

Digestion and Elimination

Bowel dysfunction

Abdominal pain

Bladder/kidney dysfunction

Endocrine System

Thyroid dysfunction

Diabetes

Reproductive System

Pregnancy

Premenstrual syndrome

Painful menses/endometriosis/fibrotic cysts

Other health concerns _____

Figure 13.2 (*Continued*)

relevant factors, such as when the remedy will be used. If a client with a respiratory infection only has time to use his blend at night, essential oils such as rosemary and eucalyptus radiata, extremely powerful respiratory oils, may not be appropriate because they are stimulants and might keep him awake, depriving him of much-needed rest.

3. *The client.* Considering a client's lifestyle, constitution, and underlying issues enables the therapist to make blends that can be fine-tuned for each person. Also, each client will like and dislike different essential oils. For example, you might think eucalyptus essential oil would be the best treatment for a client's congestion, but she might dislike the oil so much that she does not enjoy her massage and avoids using the take-home blend.

The Importance of the Client. The Swiss biochemist and aromatherapist Marguerite Maury insisted that the only effective way to treat a client was to formulate what she called an "individual prescription" for each person. "The individual mixture is designed to reflect the weaknesses and violence of an individual; it has to compensate for the deficiencies and reduce the excesses. It serves above all to normalize the rhythm of the functions."[1] Two people with the same problem, according to Maury, could not be successfully treated with the same blend of oils, as each person has a different constitution and the problem arose from different causes.

Consider two people suffering from insomnia. The first has financial concerns and lies in bed at night, worrying about how to pay the bills, her thoughts going around like a hamster in a wheel. The second is an elderly man who has just lost his wife; full of grief and loneliness, he is unable to fall asleep. The essential oils you would use for each client would be completely different. For the first client, oils such as sandalwood and frankincense, which settle the mind and calm the thoughts, would be most useful, while the second client would need oils such as rose and cypress, which help soothe the heart.

The Treatment

Once you have selected the oils to use with your client, the next thing to consider is the treatment itself. There are various options for the massage therapist who practices aromatherapy, and the problem may be too many choices in treatment modality rather than too few. Time management can become an issue for practitioners who try to complete a lot of different treatment methods in one session; it is essential to decide on the most appropriate application methods for a particular client and his issues.

Selecting a Treatment Method

The treatment method will almost certainly include massage work, and the blend you choose will probably be added to your massage oil or lotion. Aromatherapy massage differs from regular massage only in the fact that essential oils are blended into the massage lubricant. Some authorities seem to assume that aromatherapy massage is by definition a relaxation massage, with flowing strokes and mild pressure, but essential oils can enhance any form of bodywork, whether light work, deep tissue work, or treatment work. However, other treatment modalities are available to the aromatherapist, including foot baths or hand baths, steam inhalation, and diffusion.

You may choose to use none of these modalities, concentrating only on aromatic bodywork. You might use one of these techniques occasionally when it is particularly relevant, for example, a steam inhalation for someone who has a severe headache because of sinus congestion. Or you might want to include one or two with each of your massage sessions. It is completely up to the therapist to what extent he or she wishes to include different forms of aromatherapy treatment in a session.

Time Management

Managing your time during an aromatherapy massage can be challenging. You have to remember everything included in the usual routine of a massage session (consultation, case history, treatment, etc.), and you also have to decide on essential oils and make a blend (and also possibly another blend for the client to take home). Beginning aromatherapy massage students might find that out of the 75–90 minutes allotted for a session, they end up with only about 40–50 minutes of actual hands-on time. Many massage clinics allow only 60–75 minutes for a typical session, with some of that time used to prepare the room for the next client. You need to become very efficient in managing your time with aromatherapy, or massage clients will not be satisfied.

With practice, the time you will need for oil selection and blending decreases. This is the first key to successful time management of aromatherapy in a massage session: Do not try to use your essential oils professionally until you have had ample practice on friends and relatives. You will be surprised at how long this process takes the first few times, but within several sessions the routine will be much smoother and faster. However, no matter how efficient you become, an aromatherapy session will always take slightly longer than a regular massage session because of the additional questions that need to be asked and the time needed for oil selection and blending. Some aromatherapy massage practitioners will simply deduct this extra time from the hands-on part of the session, giving a massage that is perhaps 5–10 minutes shorter than the usual length. Other therapists will explain to clients that an aromatherapy massage takes slightly longer and will charge more accordingly.

Another way of managing your time more efficiently is to identify where you have small periods of spare time. For instance, I always have a few minutes free while my clients undress before the massage and then get dressed afterwards, so I use this time to do most of my blending. All my essential oils are in the massage room, so I can let clients smell them during the selection process, but my carrier oils and blending bowls are outside in a small adjoining room. When I finish the consultation, I take the essential oils we have chosen out with me while the client undresses and gets on the table, and I use this time to do the initial blending for the massage itself. At the end of the session I leave the room, having told the client to relax for a minute or two on the table before getting up slowly and getting dressed. This gives me time to make any take-home blends before the client emerges.

Thinking ahead also saves a lot of time. If you make your own appointments and a client calls to ask for an aromatherapy session, it is well worth spending a minute or two asking if she has any particular problem that might respond well to aromatherapy treatment. This gives you time to think about which essential oils may be suitable, and even to consult resources, before the client arrives for her appointment. If this is not possible, it is important to start thinking about appropriate essential oils during the consultation so that you do not get to the end of the interview and think "now what?"

Charging for Aromatherapy

If you are in practice already, you will have a scale of prices, at least for different lengths of massage, and many massage therapists also charge different rates for different techniques used. Aromatherapy requires some thought in this area because there is no standard method of charging clients. The most important factor is to make sure that at the very least you are covering the cost of the essential oils used and preferably making some profit from your blends and from any extra time spent in the session. It is essential to have a clear idea of how much your blends cost you to make, if you intend to monitor your expenses accurately. Refer to Chapter 8 for information on how to calculate the cost of a blend, and don't forget to add in the expense of any bottles and carrier oil or lotion that you use.

Blends have vastly different costs, depending on the essential oils a particular practitioner favors. Someone who prefers the moderately priced oils, such as lavender, grapefruit, fennel, and rosemary, will be making much more reasonably priced remedies than a therapist who regularly uses rose, jasmine, and chamomile. You might be surprised the first time you work out the cost of a blend; even a 2% massage blend in a 2 oz. bottle has been known to price out at over $20.00. Figuring out exactly how much a blend costs you is time-consuming, detailed work that you do not want to be doing during or after a professional massage. It is best to do several of these calculations on paper or in practice sessions with friends, to get a rough idea of your costs.

Once you have worked out your expenses, you can then decide more clearly how much to charge your clients. You want to cover your own costs and make some profit, but exactly how you do this is up to you. Some aromatherapists charge their regular rates for massage work and then add on the (approximate) cost of the blend they made, which means that one client may be paying more for an aromatherapy massage session than another. Other practitioners charge a flat rate for aromatherapy massage, reckoning that if they make less on one session because they made a very expensive blend, they will make it up in the next, when they make a much cheaper one. You might have an inclusive fee for the aromatherapy massage itself but charge extra for any take-home blends. Whatever you decide, make sure your clients clearly understand your pricing system ahead of time, perhaps explaining it when they make their appointments or before the session starts.

You may also want to decide what to charge if you get a client who doesn't want to schedule another massage yet but would like you to refill his aromatherapy blend. For these clients, I usually calculate roughly how much the blend is worth and at least double it, as I have to pay myself for the time spent blending and I also need to make some profit on the essential oils used.

SUMMARY

- The consultation with the client should cover skin sensitivity, allergies, medications, stress level, emotional issues, and scent preferences.

- Information on skin sensitivity and allergies helps the aromatherapist decide on appropriate dilution levels.

- Information about prescription medications helps the therapist assess a client's general health and avoid essential oils that are contraindicated with those medications.

- Understanding something about a client's stress level and emotional issues may influence the therapist's choice of oils, even when dealing with a physical issue.

- The client's scent preferences are important, as this may influence whether he enjoys the session or uses the take-home blends.

- Taking case histories, which record the details about each session, is important for duplicating blends later, as well as for documenting the effectiveness of the essential oils used and for stating any problems they caused for the client.

- The therapist should focus on one or two main issues when selecting essential oils for a treatment.
- Considering the client's lifestyle, constitution, and underlying problems can help determine which essential oils will be most effective.

- To manage time efficiently, the therapist should practice the aromatherapy consultation, essential oil selection, and treatment methods before using them in a professional setting.
- The price of an aromatherapy session should at least cover the cost of the essential oils used and the extra time spent on consultation and blending.

Review Questions

1. Name three areas important for an aromatherapy intake consultation that are not always covered in a standard massage intake.
2. A sensitivity to aspirin means that the practitioner should not use _____ and _____ essential oils with this client.
3. An allergy to a plant's pollen means that the client should not use the essential oil from that plant, as there is always a significant amount of pollen in the essential oil. (T / F)
4. State two reasons why it is important to take a case history.
5. What information about the essential oils should be recorded in the case history?
6. Why might two clients with the same problem be given different essential oil blends?
7. An aromatherapy massage always takes longer than a standard massage without aromatherapy, because of _____ and _____.
8. What you charge for an aromatherapy massage needs to at least cover the _____ and _____.

Notes

1. Maury M. Marguerite Maury's Guide to Aromatherapy: The Secret of Life and Youth. Essex, UK: CW Daniel, 1995:95.

14

Sending Aromatherapy Home With the Client

One of the biggest advantages of aromatherapy for a massage therapist is that treatment can be continued outside of the massage room. This is important for both acute and chronic problems. Few clients can afford to have sessions two or three times a week, even though their health would be greatly improved by doing so. However, aromatherapy massage therapists can send their clients home with a remedy that can extend the benefits of their massage session by doing such things as:

- Utilizing the "learned odor response" by using the same essential oils in a relaxation blend for both the massage session and a take-home product so that the client automatically relaxes when she smells the aroma again.

- Giving an anti-inflammatory blend to a client with an injury, to help with tissue healing and repair.

- Making up a chest rub with essential oils that help clear the respiratory system for someone with asthma who has chronic mucus in the chest.

Take-home remedies can target either physical or emotional problems, and their purpose is to continue the work done during the session. They are also useful for addressing such issues as insomnia, athlete's foot, and fear of flying, which may not be possible or appropriate to address during the massage.

Giving Remedies to the Client

There are several questions to consider when making take-home blends:

1. Which method of application will be most suitable for the client's issues? There is little point in sending home a spritzer with a client who needs a topical treatment for severe carpal tunnel syndrome, for example.

2. Which method of application is most suitable for the client's lifestyle? Extremely busy or very stressed people may have neither the time nor the energy to use a remedy that is messy, complicated, or time-consuming.

3. What dilutions will be safe and appropriate, and what instructions should be given to clients?

Applications for Home Use

The most common applications for take-home products are lotions or oils for topical application, neat blends to be used in diffusers or in steam inhalers, and spritzers. Other applications that are occasionally suitable are bath products, strong dilutions for use under compresses for acute pain, and neat blends for topical application.

Massage therapists will often give their clients blends that address the same problems that were treated during the massage session; in these cases, the essential oils in the remedies are usually the same. Sometimes the take-home blends are different from the massage session blends because they treat different problems.

Lotions and Oils. Lotions or oils with essential oils added to them are commonly given to clients for the following problems:

- Muscle or joint pain, such as carpal tunnel syndrome, arthritis, or overworked muscles.

- Skin problems, such as dermatitis or sunburn.

- Digestive issues, such as colic, irritable bowel syndrome, or constipation.

- Chest congestion or coughing.

- Varicose veins.

- Minimizing stretch marks from pregnancy.

The blend is designed to be applied by the client without any particular massage work involved. Small to moderately sized areas such as the low back, abdomen, and knees are best for this type of treatment, as the client may find it too difficult or challenging to apply the blend to much larger areas such as the entire back. Most clients prefer lotion because it tends not to stain clothes or bedding as much as oil.

Blends for Diffusers and Inhalers. Neat blends for diffusers or steam inhalers are usually given to clients to enhance emotional or mental states, or to help with respiratory difficulties. If it is a blend to relax the client, help him concentrate, or uplift his mood, then a diffuser is generally recommended. Diffusing essential oils can mean lighting an aroma lamp with a candle inside and warming essential oils and water together, or it can be as simple as putting a couple of drops of the blend onto a tissue and waving it under the nose or in front of the face. Small pottery rings that fit onto a light bulb and warm the essential oils dripped onto it are sold in many stores; you might decide to keep a stock of these to sell to clients.

Although steam inhalation is a little more trouble for the client to set up, for people with a really uncomfortable head cold or congestion in the lungs the relief is well worth the effort. This is by far the best method to loosen congestion in the respiratory system. The client places a couple of drops of the essential oil blend in a bowl of steaming water, turns her face into the steam, places a towel over her head to enclose the steam, and inhales the steaming blend.

Spritzers. Because of their simplicity and portability, spritzers are convenient take-home products. They can be carried anywhere in a purse or a pocket, they generally do not inconvenience anyone else nearby when used, and it takes only about 10 seconds to take them out and spray. For relief from stress, depression, anxiety, irritability, a foggy mind, or an inability to concentrate, spritzers are ideal.

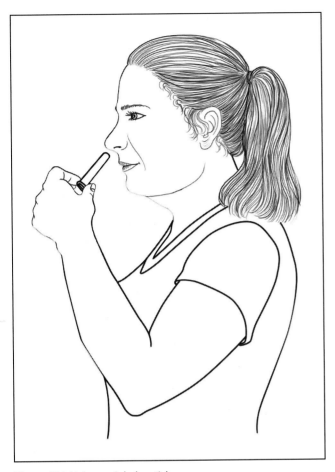

Figure 14.1 Using an inhaler stick.

Spritzers are also useful for certain types of respiratory problems, especially when triggered by stress, which is often the case with asthma, for example. The combination of a stress-relieving essential oil that also clears the chest and is possibly an antispasmodic is extremely helpful for asthmatics when they are under pressure and begin to feel their chest tightening up. Oils such as frankincense (*Boswellia carteri*) and clary sage (*Salvia sclarea*) fulfill all of these requirements.

Inhaler Sticks. Very light, portable, and easy to use, inhaler sticks are made of hard plastic with an inner cotton wick, which can be soaked in undiluted essential oils and then sealed into the tube of the inhaler. The client simply unscrews the outer shell and inhales deeply from the tube (Figure 14.1). Inhaler sticks primarily relieve sinus congestion when filled with eucalyptus, peppermint, and rosemary. They can also be used for blends to relieve stress, PMS, and anxiety. I particularly like to give inhaler sticks to clients who will be traveling by plane, as they can use their favorite essential oil remedies without disturbing their fellow passengers.

Blends for Use With Compresses. A compress is not usually a take-home remedy, but it is extremely effective for acute pain and inflammation. Typical problems that respond well to this application are recent injuries for which the client has been advised to apply ice to the area, and menstrual pain, for which many women use a hot water bottle or hot pack to ease the cramps. A fairly strong dilution (4–10% depending on the size of the area) is often used here, as the area affected is not large and the blend will simply be applied to the skin and the ice, or hot pack, placed on top.

Bath Blends. Blends designed to be used in the bath can be helpful for a range of problems, from muscle and joint pain to sunburn and other skin problems, stress, sinus and chest congestion, and headaches. Hydrotherapy, as most massage practitioners have experienced, is a powerful therapeutic tool that can easily be used by clients at home. However, few people take baths regularly, and many bathrooms contain only a shower. But for those clients who have baths and like to take them, this can be an extremely effective form of self-treatment.

I like to dilute bath blends before giving them to clients because they may prefer to skip the bother of dilution and add them directly to the bath. For most people this will not be an issue, but for those with sensitive skin, dilution in some kind of dispersant before adding the blend to the bath water is a must. Blends can be added to Epsom salts or sea salt, honey, or an unscented liquid soap, for example. Then you need to calculate how much of the carrier clients need to add to the bath water to obtain a therapeutic dose of essential oils. A therapeutic dose is usually 6–12 drops depending on the age of the client, the intensity of the essential oils used, and the problem being treated.

Neat Blends for Topical Application. Undiluted blends are used for few ailments; the most common problem is warts. Even for persistent athlete's foot, or for severe acne, it is much better to make up a blend diluted in lotion, oil, or gel because neat essential oils can cause skin irritation and they have a tendency to lead to allergic reactions if used for prolonged periods of time (see Chapter 10).

Instructions for Clients

It is very important to give clear instructions to clients about how to use their take-home remedies. Otherwise, they may not see the results they would like and they could have undesired effects from inappropriate use. When working with children, be sure to give instructions to the parents. With clients who are unable to retain or understand instructions, such as people in hospice, directions for use should be explained to a caregiver.

A Guide to Using Aromatherapy Products

Essential oils can be hazardous if used improperly. Do not ingest this blend, or put it into or near your eyes. It should be kept away from children. If any skin irritation develops, stop use immediately and contact your practitioner.

- **Lotions or oils.** Lotions or oils should be aplied in small amounts over the area you wish to treat and allowed to absorb into the skin. You do not need to do any massage on the area. If the problem is acute, such as a very painful low back, overworked muscles, or heavy chest congestion, the blend can be used several times a day. For less severe, more chronic problems, such as varicose veins or athlete's foot, you will need to apply it only once or twice a day. If you are unsure how often it is best to apply the blend, please check with your practitioner.

- **Spritzers.** Spritzers can be sprayed into the air or over the head and inhaled, but should not be sprayed directly onto the skin or into the eyes. The bottle should be shaken each time before use, because the essential oils will separate from the water. Spritzers can be used as often as you like.

- **Oil burners.** If using blends in oil burners with candles, the oils should be mixed with water, because essential oils are flammable. Place a small amount of water in the dish on top of the burner and add a few drops of essential oil. Start with about 5 drops and increase the amount if it does not seem to be enough. The amount depends on the size of your room. You can diffuse the oils for up to about 30 minutes at a time.

- **Steam inhalations.** Add 1 or 2 drops of the essential oil blend to a bowl of steaming water. (Using more will not necessarily have a greater effect, and may actually make your congestion temporarily feel worse.) Put a towel over your head and the bowl and inhale deeply for a couple of minutes. Remember to keep your eyes closed, as essential oils can irritate them. If your congestion is very uncomfortable, you can repeat this several times over the space of an hour or two. You will often get better results from short, more frequent inhalations.

- **Bath blends.** About 1 cup of bath salts, or 1/4 cup of liquid soap, is enough to give a therapeutic dose of essential oils. Make sure the salt or soap is completely dispersed in the water before you get in.

- **Ice packs.** The blend can be applied to the skin directly over the injured area, and the ice pack put immediately on top of it. This can be repeated several times a day until the condition feels better.

- **Heat packs.** The blend can be applied to the skin over the area to be treated, and the heat pack put immediately on top of it. This can be repeated several times a day until the condition feels better.

- **Neat blends.** Apply the blend directly to the wart at least once a day. Try not to touch the surrounding skin with the essential oils, because they may irritate healthy skin.

Figure 14.2 Sample take-home instructions for clients.

I try not to give more than two products to clients to take home because I have found that if they are presented with an array of remedies to use in different ways, at different times of the day, for different problems, many clients will simply give up in confusion or from lack of time and not use any of them.

Labels or typed instructions are small but important items. After a massage, most people are drowsy, slightly light-headed, or unable to concentrate. If they are taking away remedies you have made for them, it is highly unlikely they will remember clearly any instructions for use, so it is best to write these down. The most convenient method for clients is neatly written (or typed) instructions on a label stuck directly onto the container.

However, writing labels can be somewhat time-consuming for a busy practitioner who is expecting her next client any moment, so a good alternative is to type up a list of general instructions on how to use all the home remedies and hand one of these to every client who receives a blend. The instructions can be simple, clearly stating how to use the blend, together with recommendations for dosage and frequency of use. Massage therapists are not medical practitioners, so it should be emphasized to clients that these written instructions are a guide to safe and effective use, not a prescription of any kind. Figure 14.2 presents a suggested set of instructions for clients.

SUMMARY

- Blends for the client to take home help continue the effects of the massage session; they can also treat problems that cannot appropriately be treated during the session.
- The method of application should suit both the problem being addressed and the client's lifestyle.
- Aromatic lotions or oils are suitable for issues involving muscles and joints, skin, digestion, and the respiratory system.
- Blends for diffusers are suitable to help with mental or emotional states.
- Blends for steam inhalation are suitable for respiratory problems.
- Spritzers are suitable for treating stress, emotional issues, and difficulty with concentration.
- Inhaler sticks are suitable to help relieve sinus congestion, stress, and emotional issues.

- Blends for compresses are typically used for acute injuries (cold compress or ice) or menstrual cramping (heat packs).
- Bath blends are suitable for a wide range of problems, including muscle and joint pain, skin problems, stress, sinus and chest congestion, and headaches. Blends should be diluted in salts, honey, or liquid soap before being given to clients.
- Neat blends for topical application are rarely given, as diluted blends are generally safer for longer-term use.
- Instructions for use should be clear and preferably written. Limit the amount of take-home products that you give your clients, as they might not use them if they are given too many.
- Printed instruction sheets, with guidelines for dosage and frequency of use, save time for the therapist.

Review Questions

1. Give two examples of how the effects of a massage can be extended by giving clients a blend to take home.
2. Give two examples of problems that could be addressed with an aromatherapy take-home blend but would probably not be treated during a massage session.
3. Bath blends are not suitable for many people because: (a) most people do not use them correctly, (b) many people do not like to take baths, (c) they are not suitable for many problems.
4. Oils or lotions with essential oils are usually given to the client to treat large areas of the body, such as the entire back. (T/F)
5. Neat blends for diffusion can be used with a _____, or a few drops can simply be placed on a(n) _____ and waved under the nose.
6. Spritzers are popular take-home items because they are: (a) cheap, (b) effective for muscular pain, (c) easy to use and to carry.
7. Why are neat blends not typically given to clients?
8. Take-home blends are usually limited to one or two because: (a) clients will not use any remedies at all if given too many, (b) more than two remedies cancel each other out and are ineffective, (c) it becomes too costly for the therapist.
9. Instructions to clients for use of the blends should include _____, and _____, and _____.

15

Stress

The alarm clock shocks you awake in the morning. You grab a quick shower, eat something in a hurry, and head out the door to work. There has been an accident on the highway, so the traffic crawls for about 20 minutes while you phone work to tell them you might be late. Just as you start to speed up, you notice a truck changing lanes almost on top of you, so you slam on the brakes. You avoid the truck and realize your heart is beating painfully fast, you're panting for breath, and your hasty breakfast is making you feel slightly nauseous. It's only 8 o'clock in the morning and you are stressed already.

What Is Stress?

There is no strict or simple definition of stress. **Stress** is a reaction to a set of circumstances, rather than an illness or even a syndrome. In fact, anything that affects the body's homeostasis could be regarded as stressful. A recent *New York Times* article stated, "The stress response evolved as the body's way of identifying potential threats, deciding how to respond and remembering where and when the danger occurred."[1] In other words, the stress response is a survival mechanism that protects the body against threat, whether real or imagined. It involves complex mechanisms in many systems that temporarily increase physical strength and alertness. All these mechanisms and processes are integrated by the nervous system.

Stress is generating a lot of interest these days. There are television shows and self-help books on how to cut down on the stress in our lives, and legions of therapists and clinics are devoted to helping us manage it. Physicians talk about its harmful effects on the body and implicate stress in a long list of health problems, including high blood pressure, heart disease, asthma, and degenerative diseases such as arthritis. Life has always been stressful—wars, famine, epidemics, and natural disasters have devastated most countries at some point in history—but our modern lives are stressful in a unique way. They are faster changing and more hectic than at almost any other time in history. We seem to talk faster, eat faster, drive faster, and do more things all at the same time than ever before.

Stress is almost always regarded as harmful, yet evidence shows that we cannot be healthy without a certain amount of stress in our lives. This is well established in medical circles on a physical level. Broken legs are no longer put in plaster for weeks on end; instead, the patient is encouraged to walk as soon as possible because the bone will heal faster and get stronger as a result of the pressure put on it. Menopausal women are strongly encouraged to do weight-bearing exercise because the physical stress is known to increase bone density. On an emotional level, a life with no stress at all may have us literally dying of boredom and not getting very much done. In moderation, stress can actually be beneficial, often showing up as excitement and leading to a sense of achievement when we are tested under pressure. In the words of bodywork practitioner Deane Juhan:

If we are unwilling or unable to tolerate certain levels of stress—occasionally even high levels—we are probably not going to get very much accomplished in our lives. Life and work are often inherently stressful. But on the other hand, if we overload ourselves with stress in an unrelenting effort towards more and more achievements, we can literally die trying, and quite prematurely at that.[2]

Some people are more suited to today's fast-paced lifestyle than others. They thrive on the excitement of a long and demanding workday and can't wait to start again tomorrow. Others may be unable to cope even with a much less hectic workload; they become overwhelmed and depend on tranquilizers and antidepressants to get through their day. It is obvious that stress cannot be measured objectively; it is experienced individually, which is why popular quizzes entitled "How stressed are you?" cannot be really effective at assessing the amount of stress a person is handling.

The Effects of Stress

The body has certain strategies to deal with severe short-term stress or with moderate stress for longer periods. Although these responses function to protect the body, if very stressful conditions continue for too long, the effects of the body's coping mechanisms can ultimately be extremely harmful, both psychologically and physically. Illnesses resulting from stress have been recognized for thousands of years. An ancient Chinese text, *The Yellow Emperor's Classic of Internal Medicine*, dating back at least 3000 years, comments that "grief, calamity and evil cause inner bitterness."[3]

Hans Selye, an endocrinologist working in the mid-1930s, is recognized as the first scientific investigator to develop a coherent theory of how the body responds to stress, which he called the **general adaptation syndrome (GAS).**[4] According to Selye, there are three stages in the GAS stress reaction, with increasingly serious symptoms:

1. *Alarm.* This is an immediate, short-term reaction to a crisis.
2. *Adaptation.* If a crisis continues for more than a few hours, longer-term metabolic adjustments start to occur.
3. *Exhaustion.* Vital systems start to collapse.

Alarm: The Short-Term Effects
We see the effects of the alarm reaction of the GAS most clearly when something happens to shock us—for example, the truck veering toward you on the highway. This is the activation of the sympathetic nervous system, often termed the **fight-or-flight response.** In the brain, the limbic system is involved in the recognition of fear and signals to the hypothalamus that action needs to be taken. The hypothalamus

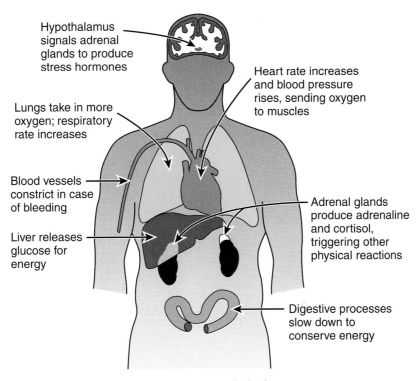

Hypothalamus signals adrenal glands to produce stress hormones

Heart rate increases and blood pressure rises, sending oxygen to muscles

Lungs take in more oxygen; respiratory rate increases

Blood vessels constrict in case of bleeding

Adrenal glands produce adrenaline and cortisol, triggering other physical reactions

Liver releases glucose for energy

Digestive processes slow down to conserve energy

Figure 15.1 The immediate effects of stress on the body.

releases hormones to alert the pituitary, which in turn signals the adrenal cortex to produce the stress hormones **adrenaline** and **cortisol,** which are pumped into the bloodstream, initiating a cascade of responses:

- Heart rate increases and blood pressure rises.
- Respiratory rate increases.
- Energy is released quickly in the form of stored sugars.
- The digestive system temporarily slows down.

These are only the most obvious effects, and every part of the body is affected strongly (Figure 15.1).

Adaptation and Exhaustion: The Long-Term Effects

The same mechanisms that give us the energy and alertness to deal with danger in an immediate situation can themselves be dangerous if left to continue for too long. Selye observed that the stage of adaptation following the immediate shock is characterized by increased adrenal activity, gastrointestinal ulceration, and atrophy of the thymus gland and lymphatic system. If prolonged, this can lead to exhaustion and even death.[5] In fact, prolonged stress has been shown in both laboratory experiments and clinical observations to lead to hypertension,[6] coronary heart disease, diabetes,[7] exhaustion,[8] irritable bowel syndrome,[9] lowered immune functioning, skin problems,[10] depression, and other psychological issues and has been implicated in many more health problems, including postoperative complications.[11]

Managing Stress

Stress is multidimensional in that it affects the body, the mind, and the emotions. However, because of its multifaceted nature, concentrating on any one of these areas can help break the cycle of the stress response. A modality such as aromatherapy massage, which positively affects both the physical body and the mind, seems to be an ideal way to treat stress-related conditions. The main ways aromatherapy can be used to improve a person's ability to manage chronic stress are in:

- Alleviating the symptoms, or the effects, of stress, giving the client a higher level of comfort and energy
- Reducing stress levels themselves, by improving mood and emotions
- Increasing resistance to stress by strengthening the nervous system and the immune system

Alleviating the Symptoms

When we think of someone who is under a great deal of stress, we tend to imagine a person who is obviously anxious, nervous, and moving quickly. Especially at the beginning of a period of heightened stress for such a person, the sedative, relaxing essential oils such as lavender (*Lavandula angustifolia*), mandarin (*Citrus reticulata*), Roman chamomile (*Chamaemelum nobile*), and ylang ylang (*Cananga odorata*) come to mind readily. This kind of client needs to slow down, at least temporarily, to move out of sympathetic nervous system functioning and conserve energy. Relaxation is one of the most effective remedies for stress-related problems. Both touch, in the form of massage, and aromatherapy can influence the heart rate and blood pressure, deepen breathing, and relax the whole body.

Aromatherapy can increase the length of time relaxation lasts when blends are given to the client as take-home remedies. Using aromatherapy at home can lead to a more balanced way of being in everyday life. To establish healthier patterns of nervous system functioning, a client may be given more than one remedy—a blend of calming yet uplifting essential oils, such as the citruses, for use in the morning and an evening blend of sedative oils such as Roman chamomile and lavender.

For people who have been experiencing an extended period of stress, the most common symptom is extreme tiredness, or even exhaustion; this is popularly known as **adrenal burnout.** Unlike our first example of someone who is entering a particularly stressful period, what Selye would call the alarm stage of the GAS, this client has been there for some time and is in either the adaptation or the exhaustion stage of the stress response. He appears quite different; he may look tired and move in a slow, lethargic manner, and he will probably complain of feeling worn out or drained. Both massage and aromatherapy in this case will be designed to relax but also to strengthen the system, which has been under strain for so long. Tonic, or strengthening, essential oils such as rosemary (*Rosmarinus officinalis*), black spruce (*Picea mariana*), and ginger (*Zingiber officinale*) might be more useful for such a client, to promote energy and boost mood and confidence.

This second client may also have a whole set of symptoms, such as digestive pain and spasm, headaches or other types of pain, constant colds or flu, tight muscles, or high blood pressure. These can all be treated symptomatically, and essential oils for these problems are explored in later chapters on the relevant body systems involved. Reducing the symptoms in stress-related conditions can change the client's experience of his or her situation so dramatically that the problem itself starts to be resolved. For example, one frequent result of chronic stress is insomnia. After long stretches of not sleeping, the tiredness and grogginess the client experiences makes her entire situation appear more daunting than it actually is. If she begins to sleep longer and more regularly, not only will she be less depressed about her situation, but she may also have the extra energy required to deal with and resolve it.

Reducing Stress Levels

It may seem that the only way to reduce the effects or symptoms of stress in a person's life is to remove the cause of the stress itself. However, this may be either extremely difficult or even impossible for most people because a lot of stress arises

---

CASE STUDY 15.1

Adrenal Burnout

Ms. R. was a 34-year-old massage therapist, seeing 20 to 25 clients per week, studying part time, and looking after her young child. She had been feeling very fatigued for about a month in spite of sleeping heavily for at least 8 hours a night. She complained of waking up exhausted and feeling that she could barely drag herself through her workday. She had no other symptoms except for generalized slight anxiety and irritability. She craved sugar and soft drinks. We discussed using aromatherapy to help with her feelings of tiredness and being overwhelmed and she was willing to use the remedies regularly on her own. The following blend of essential oils was used in a back massage, and she was given a bottle with the same blend to rub over her adrenal area at home every morning. The blend was made up in 2 oz. of carrier oil, making about a 4% dilution:

Black spruce (*Picea mariana*), 20 drops: adrenal support, immune support

Pine (*Pinus sylvestris*), 10 drops: adrenal support, immune support

Geranium (*Pelargonium graveolens*), 10 drops: adrenal support, mental stimulant

Bergamot (*Citrus x bergamia*), 10 drops: antidepressant, appetite balancer

Ms. R. returned in 2 weeks for another massage, using the same blend, and reported that she was feeling more alert in the mornings and had slightly more energy. She still craved sugar and soft drinks, but was eating better in general. Four weeks later, she phoned to say that her energy had returned almost completely and that she had managed to work a full week without feeling exhausted by the end of it. She had purchased some different essential oils to use in a diffuser to try to avoid getting overstressed and therefore overtired. She was still using the original blend, but only on occasional mornings when she felt less energized than usual.

---

from life situations that may be unavoidable. An interesting point already mentioned is that the experience of stress is an individual one; in other words, it is not the circumstances that create stress but our individual reactions to those circumstances that determine how we are affected. Anything that can help us steer our attitudes in a more positive direction will also help reduce the actual stress we are experiencing.

The Pleasure Response. When the body has a pleasurable sensation, it responds by producing a group of chemicals called **endorphins.** The body's own natural opiates, endorphins reduce pain and increase feelings of well-being. According to Candace Pert, a leading researcher in brain chemistry, endorphins are released when a person is engaged in any activity that is enjoyable, such as physical exercise, laughter, or sex. In her book *Molecules of Emotion*, she speculates that stress may possibly slow down the free flow of these essential chemicals, leading to a situation in which "the largely autonomic processes that are regulated by peptide flow, such as breathing, blood flow, immunity, digestion, and elimination, collapse down to a few simple feedback loops and upset the normal healing response."[12]

Helping the endorphins flow again may restart the healing process. One person who experienced this very directly is Norman Cousins. He used the power of laughter in his fight to recover from a crippling disease. In his book *Anatomy of an Illness*, he explains: "I made the joyous discovery that ten minutes of genuine belly laughter had an anesthetic effect and would give me at least two hours of pain-free sleep."[13]

Essential oils provide one of the quickest and easiest routes to a pleasurable experience. I have had the experience many times of watching people as they pick up a bottle of essential oil at a talk or a workshop and inhale the contents. Almost always their faces relax, a smile appears, and they say something like, "Oh, that's lovely!" This is a pure, simple enjoyment of a basic sensory experience that is very easy to achieve with aromatherapy. Some studies show that pleasing aromas are more effective in reducing pain or depression when compared with odors that are perceived as unpleasant.[14]

Strengthening the Nervous and Immune Systems

The nervous system and immune system both are immediately affected by stress. Brain chemistry changes, white blood cell levels decrease, and the body is more at risk of infection, which in turn will create more stress. Certain essential oils are regarded in aromatherapy as having a tonic effect on the body as a whole, and on these systems in particular. One study showed that long-term inhalation of lemon and oakmoss restored immune functioning in mice after it was suppressed as a result of stress.[15] Mice are often used for laboratory testing because their immune systems are similar to those of humans.

Immunostimulants: tea tree (*Melaleuca alternifolia*), eucalyptus (*Eucalyptus globulus* or *radiata*), ravensara (*Ravensara aromatica*), niaouli (*Melaleuca quinquinervia viridiflora*), bay laurel (*Laurus nobilis*), lemon (*Citrus limon*), other citruses.

Neurotonics: basil (*Ocimum basilicum*), black spruce (*Picea mariana*), pine (*Pinus sylvestris*), neroli (*Citrus aurantium* var. *amara*), marjoram (*Origanum majorana*).

Specific Problems Related to Stress

Various health problems have been directly or indirectly attributed to the amount of stress we experience in our lives. In other words, the ailments are directly caused, or worsened, or have various symptoms triggered by stress. Most of these problems and the ways in which aromatherapists can address them are discussed in the body systems chapters (Chapters 16–24). However, some stress-related problems do not correspond clearly to any one system, and these are discussed in depth here.

Insomnia

Causes and Symptoms. A lack of sleep is regarded as both a result and a cause of stress. In daily life, many people try to sleep less and do more, taking herbal supplements, prescription medication, or caffeine in an effort to stay awake. Whether they have insomnia or are deliberately depriving themselves of sleep, the results are the same. A short-term lack of sleep can make a person groggy, unable to concentrate, depressed, and irritable. Long-term insomnia can have serious health implications. According to Dr. Kavey, director of the Sleep Disorders Center at Columbia Presbyterian Medical Center in New York, sleep affects performance, blood pressure, heart rate, insulin levels, and various hormone secretions.[16]

Essential Oils. Many essential oils have been shown to have sedative or calming effects, promoting natural, restful sleep. Lavender (*Lavandula angustifolia*) has been the most extensively researched, and is a good general **soporific,** or sleep enhancer, that appears to help with sleeplessness no matter what the cause.[17] Another study found bitter orange (*Citrus aurantium* var. *amara*) essential oil to be especially effective, increasing sleeping time significantly and making it easier for subjects to sleep even under conditions of mental stress.[18]

In addition to addressing only the symptom, it is even more effective to look into the issues underlying insomnia and to choose the most appropriate essential oil for the problem. Frankincense (*Boswellia carteri*) is reputed to calm the mental processes and can be useful for clients who lie awake for hours with their mind racing. Mandarin (*Citrus reticulata*) and neroli (*Citrus aurantium* var. *amara*) are often used for worry and anxiety, which can cause insomnia, while marjoram (*Origanum majorana*) seems to be effective for those who are too tired to sleep, tense yet exhausted. Rose (*Rosa damascena*) is extremely useful for insomnia caused by emotional upset.

Methods of Application. The most effective way to use the oils for sleep is in some form of inhalation just before bedtime. Methods include a few drops of an essential oil in a bath or in a diffuser of some kind. The simplest method is placing a few drops on a tissue and tucking the tissue under the pillow or in the bed sheets.

Chronic Pain

Causes and Symptoms. It may seem strange to include pain in a section on stress, but research shows that stress sensitizes us to pain, making it feel more intense. Chronic pain can itself be emotionally stressful, leading to a vicious cycle of pain-stress-pain. Like stress, pain is a subjective experience, with no objective way to measure how severe it is. Many hospitals use a scale for pain from 0 to 10, with 0 representing a pain-free state and 10 being unbearable. Patients assess their own pain, and painkillers are generally prescribed for a score of 3 and above. Chronic pain can lead to significant physical, emotional, and social dysfunction, with depression, anxiety, sleep deprivation, and inability to work being among the effects.

Essential Oils. The ability of aromatherapy to access the parasympathetic nervous system makes it helpful in easing chronic pain. The pleasure of the aroma and the relaxation induced by both the essential oils and gentle touch therapies can enable clients to change their pain perception, even without addressing the original cause of the pain. Essential oils with analgesic properties are particularly helpful in dealing with chronic pain. One study confirmed that "a significant analgesic effect with reduction in sensitivity to headache was produced by peppermint oil."[19] Another showed analgesic effects from three different species of eucalyptus (*E. globulus, E. citriodora,* and *E. tereticornis*).[20]

Other essential oils frequently used in aromatherapy for their pain-relieving effects include clove bud (*Syzygium aromaticum*), sweet birch (*Betula lenta*), wintergreen (*Gaultheria procumbens*), lavender (*Lavandula angustifolia*), spike lavender (*Lavandula latifolia*), nutmeg (*Myristica fragrans*), and myrrh (*Commiphora myrrha*). The calming and sedative oils are also helpful for chronic pain.

Methods of Application. Methods of application vary for pain, depending on the severity and location. Gentle touch almost always has a beneficial effect, and light massage with essential oils is frequently used. Some clients may respond better to warmth, with essential oils added to foot baths or used under warm compresses. Using the essential oils in diffusion may provide enough of a pleasant distraction to break the pain-stress-pain cycle.

Emotional Issues

Causes and Symptoms. A person who is under stress for a period of time will frequently show some form of psychological distress, with anxiety, irritability, and depression being common states. The inability to cope with a hectic lifestyle has led to a growing number of people taking antidepressant medications. Of course, emotional ups and downs are a part of life, but under continued stress a person may find it difficult or impossible to move out of a particular emotional state.

Essential Oils. One study on the effects of citrus fragrances shows that they can be particularly useful in helping with depressive states. The researchers made a blend of lemon, orange, and bergamot oils with cis-4-hexanol, and exposed a group of depressed male inpatients to the fragrance, while reducing their antidepressant medication gradually. Most of the patients inhaling the citruses reduced their antidepressant drug intake to zero by the end of 11 weeks, and their cortisol and dopamine (another important brain chemical) levels were also significantly lower than the levels in a control group. The report stated that "citrus fragrance may improve the homeostatic balance more than treatment with antidepressants."[21] Citrus essential oils are frequently used in aromatherapy work to help with depression and other emotional states, as they are regarded as both uplifting and emotionally balancing.

Other essential oils that are often named in aromatherapy books or scientific studies as useful for depression include frankincense (*Boswellia carteri*), fennel (*Foeniculum vulgare*),[22] basil (*Ocimum basilicum*), geranium (*Pelargonium graveolens*), rose (*Rosa centifolia* or *R. damascena*), marjoram (*Origanum majorana*), and ylang ylang (*Cananga odorata*).

Fragrances have also been shown as useful for relieving states of anxiety. One study diffused heliotropin (a vanilla-like scent) to reduce anxiety during magnetic resonance imaging (MRI), a process many people find claustrophobic, producing panic attacks in some patients. A decrease of 63% in average anxiety was recorded, using a visual analog scale.[23] Another study found lavender to be **anxiolytic,** or anxiety-reducing, and reported that "aromatherapy was found to produce favorable psychological effects in dialysis patients without the side effects associated with pharmacotherapy."[24] Other oils commonly used for anxiety in aromatherapy include neroli (*Cananga odorata*), petitgrain (*Citrus aurantium* var. *amara*), bergamot (*Citrus x bergamia*), basil (*Ocimum basilicum*), marjoram (*Origanum majorana*), cypress (*Cupressus sempervirens*), and ylang ylang (*Cananga odorata*).

Another emotional state often found in people under stress is anger or irritability. Neither has been thoroughly researched, presumably because as an emotion anger or irritability does not tend to last as long as depression or anxiety and is more difficult to analyze. However, several essential oils are frequently recommended in aromatherapy to reduce anger, including bergamot (*Citrus x bergamia*), mandarin (*Citrus reticulata*), Roman chamomile (*Chamaemelum nobile*), lavender (*Lavandula angustifolia*), and frankincense (*Boswellia carteri*).

Panic Attacks

Mr. B. was a professional man in his late thirties. He had recently broken up with his girlfriend and was worried about his visitation rights to their infant son. He had also recently started his own business and had concerns about money. He was not sleeping well and had lost some weight. He had his first panic attack on vacation at the beach. He started hyperventilating, his heart rate increased significantly, and he felt tightness in his chest. He started to sweat and felt nauseous. He assumed he was having a heart attack and went to the emergency section of the hospital, where they assured him that there was no problem with his heart. Since that episode, he had three further panic attacks within 4 months.

It seemed most important to decrease the levels of stress in Mr. B.'s life. He agreed to have weekly relaxation massages, in which the following blend was used. The blend was made up in 2 oz. of carrier oil, making about a 1.5% dilution:

Lavender (*Lavandula angustifolia*), 5 drops: anxiolytic, sedative

Neroli (*Citrus aurantium* var *amara*), 4 drops: anxiolytic, sedative

Cardamon (*Elettaria cardamomum*), 5 drops: antidepressant, appetite stimulant

Cypress (*Cupressus sempervirens*), 3 drops: nervine, promotes acceptance of change

Marjoram (*Origanum majorana*), 3 drops: hypotensive, helps with grief

Mr. B. also received a spritzer with the same oils to use in the evening after work and before bedtime to promote restful sleep. He reported one panic attack in the 3 weeks following the initial session, but of shorter duration. Since then he has had no episodes and uses varying blends of anxiolytic, sedative essential oils to help him relax in the evenings, to sleep, and to remain calm during particularly upsetting times.

Methods of Application. For emotional issues, some form of diffusion is generally used, as essential oils affect mood and emotion by influencing the brain via the olfactory system. However, since massage therapy also positively affects mood, aromatherapy massage would be an excellent application method.

Unhealthy Coping Behaviors

Causes and Symptoms. People under stress find many strategies to help them cope, including smoking, overeating, drinking alcohol, excessively consuming caffeine, or taking recreational or prescription drugs. These coping mechanisms may not cause any problems when used in moderation and for a short time, but over the longer term they can lead to addiction, social withdrawal, weight gain or loss, and a long list of health problems.

Overeating and obesity are subjects of great concern to medical practitioners, as approximately 60% of the population in the United States is currently estimated to be overweight. Obesity is an extremely complex problem, with factors including genetics, environment, and exercise, as well as diet, and for most people there is probably no single remedy.

Essential Oils. Aromatherapy may help people avoid unhealthy coping behaviors in the first place, as a direct result of alleviating the emotions and symptoms associated with stress. Some studies suggest that essential oils may help people reduce their dependency on addictive substances, such as tobacco. One trial used an inhaler device with black pepper to lessen the cravings for cigarettes, and researchers stated that "reported cravings for cigarettes was significantly reduced. . . . In addition, negative affect and somatic [physical] symptoms of anxiety were alleviated."[25] Another study reported simply that sniffing either a pleasant or an unpleasant odor reduced the urge to smoke.[26] In my practice, I have had considerable success using frankincense (*Boswellia carteri*) to help clients who wish to stop smoking. Frankincense is named in several aromatherapy sources as being helpful in breaking unhealthy attachments to the past.

With regard to overeating, researchers have become interested in the connections between taste, smell, and appetite. At the Smell and Taste Treatment and Research Foundation in Chicago, the effects of odor on weight loss are being studied. The neurologist and psychiatrist Alan Hirsch has written a self-help book based on his research using mint-, apple-, and banana-flavored inhalers.[27] Essential oils traditionally used in aromatherapy to lessen food cravings include peppermint (*Mentha piperita*), the citruses, especially lemon (*Citrus limon*) and bergamot (*Citrus x bergamia*), rosemary CT verbenone (*Rosmarinus officinalis* CT verbenone), and fennel (*Foeniculum vulgare*).

Methods of Application. Aromatherapy massage is an excellent form of treatment because of its highly relaxing nature. However, clients should be given a take-home blend, either a spritzer or an inhaler stick, they can use whenever they experience cravings. Hirsch reported that the best results for weight loss in his studies were found with participants who used an aromatic inhaler device up to 250 times per day.[28]

SUMMARY

- Stress is a reaction to circumstances that are perceived as threatening in some way. The effects involve complex mechanisms in many body systems, coordinated by the nervous system.

- Stress can be both healthful and harmful. Beneficial stress can create excitement and a feeling of challenge; in the case of physical stress, it can strengthen the body.

- Three stages have been identified in the stress response: alarm, adaptation, and exhaustion.

- The alarm stage is short-term and includes the release of adrenaline and cortisol, which increase heart rate and pressure, respiration rate, and blood sugar levels, and decrease digestive processes.

- The adaptation and exhaustion stages are responses to long-term stress and include increased adrenal activity and lowered immune functioning. Many chronic health problems are linked to these stages.

- Aromatherapy can help clients under stress by alleviating the symptoms of stress, reducing stress levels by improving mood and emotions and by strengthening the nervous and immune systems.

- Increasing pleasurable sensations, such as by inhaling essential oils, can encourage the body to produce endorphins, the body's own natural painkillers and antidepressants.

- Some health problems directly caused by stress have been shown to be relieved by aromatherapy, including insomnia, chronic pain, anxiety, depression, and cravings of all kinds.

Review Questions

1. The stress response is a reaction by the _____ system to a threatening situation.
2. Stress is always harmful because it disrupts homeostasis. (T/F)
3. The alarm stage of the stress response involves the release of hormones from which three glands?
4. Adrenaline and cortisol raise _____, _____, and _____ and depress _____.
5. Give three examples of essential oils that lower short-term stress by relaxing the sympathetic nervous system.
6. Give three examples of essential oils that are strengthening for a client who is feeling exhausted after a long period of stress.
7. Pleasant scents may help stimulate the production in the brain of _____, which are the body's own painkillers and antidepressants.
8. To be most effective for insomnia, essential oils should be used as a(n) _____, just before _____.
9. One group of essential oils is particularly helpful in working with depression: (a) the woods, (b) the citruses, (c) the roots, (d) the seeds.
10. Oils with _____ properties are most useful in directly dealing with chronic pain. Relaxing essential oils can help to access the _____ nervous system, which can alter pain perception.
11. Why should clients using essential oils to help with cravings be given a take-home blend?

Notes

1. Goode E. The heavy cost of chronic stress. New York Times, Science section, December 17, 2002:D1.
2. Juhan D. Job's Body. New York: Station Hill Press, 1987:302.
3. Veith I. The Yellow Emperor's Classic of Internal Medicine. Berkeley, Los Angeles: University of California Press, 1972:149.
4. Selye H. The Stress of Life. New York: McGraw Hill, 1956.
5. Griffin JF, Thomson AJ. Farmed deer: a large animal model for stress. Domest Anim Endocrinol 1998;15(5):445–456.
6. Raikkonen K, Hautanen A, Keltikangas-Jarvinen L. Feelings of exhaustion, emotional distress, and pituitary and adrenocortical hormones in borderline hypertension. J Hypertens 1996;14(6):713–718.
7. Keltkangas-Jarvinen L, Ravaja N, Raikkonen K, et al. Relationships between the pituitary-adrenal hormones, insulin, and glucose in middle-aged men: moderating influence of psychosocial stress. Metabolism 1998;47(12):1440–1449.
8. Patacchioli FR, Angelucci L, Dellerba G, et al. Actual stress, psychopathology and salivary cortisol levels in the irritable bowel syndrome (IBS). J Endocrinol Invest 2001;24(3):173–177.
9. Berezi I. The stress concept and neuroimmunoregulation in modern biology. Ann NY Acad Sci 1998;851:3–12.
10. Consoli S. Skin and stress. Pathologie-biologie 1996;44(10):875–881.
11. Genzdilov AV, Alexandrin GP, Simonov NN, et al. The role of stress factors in the postoperative course of patients with rectal cancer. J Surg Oncol 1977;9(5):517–523.

12. Pert C. Molecules of Emotion. New York: Scribner, 1997:243.
13. Cousins N. Anatomy of an Illness. New York: Bantam Books Inc., 1981:39.
14. Marchand S, Arsenault P. Odours modulate pain perception. A gender specific effect. Physiol Behav 2002;76:251–256.
15. Fujiwara R, Komori T, Noda Y, et al. Effects of a long-term inhalation of fragrances on the stress-induced immunosuppression in mice. Neuroimmunomodulation 1998;5(6):318–322.
16. O'Connor A. Wakefulness finds a powerful ally. *New York Times* June 29, 2004:D1.
17. Hardy M, Kird-Smith MD, Stretch DD. Replacement of drug treatment for insomnia by ambient odor. Lancet 1995;346:701.
18. Miyake Y, Nakagawa M, Asakura Y. Effects of odours on humans (I). Effects on sleep latency. Chem Senses 1991;16:183.
19. Gobel H, Schmidt G, Soyka D. Effect of peppermint and eucalyptus oil preparations on neurophysiological and experimental algesimetric headache parameters. Cephalalgia 1994;14:228–234.
20. Silva J, Abebe W, et al. Analgesic and anti-inflammatory effects of the essential oils of Eucalyptus. Journal of Ethnopharmacology, 2003, Issue 89, pp. 277–283.
21. Komori T, Fujiwara R, Tanida M, et al. Effects of citrus fragrance on immune function and depressive states. Neuroimmunomodulation 1995;2:174–180.
22. Nagai H, Nakagawa M, Fujii W, et al. Effects of odors on humans (II). Reducing effects of mental stress and fatigue. Chem Senses 1991;16:198.
23. Redd WH, Manne SL, Peters B, et al. Fragrance administration to reduce anxiety during MR imaging. J Magn Reson Imaging 1994;4:623–626.
24. Itai T, Amayasu H, Kuribayashi M, et al. Psychological effects of aromatherapy on chronic hemodialysis patients. Psychiatry Clin Neurosci 2000;54:393–397.
25. Rose JE, Behm FM. Inhalation of vapor from black pepper extract reduces smoking withdrawal symptoms. Drug Alcohol Depend 1994;34(3):225–229.
26. Sayette MA, Parrott DJ. Effect of olfactory stimuli on urge reduction in smokers. Experiential Clin Psychopharmacol 1999;7(2):151–159.
27. Hirsch A. Dr Hirsch's Guide to Scentsational Weight Loss. Rockport, MA: Element Books, 1997.
28. Hirsch A. Dr Hirsch's Guide to Scentsational Weight Loss. Rockport, MA: Element Books, 1997:36.

16

The Musculoskeletal System

Our musculoskeletal system gives us our shape, protects our internal organs, and enables us to move. It is extremely resilient, putting up with hours of sitting, repetitive work, extreme sports, or plain inactivity. But when we have a problem with our muscles or bones or joints, it is difficult, if not impossible, to ignore. Every movement we make seems to worsen the pain, and it is hard to find a comfortable position.

Most clients come to a massage therapist's office because they have some form of soft tissue problem and they have heard that massage is an especially good treatment. Aromatherapy combines well with massage for musculoskeletal problems. It is remarkably effective for muscular and joint problems, often providing quick relief from pain and inflammation.

An Overview of the Musculoskeletal System

The musculoskeletal system is composed of muscles and connective tissues: bones, ligaments, tendons, and fascia (Figure 16.1). Bone is one of the hardest tissues in the body. It possesses both toughness and resilience to stand up to the pressures and minor accidents of everyday life. Our bony skeleton provides a framework for soft tissues, protects the internal organs, and stores minerals, especially calcium. Red bone marrow produces blood cells. Bones also provide attachment sites for muscles and tendons. When muscles contract, the joints provide levers to move the entire body. Bones are joined to each other by ligaments, and joints are stabilized by ligaments.

Although the body has three types of muscle, our focus here is skeletal muscle, which we can move voluntarily. It can contract rapidly and with a significant amount of force. Skeletal muscles are attached to bones by tendons, tough tissues made up largely of collagen fibers. Muscles give shape and stability to the body and work together to move the bones. They also provide warmth as a by-product of movement.

Fascia, or fascial tissue, covers the entire body at the level of the muscles. It holds the muscles together, divides them into working groups, and provides a space for nerve, blood, and lymph vessels. It also prevents heat loss and stores water and fat.

Risk Factors

Factors that have a negative effect on the musculoskeletal system include:

- *Lack of exercise.* Inactivity leads to weakness and atrophy of the muscles, making injury more likely. It also leads to a loss of bone strength.

- *Smoking.* Smoking cuts down significantly on oxygen intake, thereby slowing the tissue healing process.

- *Poor nutrition.* Improper diet can result in weakness in the muscles, or a loss of minerals from the bones, leading to osteoporosis.

- *Inadequate hydration.* A lack of water leads to toxin buildup in the muscles.

- *Poor posture or body mechanics.* Incorrect posture or alignment places stress on particular structures, making them more prone to injury.

How Aromatherapy Affects the Musculoskeletal System

Essential oils permeate the skin and can affect underlying muscles and other tissues. This is regarded in aromatherapy as a local effect, because the best results occur when the essential oils are applied directly over the affected area. Some essential oils are cooling and anti-inflammatory, ideal for acute inflammation in any form. Others warm the tissue and increase blood flow to the area, but because they suppress hormones usually released by the body when trauma occurs, they are also classed as anti-inflammatory and work well for chronic inflammation. Many of the anti-inflammatory oils, both warm and cool, also have analgesic properties. Essential oils with an antispasmodic effect can also be useful for many muscular problems.

Analgesics: bay laurel (*Laurus nobilis*),[1] black pepper (*Piper nigrum*), eucalyptus (*Eucalyptus globulus* or *E. citriodora*),[2] German chamomile (*Matricaria recutita*), ginger (*Zingiber officinale*), lavender (*Lavandula angustifolia*),[3] lavandin (*Lavandula x intermedia*), nutmeg (*Myristica fragrans*), peppermint (*Mentha piperita*),[4] sweet birch (*Betula lenta*), wintergreen (*Gaultheria procumbens*)

Cooling anti-inflammatories: blue cypress (*Callitris intratropica*), German chamomile (*Matricaria recutita*),[5] helichrysum (*Helichrysum italicum*), lavender (*Lavandula angustifolia*),[6] palmarosa (*Cymbopogon martinii*),[7] sweet birch (*Betula lenta*), turmeric (*Curcuma longa*),[8] wintergreen (*Gaultheria procumbens*), yarrow (*Achillea millefolium*)

Warming anti-inflammatories: black pepper (*Piper nigrum*), cardamon (*Elettaria cardamomum*),[9] clove (*Syzygium aromaticum*), cumin (*Cuminum cyminum*),[10] ginger (*Zingiber officinale*),[11] nutmeg (*Myristica fragrans*)[12]

Antispasmodics: basil (*Ocimum basilicum*), black pepper (*Piper nigrum*), cardamon (*Elettaria cardamomum*),[13] clary sage (*Salvia sclarea*),[14] lavender (*Lavandula angustifolia*), marjoram (*Origanum majorana*), petitgrain (*Citrus aurantium* var. *amara*), Roman chamomile (*Chamaemelum nobile*), tarragon (*Artemesia dracunculus*)

Common Problems of the Musculoskeletal System

Most soft tissue problems that massage therapists regularly encounter in their practices can be categorized into a few main areas:

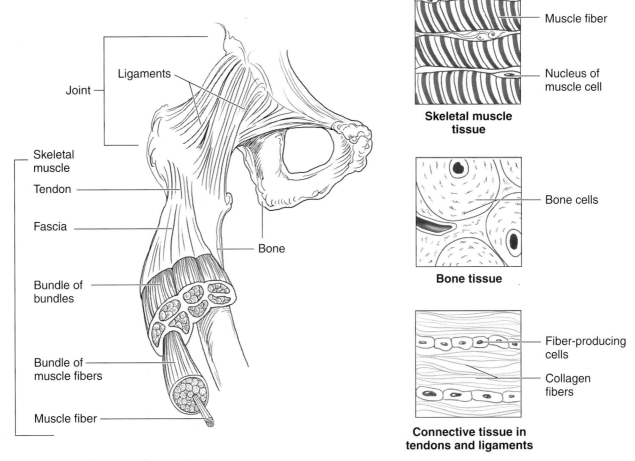

Figure 16.1 Various types of connective tissue.

- Sudden injuries, in which the client has gone beyond his or her physical capabilities
- Overuse injuries, in which the problem has been building up from repetitive, continuous activity, sometimes for a long time
- Hypertonic muscles, which can lead to structural problems and pain
- Arthritis, which affects the joints
- Fibromyalgia
- Cramps and spasms

The issues within each of these sections have similarities in both presenting symptoms and treatment methods.

Levels of Inflammation

Massage treatments for problems of the musculoskeletal system are often chosen based on the level of inflammation present, and aromatherapy treatments and essential oils can be selected using the same criteria. The main treatment goal for acute inflammation is to reduce the heat and inflammation, often using the methods summed up by the acronym RICE: rest, ice, compression, and elevation.

The most useful oils in this case are the cooling anti-inflammatories. ("Cooling" and "anti-inflammatory" do not always mean the same thing, as some essential oils have an anti-inflammatory effect by suppressing certain hormones involved in the inflammation process.)

Massage treatment for subacute inflammation includes cold/hot contrast to increase drainage and venous return. Using both cooling and warming anti-inflammatories to increase blood flow will improve this process. Treatment for chronic inflammation includes deep moist heat or contrast therapy to increase local circulation and soften any adhesions. Warming anti-inflammatories will have a similar effect.

These principles can be applied to many of the ailments in the sections that follow. Treatment selection often is based on the level of inflammation, whether the problem is a recently sprained wrist or chronic rheumatoid arthritis.

Sudden Injuries

This section addresses problems that usually result when clients do something that goes beyond their physical capabilities. Sudden injury treatment involves working with acute, subacute, and chronic stages of injury.

Post-Exercise Muscle Soreness

Although it might not sound like an injury, muscle soreness following exercise is a sign of overexercise, particularly if the tenderness is so extreme that range of motion is limited. The first time I went to a gym, I overworked my quadriceps muscles. I had such extreme muscle soreness the next day that I could only walk down the subway steps backwards!

Causes and Symptoms. Soreness generally appears up to 24 hours after excessive or unaccustomed exercise, and it usually disappears completely within a week at most. The muscle is tender to the touch, is painful to move, and may be swollen.

Essential Oils. The main issue is inflammation, so any of the anti-inflammatory oils will be helpful. However, it is possible that the warming anti-inflammatories, such as nutmeg (*Myristica fragrans*), ginger (*Zingiber officinale*), and black pepper (*Piper nigrum*), may produce more rapid healing because of their tendency to increase blood flow, bringing oxygen and nutrients to the tissues.

Methods of Application. The traditional method in Western massage work for any acute muscle inflammation is ice, and essential oils can be applied in strong dilutions (3–10% depending on the size of the affected area) under a cold compress. After a few days, the same essential oils may be applied in a slightly milder dilution (2–3%) with massage to loosen the muscles and avoid any long-term spasm or tightness.

Strains, Sprains, and Dislocations

Although the type of tissues involved in these three injuries differs, the symptoms and treatment are similar. A **strain** is an injury caused by overstretching a muscle–tendon unit, a **sprain** is an injury caused by overstretching a ligament, and a **dislocation** is a dissociation of the articulating surfaces of a joint, which generally includes injury to surrounding ligaments and tendons. Sprains and strains are extremely common injuries. According to the U.S. Bureau of Labor Statistics, "sprains and strains, most often involving the back, accounted for 43 per cent of injuries and illnesses resulting in days away from work in 2002."[15]

Causes and Symptoms. Strains are caused by a sudden overstretching of the muscle, or a sudden contraction against heavy resistance. Sprains and dislocations are caused by sudden wrenching or twisting movements of a joint, and dislocations may also be caused by an outside force, such as a heavy blow. Poor body mechanics, congenital hypermobility, and a history of previous similar injuries also contribute.

All three injuries are accompanied by local heat, edema, and bruising, as well as pain, decreased range of motion, and muscle weakness or loss of function in the area affected. These symptoms will be more or less evident depending on the severity of the injury.

Essential Oils. In the acute stage, the use of cooling anti-inflammatory essential oils that are also analgesic is ideal. Examples are lavender (*Lavandula angustifolia*) and German chamomile (*Matricaria recutita*). Essential oils that are astringent and help move lymph can start to relieve swelling. These include cypress (*Cupressus sempervirens*), grapefruit (*Citrus paradisii*), and juniper (*Juniperus communis*). If there is bruising, helichrysum (*Helichrysum italicum*) and hyssop (*Hyssopus officinalis*) are particularly helpful.

In the subacute stage, combining the cooling and the warming anti-inflammatory oils will help remove toxins and bring nutrients and oxygen to the area by creating a vascular flush. In the late subacute stage, gentle friction and muscle stripping are often used to prevent excessive adhesions. Any of the cooling anti-inflammatory oils can be used after these techniques to help decrease any subsequent inflammation. German chamomile (*Matricaria recutita*) and helichrysum (*Helichrysum italicum*) are particularly good for this treatment.

In the chronic stage, the main goals are to increase range of motion and reduce adhesions and hypertonicities. Here, essential oils that warm the tissues and increase blood flow are useful additions to the treatment. If any scar tissue is present, either from the injury itself or from surgery to correct the injury, certain essential oils can be used to help correct tissue alignment. These are known as cicatrizant oils and include helichrysum (*Helichrysum italicum*), juniper (*Juniperus communis*), rosemary (*Rosmarinus officinalis*), and lavender (*Lavandula angustifolia*).

Methods of Application. In the acute stage, essential oils can be used on the injury site, provided that the skin is unbroken, either under a cold compress or in lymphatic drainage techniques. Dilutions are usually strong, and the milder essential oils can even be used undiluted on small areas, such as a sprained wrist, on otherwise healthy adults. Sweet birch (*Betula lenta*) and wintergreen (*Gaultheria procumbens*) are extremely useful in this stage but should not be used at more than a 5% dilution, even for acute injuries.

In the subacute and chronic stages, essential oils can be used in massage work on the affected area in dilutions of 3–10% depending on the size of the area involved. Warm baths with essential oils are extremely effective, especially with chronic injuries. For a healthy adult, 10–15 drops in the bath should be used. Essential oils with a warm compress can also be helpful in the chronic stage.

Achilles Tendon Rupture

Ms. I. was a massage therapist in her mid-forties who had recently had surgery to repair a ruptured Achilles tendon. The surgical incision had initially been covered with a hard cast for about 10 days to restrict movement, so no direct aromatherapy application to the area was possible. She had applied lavender (*Lavandula angustifolia*) and helichrysum (*Helichrysum italicum*) essential oils in a strong dilution (about 5%) for 3 days before the surgery to help reduce pain and swelling from the injury, and continued to apply the blend to the exposed part of the leg and foot postsurgery for the same reasons. She was able to stop taking painkillers about 36 hours after the surgery, and both swelling and bruising were minimal when the cast was removed.

A walking cast was prescribed for the next 2 months, during which manual lymphatic techniques with grapefruit (*Citrus x paradisii*) and juniper (*Juniperus communis*) essential oils were used to improve lymphatic flow, which seemed to be sluggish. Calophyllum (*Calophyllum inophyllum*) and rosehip seed (*Rosa rubiginosa*) oils were applied regularly to the surgical scar and the area around it. Blends with rosemary (*Rosmarinus officinalis*), black pepper (*Piper nigrum*), lavender (*Lavandula angustifolia*), and cardamon (*Elettaria cardamomum*) were used on the rest of the leg and foot to improve blood circulation and tone muscles, as the lower leg muscles were atrophying from the enforced lack of movement.

After about 3 months, the walking cast was removed and physiotherapy was started. Both the surgeon and the physiotherapist remarked that the ankle had a surprisingly large range of motion and lack of edema. Massage was continued regularly with essential oils to tone muscles and improve circulation. A combination of lavender (*Lavandula angustifolia*) and helichrysum (*Helichrysum italicum*) was used over the scar area with massage techniques to reduce scar tissue and adhesions. Ten months postsurgery, the ankle and leg had regained 100% strength and range of motion.

Fractures

Fractures are classified according to the nature of the break. If the skin is unbroken, it is called a simple fracture, but if the bone has broken through the skin, it is called a compound fracture. Compound fractures are more prone to infection because of the break in the skin. The break may be complete, in which the two parts of the bone are completely separated, or incomplete, in which the bone is twisted or cracked. Soft tissue injuries always accompany fractures of the bone, and muscles, tendons, ligaments, nerves, and blood vessels may all be damaged.

Causes and Symptoms. The cause is usually a sudden, direct shock that the bone cannot absorb. However, overuse can also result in cracks or stress fractures in a bone. A contributing factor can be an existing disorder or disease that weakens the bone, such as osteoporosis, bone infection, or a tumor.

Essential Oils. The cooling anti-inflammatory oils can be used to help with swelling and heat while the injured limb is in a cast. Essential oils that help drain lymph may also be indicated. Once the cast is removed, gentle massage over the area with sandalwood (*Santalum album*), rose (*Rosa damascena*), or geranium (*Pelargonium graveolens*) in an emollient cream or carrier oil will help nourish the skin. Essential oils such as eucalyptus (*Eucalyptus globulus*) or rosemary (*Rosmarinus officinalis*) will help increase local circulation.

Methods of Application. A fracture is generally treated medically by bringing the ends of the bone together, by surgery or traction, and placing it in a cast. A non-weight-bearing bone, such as a rib, with a simple crack may not require medical treatment beyond painkillers. Massage therapists and aromatherapists can support the healing process by helping to reduce swelling and pain directly related to the fracture and by treating the accompanying soft tissue injuries. Applying essential oils with lymphatic drainage techniques or a cold compress in strong dilutions (5% and higher) is always suitable for injuries in the acute stage. Later, the essential oils can be used in milder dilutions (2–3%) in massage, or in moderate amounts (10–15 drops) in the bath to ease symptoms of pain and stiffness.

Aromatherapy may also help with problems relating to the cast, such as dermatitis caused by poor ventilation of the skin under the cast or by allergic reaction to the materials. Essential oils should be used in mild dilutions (1–2%) in a soothing carrier such as aloe vera gel.

Prolapsed or Herniated Disc

Intervertebral discs act as shock absorbers between the hard bones of the vertebrae themselves. They consist of an outer casing of tough collagenous fibers, filled with a gel-like watery substance.

Causes and Symptoms. When subjected to high stress, particularly a combination of bending and twisting movements, perhaps combined with lifting a heavy object, the disc can rupture. The chance of rupture is increased through gradual disc degeneration caused by years of poor posture, inadequate back support, and a lack of flexibility or muscle strength. Discs can rupture anywhere along the spine, but lumbar disc ruptures are the most common because of the amount of pressure put on this area. A protruding disc means that the collagenous outer casing bulges out of shape, pressing on surrounding nerves and ligaments, while a herniated disc is one that has completely ruptured, allowing the inner gel to escape.

In both cases there is a significant amount of nerve pain, especially in the morning and after sitting. Often there is swelling and muscle spasm. Pain may affect the area innervated by the spinal nerves emerging from the point of the disc rupture. Lumbar disc rupture may lead to pain radiating down the leg, while cervical disc protrusion may lead to shoulder and arm pain.

Essential Oils. Essential oils for nerve pain and muscle spasm are indicated to break the pain-spasm-pain cycle that usually accompanies disc problems. Oils that are analgesic and particularly helpful for nerve pain include lavender (*Lavandula angustifolia*), ginger (*Zingiber officinale*), nutmeg (*Myristica fragrans*), and peppermint (*Mentha piperita*). Good antispasmodics include basil (*Ocimum basilicum*), clary sage (*Salvia sclarea*), and tarragon (*Artemesia dracunculus*).

Methods of Application. In acute cases, essential oils can be used in baths, under compresses, or in gentle effleurage work to relieve the pain and spasms. Dilutions will depend on the size of the area involved, but for acute pain they can be at 3–8%.

Overuse Injuries

Overuse injuries result from repetitive movements and poor body mechanics, which lead to muscle fatigue and soft tissue damage. If the condition is untreated and the activities are continued, the injury can eventually lead to a loss of motor control and a situation of chronic pain and inflammation.

Friction and Chronic Inflammation

Inflammation may be present in any overuse injury but, generally, chronic inflammation, together with reduced range of motion and possibly a loss of muscle function, characterizes several musculoskeletal problems. These problems include bursitis, tendonitis, shin splints, plantar fasciitis, and carpal tunnel syndrome.

Causes and Symptoms. The immediate cause is simple overuse, resulting in friction and inflammation of the tendons and muscles. Especially in the workplace and when playing sports, repetitive movements are common, often performed at high speed. Other factors include poor posture and body mechanics, muscle tension, a lack of flexibility, and nonergonomic working conditions. There may be episodes of acute inflammation and pain and long periods of mild, nagging pain or discomfort. If nerves are compressed, there might be tingling, numbness, and a loss of muscular control.

Essential Oils. Reducing the pain and inflammation is the main concern, and essential oils that are strongly analgesic and cooling are recommended. These include lemon eucalyptus (*Eucalyptus citriodora*), peppermint (*Mentha piperita*), and wintergreen (*Gaultheria procumbens*) or sweet birch (*Betula lenta*). Also valuable are German chamomile (*Matricaria recutita*), lavender (*Lavandula angustifolia*), and helichrysum (*Helichrysum italicum*), as these oils are mild enough on the skin that they can be used undiluted, or in very strong dilutions, on small areas. With chronic problems, which may involve less pain but more stiffness, the warming analgesics such as black pepper (*Piper nigrum*), nutmeg (*Myristica fragrans*), and ginger (*Zingiber officinale*) may be more appropriate to help with stretching and increasing range of motion.

Methods of Application. Using essential oils under cool compresses provides relief in acute cases. For chronic problems, warming essential oils may be used in a 3–5% dilution over the affected area, with massage techniques designed to stretch fascia and improve circulation.

Low-Back Pain

This is a generalized phrase used to describe the subjective feelings of pain in the area of the lumbar spine. It is regarded as a syndrome, with a range of possible symptoms. It is extremely common.

Causes and Symptoms. Low-back pain can result from any repeated activity or movement that places strain on the lumbar area. Lifting excessively heavy weights, bending from the waist, the sharp twisting movements of golf and tennis, or reaching and rotating are all possible causes. Contributing factors are muscle weakness in both the low back and the abdomen, and poor posture and body mechanics. Symptoms include generalized pain and tenderness in the lumbar area, stiffness, and decreased range of motion.

Essential Oils. For chronic pain and tenderness in this area, the warming essential oils, such as ginger (*Zingiber officinale*), black pepper (*Piper nigrum*), and bay laurel (*Laurus nobilis*), can be helpful. They seem to work particularly well for low-back pain when combined with a lymphatic mover, such as lemon (*Citrus limon*), grapefruit (*Citrus paradisii*), or cypress (*Cupressus sempervirens*).

Methods of Application. For chronic low-back pain, using essential oils under warm compresses or in gentle massage in about a 3% dilution is a good treatment. These oils can also be used in moderate amounts (10 drops) in the bath to loosen muscles and provide pain relief.

Hypertonic Muscles

Muscles with unusually high tone can cause a wide range of problems in the body, as well as simply being uncomfortable in themselves, as a result of restricted movement and pressure on nerves. **Hypertonicity,** the state in which muscles are abnormally tight and often painful, is associated with stress and/or with repetitive movements, such as those found in computer work or driving. If stress seems to be a major factor, the essential oils that are commonly indicated as calming or sedative are often useful (see Chapter 15).

Tension Headaches

Headaches are caused by many conditions. According to the International Headache Society, there are two main categories of headaches. A primary headache, such as a tension headache, is the main condition by itself. A secondary headache is caused by another condition, such as an injury, high blood pressure, infection, or a tumor.[16] It is important that the massage therapist be aware that a headache may have a more serious underlying cause. It is advisable to refer a client to a doctor if the therapist suspects this is the case.

Causes and Symptoms. Tension headaches are primarily caused by muscle contraction in the neck and shoulders. The causes of the muscle contraction usually include stress, teeth clenching, postural imbalances such as scoliosis, and poor posture. However, the World Headache Association suggests that the muscle tightness may be "a result of chemical changes that initiated the headache, not the cause of the headache."[17] The main symptom is pain in various parts of the head and neck, which can be acute or diffuse. Headaches can occur occasionally or daily, and they last from half an hour to several days.

Essential Oils. The analgesic oils are the most effective treatment for headaches, and peppermint (*Mentha piperita*) seems to give the most rapid relief. One study showed that a 10% dilution of peppermint oil spread across the forehead and temples was as effective as 1000 mg of acetaminophen (paracetamol) and significantly reduced headache pain after 15 minutes.[18] Other essential oils that can be useful include basil (*Ocimum basilicum*), lavender (*Lavandula angustifolia*), rosemary (*Rosmarinus officinalis*), and Roman chamomile (*Chamaemelum nobile*).

Methods of Application. Inhalation from a tissue or a strong dilution (5–10%) used on the forehead and temples is the quickest form of treatment. In my experience, peppermint is the most effective of the above oils when used in these ways. Many clients also benefit from a gentle massage of the neck, shoulders, and head (if it is not too tender), with any combination of the above oils in a 3% dilution.

Temporomandibular Joint Dysfunction

Temporomandibular joint dysfunction (TMJD) is a disorder of the temporomandibular joint and the muscles of mastication (chewing). It is estimated that approximately 10 million people in the United States suffer from TMJD.[19]

Causes and Symptoms. TMJD is caused by an increase in tension in the muscles controlling the mandible. Teeth grinding or clenching is often involved, leading to spasm and pain. Stress is believed to be a primary trigger, but other triggers include trauma, poor posture of the head and neck, and sinus infection. The main symptom is dull jaw pain, which increases while chewing. Other symptoms include jaw clicking or popping, earache, headache, and limitation of mouth opening.

Essential Oils. If there is a stress component, that should be addressed with the essential oils discussed in Chapter 15. Direct treatment for the painful jaw itself should include analgesic oils, such as wintergreen (*Gaultheria procumbens*), sweet birch (*Betula lenta*), German chamomile (*Matricaria recutita*), or black pepper (*Piper nigrum*). Antispasmodics such as marjoram (*Origanum majorana*), basil (*Ocimum basilicum*), or cardamon (*Elettaria cardamomum*) will also be helpful.

Methods of Application. Treatment for stress will concentrate on essential oils in a mild dilution (1–2%) used in a full-body relaxation massage to calm the sympathetic nervous system. Treatment for the jaw itself often concentrates on the muscles of the neck and shoulder and on the muscles of mastication. Essential oils can be used in a stronger dilution (3%) on these muscles and on trigger points, which often accompany TMJD.

Arthritis

The name of this disorder is derived from *arthro*, meaning joint, and *itis*, indicating inflammation. Arthritis is a general term used to describe many inflammatory diseases affecting connective tissue, particularly the joints of the body. Arthritis is an extremely common, chronic health problem. In 2002, 70 million people in the United States were affected. According to the Arthritis Foundation, it is the leading cause of disability among Americans older than age 15, results in 39 million physician visits annually, and costs the U.S. economy more than $86.2 billion per year.[20] Although it is often regarded as an older person's disease, it can occur at any age. There are more than 100 types of arthritis, including rheumatoid arthritis, osteoarthritis, gout, scleroderma, lupus, and ankylosing spondylitis. The symptoms of and treatment for each of the different types vary widely.

Rheumatoid Arthritis

Rheumatoid arthritis (RA) is an autoimmune disease, but as many of the symptoms affect the musculoskeletal system and it is generally treated symptomatically, it is discussed in this chapter. RA is one of the more serious and disabling types of arthritis, affecting mostly women.

Causes and Symptoms. The causes of RA are unknown, although some people seem genetically predisposed. The activity of the immune system causes the lining of the joint to become inflamed, leading to granulation and adhesions that restrict range of motion and can cause the joint to

Rheumatoid Arthritis

Mrs. M. was in her early eighties. She had had rheumatoid arthritis for about 18 years, starting in her hands and progressing to her knees, back, and neck. She was taking prescription medications for the arthritis and for high blood pressure. The arthritis was most painful in her neck and hands.

As the client was currently in a flare-up, a blend of geranium (*Pelargonium graveolens*), lavender (*Lavandula angustifolia*), and German chamomile (*Matricaria recutita*) was made in a 2% dilution and applied gently to the hands, neck, and knees. The client took the remainder home for self-application. After about 10 days, she returned for a half-hour massage session, as the inflammation had subsided. The following oils were used in a massage in a 2% dilution:

Spike lavender (*Lavandula latifolia*), 5 drops: analgesic, antirheumatic

Bay laurel (*Laurus nobilis*), 3 drops: warming, anti-inflammatory

Ginger (*Zingiber officinale*), 2 drops: warming, anti-inflammatory, analgesic

Cardamon (*Elettaria cardamomum*), 3 drops: warming, antidepressant

Mrs. M. returned for weekly half-hour sessions, reporting a general relief in pain and increased ease of movement for at least 2 or 3 days after each session.

deviate and become deformed. The inflammation flares up episodically, causing swelling, heat, and pain in the joint. As RA is a systemic disease, there are many other symptoms, including fatigue, low-grade fever, weight loss, and anemia. The disease can progress very quickly or extremely slowly.

Essential Oils. RA is treated symptomatically, and the symptoms vary depending on whether the client is having a flare-up. During flare-ups the joints become hot, swollen, and extremely tender to the touch. The cooling anti-inflammatory and analgesic oils are the most beneficial at this time. Sweet birch (*Betula lenta*), wintergreen (*Gaultheria procumbens*), German chamomile (*Matricaria recutita*),[21] peppermint (*Mentha piperita*), spike lavender (*Lavandula latifolia*),[22] turmeric (*Curcuma longa*),[23] and lemon eucalyptus (*Eucalyptus citriodora*) can bring significant relief. When RA is not in a flare-up, it is important to maintain range of motion and strength. The

more warming essential oils, such as nutmeg (*Myristica fragrans*), black pepper (*Piper nigrum*), ginger (*Zingiber officinale*),[24] and bay laurel (*Laurus nobilis*), will make connective tissue easier to loosen and stretch.

Methods of Application. Essential oils under cool compresses provide the most rapid relief during flare-ups when massage is not possible. Dilution depends on the size of the area affected and on the client's overall health and can range from 10% for small areas such as the hands only to 1% for larger areas and frailer clients.

Osteoarthritis

Osteoarthritis (OA) is a degenerative joint disease that affects the articular cartilage and bone in synovial joints. It is the most common form of arthritis, and can be seen in ancient remains, such as Egyptian mummies.

Causes and Symptoms. The cartilage covering the ends of the bones in synovial joints starts to deteriorate, leaving the bones unprotected. As bone begins to rub on bone, pain ensues, the exposed surface thickens, and bone spurs may grow, altering the shape of the joint and restricting movement. OA is often called degenerative joint disease, or osteoarthrosis, as inflammation is minimal and only found in later stages. The underlying causes may include injury or chronic overuse of the joint, hypermobility, or diabetes. Pain and stiffness are the main symptoms.

Essential Oils. Because of the relative lack of inflammation, the most important focus in treatment is improving mobility and range of motion, and decreasing pain. Oils that are warming and analgesic, such as nutmeg (*Myristica fragrans*), ginger (*Zingiber officinale*), bay laurel (*Laurus nobilis*), and black pepper (*Piper nigrum*), will be most effective.

Methods of Application. Essential oils with moist heat, such as warm compresses or warm baths, will enable connective tissue to be stretched to improve range of motion. Dilutions for local application and for soothing full-body massage should be mild to moderate (about 2% for massage, 3–5% for local application) because OA is a chronic problem that will require regular treatment, and also because the majority of clients with OA are older.

Gout

Gout mostly affects men, and typically those aged 40 to 50. It often affects only the big toe joint but is disproportionately painful to its size, making it difficult to walk or even endure the weight of bedclothes.

Causes and Symptoms. The cause is a defect of the chemical process in the body that breaks down purines, substances found in the cells of the body and in meat and fish. This defect leads to the deposit of uric acid crystals in a small joint, usually the metatarsophalangeal joint of the big toe. There may be a genetic predisposition, but attacks can also be triggered by obesity, eating certain foods, drinking alcohol, and injury or surgery. Flare-ups are episodic and extremely painful; the joint is very hot to the touch, as well as red and swollen. If untreated, inflammation can spread to other areas, and chronic gout is associated with kidney stones, diabetes, and hypertension.

Essential Oils. The cooling anti-inflammatory oils are the only ones that will provide a measure of relief during a flare-up. These include lavender (*Lavandula angustifolia*), peppermint (*Mentha piperita*), German chamomile (*Matricaria recutita*), yarrow (*Achillea millefolium*), and helichrysum (*Helichrysum italicum*). Some clients have also found detoxifying essential oils such as grapefruit (*Citrus x paradisii*), carrot (*Daucus carota*), and juniper (*Juniperus communis*) to be helpful, especially when used in combination with a detoxifying diet.

Methods of Application. As for other forms of inflammatory arthritis, essential oils with cool compresses are the best form of treatment during a flare-up. For this small toe joint, strong dilutions or undiluted essential oils can be used for rapid pain relief.

Scleroderma

Scleroderma is a disease affecting collagen that causes a thickening and hardening of the skin and other connective tissue.

Causes and Symptoms. The cause is unknown and scleroderma is relatively rare, mostly striking women between the ages of 30 and 50. It can be localized, affecting skin, fascia, muscle, and possibly bone in particular areas, or more generalized, affecting many systems of the body, including the skin, cardiovascular system, kidneys, and gastrointestinal tract. Thickening of the skin, loss of range of motion, and muscle weakness are the first symptoms. Scleroderma can lead to serious symptoms and even death from heart failure.

Essential Oils. The focus, especially in early scleroderma, is on retaining softness and flexibility in skin and muscle. Calendula-infused oil (*Calendula officinalis*) appears to have a good effect, and other carrier oils with skin healing and emollient properties, such as calophyllum (*Calophyllum inophyllum*) and rose hip seed oil (*Rosa rubiginosa*), also are beneficial. Essential oils with similar properties include rose (*Rosa damascena* or *centifolia*), sandalwood (*Santalum album*), geranium (*Pelargonium graveolens*), palmarosa (*Cymbopogon martinii*), and rock rose (*Cistus ladaniferus*).

Methods of Application. Essential oils should be in a fairly mild dilution (1–2%) because frequent application, either in full-body massage or by the client, will be most helpful. Carrier oils are as helpful in this case as the essential oils. Calendula-infused oil can be used at 100%, but both calophyllum and rose hip seed oil will need to be mixed with another carrier because of the price and the strong smell. Usually a dilution of 10–20% of these fixed oils is used in a blend.

Other Musculoskeletal Problems
Fibromyalgia

Some authorities include fibromyalgia in the arthritic diseases. However, since the accepted definition of fibromyalgia is that it is a painful but nondeforming, nonarticular soft tissue musculoskeletal condition, it does not conform to the definition of arthritis, which is described as an articular and/or deforming disease. As with rheumatoid arthritis, fibromyalgia has many symptoms beyond those affecting the musculoskeletal system, but since the majority are in this system I have included it in this chapter. Some experts believe that fibromyalgia and chronic fatigue syndrome are the same thing, while others point out distinct differences between the two, especially with regard to regular exercise, which tends to benefit fibromyalgia but worsen chronic fatigue.

Causes and Symptoms. Recognized since 1987 by the American Medical Association, fibromyalgia is probably an ancient condition. It is common, affecting 2–6% of the adult population, and of those, mostly women. A client is considered to have fibromyalgia when she has had a history of widespread pain for at least 3 months and if she has pain when pressure is applied to particular point sites. Of these 18 points, 11 need to be painful to confirm fibromyalgia. The causes are not clear, but immune dysfunction could be a factor. Symptoms can be triggered by stress, lack of sleep or exercise, trauma, weather, and infections. The main symptoms are muscular pain and fatigue, poor sleep, and tingling or other irritating sensations in the soft tissues.

Essential Oils. The warming, analgesic essential oils seem to be the most effective in helping with the muscular pain associated with fibromyalgia. These include bay laurel (*Laurus nobilis*), eucalyptus (*Eucalyptus radiata* or *globulus*), ginger (*Zingiber officinale*), and black pepper (*Piper nigrum*). Leon Chaitow, a British doctor of osteopathy and naturopathy, recommends basil for fatigue, chamomile for sleep and digestive disturbances, cypress for muscular conditions, lavender for nervous system problems, and neroli for depression and insomnia.[25]

Methods of Application. Fibromyalgia tends to be somewhat unpredictable in responding to treatment methods. However, for most clients warm hydrotherapy seems to help, with essential oils used either in baths (10–15 drops) or under compresses (about 2–3%). When used in massage, dilutions are variable depending on the focus. For full-body relaxation work, 1–3% is suitable, while for work on smaller areas of the body to stretch muscles or treat trigger points, dilutions can be up to 5%.

Cramps and Spasms

A **spasm** is a persistent muscle contraction that cannot be released at will. A **cramp** is a popular term for a painful spasm.

Causes and Symptoms. An electrical charge from a motor neuron stimulates the release of calcium in a muscle cell, which initiates contraction of the muscle. When the electrical charge stops, the calcium is recovered and the contraction also stops. When a muscle is in spasm, the contraction does not stop. Spasms can be triggered by pain, stress, fatigue, medications, cold, poor circulation, dehydration, and a lack of calcium, sodium, or vitamin D. Muscles that more commonly spasm are those of the leg, low back, and sternocleidomastoid. Pregnant women often get cramps in the gastrocnemius. The symptoms are pain and reduced range of motion due to the hypertonicity of the muscle.

Essential Oils. Antispasmodic essential oils include marjoram (*Origanum majorana*), basil (*Ocimum basilicum*), tarragon (*Artemesia dracunculus*), cardamon (*Elettaria cardamomum*), clary sage (*Salvia sclarea*), and Roman chamomile (*Chamaemelum nobile*).

Methods of Application. The main focus is to break the pain-spasm-pain cycle. Essential oils can be applied in a 3–10% dilution, depending on the area involved and the severity of the cramp, under a compress. Cold compresses are best for spasm caused by injury, while warm or contrast compresses are preferable for muscles that are chronically hypertonic. Aromatherapy can also be used with massage when the spasm has been reduced sufficiently that the therapist can work directly on the area.

SUMMARY

- The musculoskeletal system is composed of muscles and connective tissues: bones, ligaments, tendons, and fascia. It enables the body to move and provides protection for internal organs, shape and stability, and warmth.

- Factors that affect the system negatively include lack of exercise, smoking, poor nutrition, inadequate hydration, and poor posture.

- Essential oils can permeate the skin and directly affect underlying muscle and other soft tissue.

- Groups of essential oils that are beneficial to the system include analgesics, anti-inflammatories, and antispasmodics.

- Levels of inflammation will affect which essential oils are used. Generally, cooling anti-inflammatories are used with acute inflammation, while warming anti-inflammatories are used with chronic inflammation.

- For sudden injuries, anti-inflammatory essential oils are beneficial. Essential oils that move lymph can be used to relieve swelling, and helichrysum and hyssop are useful for bruising.

- For overuse injuries, it is important to monitor the level of inflammation and treat accordingly.

- Analgesic essential oils such as peppermint should be used with headaches to relieve symptoms. Antispasmodic oils can be used to massage the head, neck, and shoulders to avoid headaches.

- Other problems caused by hypertonic muscles, such as TMJD, respond well to antispasmodic essential oils. Stress is often a factor and should be addressed using the essential oils mentioned in Chapter 15.

- Arthritis incorporates many syndromes. For RA, cooling and analgesic oils should be used during inflammatory flare-ups and warming oils when the condition is stable. For osteoarthritis, analgesic and warming essential oils are beneficial. Essential oils for gout are similar to those for RA and should also include detoxifying oils. For scleroderma, skin softening and soothing carrier oils and essential oils work best.

- Fibromyalgia is best treated with warming, analgesic essential oils. Oils should also be chosen to treat symptomatically the various nonmusculoskeletal issues that are present.

- Cramps and spasms respond well to the antispasmodic essential oils.

Review Questions

1. How do cooling anti-inflammatory and warming anti-inflammatory essential oils differ in action?
2. Name two cooling anti-inflammatory and two warming anti-inflammatory oils.
3. Essential oils that are commonly used for bruising include: (a) geranium and rose, (b) helichrysum and hyssop, (c) sweet birch and wintergreen, (d) lemon and grapefruit.

4. For acute soft tissue injuries, sweet birch and wintergreen essential oils are very useful and should be used at a dilution of: (a) 100%, (b) 20–50%, (c) 5–10%, (d) not more than 5%.

5. How do astringent essential oils help reduce swelling?

6. Aromatherapy can help with bone fractures by reducing the _____ and _____, and helping with problems relating to the _____.

7. Essential oils that are _____ and _____ are most helpful with protruding disc problems (choose two of the following): anti-inflammatory, antispasmodic, antiseptic, analgesic, cicatrizant, antidepressant.

8. Which essential oil seems to be most effective in reducing pain from a tension headache?

9. Some headaches may be relieved simply by sniffing an essential oil. (T/F)

10. Cooling anti-inflammatory and warming anti-inflammatory essential oils are both used with rheumatoid arthritis. In what different situations would each be used?

11. Why are anti-inflammatory essential oils not especially useful for osteoarthritis?

12. For fibromyalgia, _____ essential oils are often the most effective.

13. For scleroderma, the main emphasis is on maintaining flexibility and softness in skin and muscle, so _____ are as important as essential oils.

Notes

1. Sayyah M, Saroukhani G, Peirovi A, et al. Analgesic and anti-inflammatory activity of the leaf essential oil of Laurus nobilis Linn. Phytother Res 2003;17(7):733–736.

2. Silva J, Abebe W, Sousa SM, et al. Analgesic and anti-inflammatory effects of the essential oils of Eucalyptus. J Ethnopharmacol 2003; 89:277–283.

3. Ghelardini C, Galeotti N, Salvatore G, et al. Local anaesthetic activity of the essential oil of *Lavandula angustifolia*. Planta Med 1999;65(8): 700–703.

4. Gobel H, Schmidt G, Dworshak M, et al. Essential plant oils and headache mechanisms. Phytomedicine 1995;2(2):93–102.

5. Carle R, Gomaa K. The medicinal use of *Matricariae* flos. Br J Phytother 1992;2(4):147–153.

6. Hajhashemi V, Ghannadi A, Sharif B. Anti-inflammatory and analgesic properties of the leaf extracts and essential oil of *Lavandula angustifolia* Mill. J Ethnopharmacol 2003;89(1):67–71.

7. Krishnamoorthy G, Kavimani S, Loganathan C. Anti-inflammatory activity of the essential oil of *Cymbopogon martini*. Ind J Pharm Sci 1998; 60(2):114–116.

8. Chandra D, Gupta SS. Anti-inflammatory and antiarthritic activity of volatile oil of *Curcuma longa* (Haldi). Ind J Med Res 1972;60(1): 138–142.

9. Al-Zuhari H, El-Sayeh B, Ameen HA, et al. Pharmacological studies of cardamom oil in animals. Pharmacol Res 1996;34(12):79–82.

10. Afifi NA, Ramadan A, El-Kashoury EA, et al. Some pharmacological activities of essential oils of certain umbelliferous fruits. Vet Med J Giza 1994;42(3):85–92.

11. Sharma JN, Ishak FI, Yusof APM, et al. Effects of eugenol and ginger oil on adjuvant arthritis and kallikreins in rats. Asia Pac J Pharmacol 1997;12(1–2):9–14.

12. Bennett A, Stamford IF, Tavares IA, et al. The biological activity of eugenol, a major constituent of nutmeg (*Myristica fragrans*): studies on prostaglandins, the intestine and other tissues. Phytother Res 1988; 2(3):124–130.

13. al-Zuhair H, el-Sayeh B, Ibid.

14. Lis-Balchin M, Hart S, A preliminary study of the effect of essential oils on skeletal and smooth muscle *in vitro*. J Ethnopharmacol 1997; 58:183–187.

15. United States Department of Labor, Bureau of Labor Statistics. Available at: www.bls.gov/iif/home.htm. Accessed November 25, 2004.

16. The International Headache Society. Available at: www.i-h-s.com. Accessed December 14, 2004.

17. The World Headache Association. Available at: www.w-h-a.org. Accessed December 14, 2004.

18. Gobel H, Fresenius J, Heinze A, et al. Effectiveness of *Oleum menthae piperitae* and *paracetamol* in therapy of headache of the tension type. Nervenarzt 1996;67(8):672–681.

19. Heffer S. Temporomandibular joint syndrome. Available at: www.emedicine.com/EMERG/topic569.htm. Accessed November 3, 2004.

20. The Arthritis Foundation. Available at: www.arthritis.org. Accessed November 3, 2004.

21. Jakovlev V, Isaac O, Thiemer K, et al. Pharmacological investigations with compounds of chamomile. Planta Med 1979;35:125–140.

22. Von Frohlich E. A review of clinical, pharmacological and bacteriological research into *Oleum spicae*. Weiner Medizinische Wochenschrift 1968;15:345–350.

23. Chandra D, Gupta SS. Anti-inflammatory and antiarthritic activity of volatile oil of *Curcuma longa*. Ind J Med Res 1972;60(1):138–142.

24. Sharma JN, Ishak FI, Yusof APM, et al. Effects of eugenol and ginger oil on adjuvant arthritis and kallikreins in rats. Asia Pac J Pharmacol 1997; 12(1–2),:9–14.

25. Chaitow L. Fibromyalgia Syndrome. London, UK: Churchill Livingstone, 2000:176.

17

The Cardiovascular System

The cardiovascular system is also called the circulatory system. The body's circulatory mechanisms include the lymphatic system, which captures fluid from the blood at the cell level and returns it to the cardiovascular system. It is the only system that has access to every cell in the body, constantly delivering vital supplies and taking away wastes. The importance of the heart has been recognized for many thousands of years, but a thorough explanation of how the circulatory system works is fairly recent.

Cardiovascular disease is a major problem in the United States and in other Western countries. According to the American Heart Association, coronary heart disease is America's number one killer, with strokes at number three.[1]

An Overview of the Cardiovascular System

The cardiovascular system consists of the heart, arteries, veins, capillaries, and blood. The heart is about the size of a person's fist and lies in the thoracic cavity, between the lungs and resting on the diaphragm. It is the working organ of the system, pumping blood at the rate of about 6000 quarts a day. Unlike skeletal muscle, cardiac muscle is involuntary; the heartbeat is controlled by an intrinsic conduction system within the heart tissue that regulates a contraction rate of about 75 beats per minute. Heart rate is also regulated by the autonomic nervous system, which means that the heart beats faster when we are under physical or emotional stress.

Blood is a liquid connective tissue, made up mainly of erythrocytes (red blood cells) and plasma, the watery part of the blood. Other components include leucocytes (white blood cells), platelets for blood clotting, and various electrolytes (positively and negatively charged ions) and proteins. The blood is pumped from the heart to the lungs, where it picks up oxygen. It is then returned to the heart and pumped around the rest of the tissues of the body, where oxygen is deposited before the blood returns to the heart once again (Fig. 17.1).

The vessels that carry blood away from the heart are called arteries, and those that carry blood back to the heart are called veins. Arteries have thicker, more elastic walls to withstand the pressure from the pumping action of the heart, while veins have thinner walls and valves, to prevent backflow of the blood. Since the heart only pumps blood away from itself, the blood returns to the heart through a combination of pressure from skeletal muscles and the slight vacuum created in the thorax by respiration.

Because arteries and veins are too thick to allow the exchange of fluids and gases necessary for cells, this process occurs in the capillaries. Capillaries are the thinnest, hair-like blood vessels, with walls only one cell layer thick, making exchanges between the blood and the cells possible.

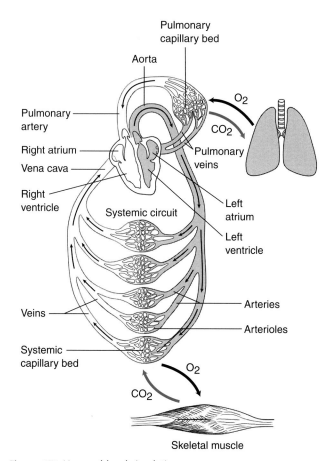

Figure 17.1 Human blood circulation.

The main function of the cardiovascular system is the transport of oxygen, hormones, nutrients, and waste products, such as carbon dioxide. Blood also helps regulate body temperature and the pH (relative acidity) of body fluids. The cardiovascular system is also part of the immune function of the body, since it contains white blood cells, antibodies, and interferons, or messenger proteins of the immune system.

Risk Factors

Factors that have a negative effect on the cardiovascular system include:

- *Lack of exercise.* Regular aerobic exercise is essential for the well-being of the heart and the rest of the body. The heart pumps harder, increasing its capacity over time and making it more efficient and also increasing the rate at which fresh blood (along with more oxygen and nutrients) reaches the body's cells. Moderate exercise of 30 minutes every day seems to be the most often recommended minimum.

- *Smoking.* Tobacco smoke causes the formation of plaque in the arteries, which could eventually result in a heart attack or stroke. Also, smokers have a much higher blood content of carbon monoxide, robbing their tissues of needed oxygen.

- *Excessive stress.* Stress activates the sympathetic nervous system, increasing heart rate and, over time, leading to hypertension.
- *Obesity and excessive alcohol intake.* Both of these factors increase blood pressure and put a strain on the heart muscle.
- *Poor nutrition.* A diet high in saturated fats is considered by many physicians to contribute to a high blood cholesterol level, which could lead to atherosclerosis and heart attack.

How Aromatherapy Affects the Cardiovascular System

Aromatherapy affects the cardiovascular system in several different ways. Some essential oils are classified as **hypotensive,** meaning that they lower blood pressure. They achieve this effect by dilating blood vessels (vasodilation), relaxing the smooth muscle of the vein's walls (vasorelaxation), or increasing parasympathetic nerve activity and decreasing sympathetic nerve activity. Some essential oils, such as lavender, have been shown to do both.[2]

Other essential oils are considered **hypertensive,** meaning that they raise blood pressure. However, evidence shows that they will raise blood pressure for people with hypotension but will have no effect on normal or high blood pressure. According to Tisserand and Balacs, "there is no need for contraindication of essential oils in either hypertension or hypotension."[3] In fact, one of the essential oils most often contraindicated in aromatherapy for hypertensive clients, rosemary (*Rosmarinus officinalis*), is more likely to help lower blood pressure because of its high content of 1,8 cineole. One study showed that treatment with 1,8 cineole "elicits hypotension."[4]

Some essential oils are **rubefacient,** meaning that they increase local peripheral circulation, which can be helpful for cold hands and feet or for problems such as diabetes, in which circulation may be impaired. The effect seems to be caused by slight skin irritation, which releases chemicals that cause vasodilation.

A few essential oils such as clove have been shown to have **anticoagulant** properties.[5] This therapeutic effect can be helpful for people who are at risk for blood clots, which could lead to more serious problems.

Hypotensives: lavender (*Lavandula angustifolia*),[6] celery seed (*Apium graveolens*),[7] basil (*Ocimum gratissimum*),[8] cedarwood (*Cedrus atlantica* or *deodara*),[9] geranium (*Pelargonium graveolens*), nigella (*Nigella sativa*),[10] ylang ylang (*Cananga odorata*), sweet marjoram (*Origanum majorana*), spikenard (*Nardus jatamansi*), neroli (*Citrus aurantium* var. *amara*)

Vasoconstrictors: cypress (*Cupressus sempervirens*), geranium (*Pelargonium graveolens*), lemon (*Citrus limon*), juniper (*Juniperus communis*)

Rubefacients: rosemary (*Rosmarinus officinalis*), juniper (*Juniperus communis*), eucalyptus (*Eucalyptus globulus*), ginger (*Zingiber officinale*), bay laurel (*Laurus nobilis*), black pepper (*Piper nigrum*), cinnamon (*Cinnamomum zeylanicum*)

Anticoagulants: helichrysum (*Helichrysum italicum*), clove (*Syzygium aromaticum*),[11] West Indian bay (*Pimenta racemosa*), cinnamon leaf (*Cinnamomum zeylanicum*), basil (*Ocimum gratissimum*), pimento (*Pimenta dioica*)

Common Problems of the Cardiovascular System

It is not within the scope of practice of massage therapists to treat most serious conditions of the heart or blood vessels. However, it is well documented that both massage and aromatherapy are helpful in the treatment of hypertension, which is a potentially dangerous problem itself as well as the cause of other serious cardiovascular issues. Aromatherapy massage can be a useful adjunct therapy for clients who are receiving treatment for these problems from primary care providers. Other, less dangerous but annoying issues, such as varicose veins or chronically cold hands and feet, can definitely improve with the regular use of aromatherapy treatments.

Hypertension

According to the National Institutes of Health, more than 50 million American adults (or one in four) suffer from high blood pressure. Many are not aware that they have the condition, and thus **hypertension** has become known as "the silent killer" because of the tendency of people with high blood pressure to become ill quite suddenly with no warning symptoms. A person is considered to have hypertension with a blood pressure reading consistently higher than 140/90.

Causes and Symptoms. Hypertension may be the result of an underlying pathology, such as kidney disease or a tumor. This type is known as secondary hypertension. Primary hypertension has no obvious direct cause but is associated with various risk factors, such as smoking, obesity, stress, lack of exercise, excessive alcohol consumption, and oral contraceptive use. It seems to occur more in men older than age 55, women older than age 45, African Americans, and those with a family history of hypertension.

Because the heart is forced to work harder, in time the muscle of the heart enlarges and finally weakens. The pressure also causes small tears in the walls of the blood vessels, which increase the risk of developing atherosclerosis, aneurysms, and strokes.

Essential Oils. Any of the oils listed as a hypotensive will be useful in treating this problem. If stress appears to be a contributing factor, the essential oils discussed in Chapter

15 should be considered. In my experience, lavender (*Lavandula angustifolia*), ylang ylang (*Cananga odorata*), sweet marjoram (*Origanum majorana*), and neroli (*Citrus aurantium* var. *amara*) have been particularly effective in helping with hypertension.

Methods of Application. Massage, especially of the arms and legs to encourage peripheral vasodilation, is helpful in treating high blood pressure. It can be combined with essential oils in a 1–3% dilution. Because this is a chronic problem, it is best addressed by using take-home remedies, such as spritzers with a 2–3% dilution of appropriate essential oils.

Angina Pectoris

Angina is a symptom, rather than a disease in itself. Physicians often consider it a warning signal of potential heart disease, and medications and/or lifestyle and dietary changes are often recommended for people who experience angina.

Causes and Symptoms. Angina is a result of inadequate blood flow to the walls of the heart, often because of a chronically accelerated heart rate as a result of stress or blocked arteries. It is experienced as mild to moderate chest pain or pressure, usually lasting up to 10 minutes. It is usually treated with rest or by taking nitroglycerin. The pain should not be ignored because angina can eventually lead to myocardial infarction (heart attack) if left untreated.

Essential Oils. As this painful condition is often triggered by physical or emotional stress, essential oils that are relaxing and analgesic will be helpful. Oils that have both properties include lavender (*Lavandula angustifolia*), Roman chamomile (*Chamaemelum nobile*), and myrrh (*Commiphora myrrha*). One study used an aerosol, including essential oils of "long pepper" (*Piper longum*) and sandalwood (*Santalum album*), and found it to be as effective as nitroglycerin for the quick relief of anginal pain.[12] Another study found that valerian essential oil (*Valeriana officinalis* var. *latifolia*) decreased the frequency of angina episodes and shortened their duration.[13]

Methods of Application. The use of essential oils in a low dilution (1–2%) in relaxation massage is most appropriate for clients who have angina, to help prevent attacks by lowering stress levels. A take-home blend can be given as a spritzer (1–2%) to be used as a preventative, or during an attack, to help relax the client.

Arrhythmia and Tachycardia

Arrhythmia is an irregular heartbeat, and **tachycardia** is an unusually rapid heartbeat. Both usually last for a very short time and are not generally regarded as dangerous from a medical standpoint, unless they continue for a long time. However, they can be extremely distressing for clients, especially when they do not know the cause and feel that their heart is out of control in some way. Both conditions are common and are popularly known as "palpitations."

Causes and Symptoms. An unusually fast heartbeat can occur for a variety of reasons, including exercise, stress, and physical trauma. However, tachycardia and arrhythmia might occur for no obvious reason, although stress does seem to be a factor. There are no symptoms beyond the uncomfortable sensation of an unusual heartbeat, but the sensations can produce considerable stress for the client.

Essential Oils. Oils commonly recommended in aromatherapy for arrhythmia or tachycardia include rose (*Rosa damascena* or *centifolia*), neroli (*Citrus aurantium* var. *amara*), lavender (*Lavandula angustifolia*), marjoram (*Origanum majorana*), and ylang ylang (*Cananga odorata*).

Methods of Application. Relaxation massage with essential oils in a low dilution (1–2%) can be helpful for clients who are prone to arrhythmia or tachycardia, to reduce the stress that may be a cause or a result. Because the onset of symptoms is extremely unpredictable, some kind of inhaler or spritzer that can be used rapidly would be useful, to relax the client and also to give him or her some sense of control over the issue.

Impaired Circulation

Impaired circulation can be a minor irritation when someone's hands are chronically cold. But it can represent a major health problem, leading to a lack of nutrition and oxygen being sent to important body tissues.

Causes and Symptoms. Impaired circulation can be the result of illnesses such as diabetes or Raynaud's disease. It can also be caused by compression of the blood vessels, as in thoracic outlet syndrome. However, it is most often caused by a sedentary lifestyle, lacking in the physical exercise that makes the heart pump faster and more efficiently, and lacking in the contraction of skeletal muscle to squeeze the blood back to the heart. Poor circulation often results in feelings of chilliness, cold hands and feet, and problems such as chilblains, which are red itchy bumps on the toes and fingers. It may also mean that tissues heal more slowly, because they receive less oxygen. In the worst cases, such as severe complications of diabetes or paralysis, impaired circulation can lead to tissue death, which may develop into gangrene and the resulting loss of that part of a limb. It is extremely important for people who cannot exercise or who have diseases such as diabetes to get regular massage and to use hydrotherapy and essential oils to improve circulation as much as possible.

Essential Oils. The rubefacient oils, such as ginger (*Zingiber officinale*), black pepper (*Piper nigrum*), rosemary (*Rosmarinus officinalis*), and juniper (*Juniperus communis*), tend to be most helpful. They are warming, which is always comforting for those with cold hands and feet, and they produce a mild irritation that draws blood to the area, improving local circulation. Studies show that a mixture of eucalyptus oil and menthol (found in high quantities in peppermint essential oil) applied to the skin on the forearm resulted in "significant increases in cutaneous blood flow, skin temperature, and muscle temperature."[14] In Russia the use of baths with white or yellow turpentine (usually derived from pine) was shown to improve capillary blood flow in patients with insulin-dependent diabetes.[15]

Methods of Application. Essential oils used in a full-body massage can help improve circulation. Using the oils in a warm bath will also be beneficial. However, the warming rubefacient oils will be more skin irritating when heat is added, so fewer drops of essential oil should be used. Strong heat is contraindicated for severely impaired circulation with poor tissue health, such as in diabetes.

Arteriosclerosis

Causes and Symptoms. **Arteriosclerosis** is the end stage of a disease that starts as **atherosclerosis,** which is a narrowing of the arteries caused by a thickening of the artery walls. As the thickening progresses, the elastic fibers of the arteries are replaced by scar tissue, making the vessels rigid and leading to hypertension. The arterial wall ulcerates, making the formation of a thrombus, or clot, more likely and increasing the risk of a heart attack, stroke, or kidney failure. Lifestyle factors such as stress, smoking, obesity, poor diet, and lack of exercise contribute to the progress of the disease.

Essential Oils. Arteriosclerosis is a serious disease, usually treated by cholesterol-lowering drugs, angioplasty, and even bypass surgery, and I am not suggesting that aromatherapy can take the place of these treatments. However, as part of a healthy lifestyle designed to prevent the more severe problems associated with arteriosclerosis, aromatherapy can definitely play a part. Stress-relieving essential oils (see Chapter 15) can help as part of a relaxation routine, and other oils may help with the hypertension that accompanies arteriosclerosis.

There have been a few studies on the direct effects of essential oils on the arteries and on clots. One study showed that inhaling the essential oils of lavender, basil, and monarda reduced the concentration of cholesterol in the aorta and reduced the effects of atherosclerotic plaques, giving an "angioprotective effect."[16] Other studies show that essential oils such as clove may help prevent the clotting that can result in a heart attack or stroke.[11]

Methods of Application. Applications are similar as for hypertension, with mild dilutions of essential oils in relaxation massage and take-home blends designed to help the client cope with stress.

CASE STUDY 17.1

Impaired Circulation

Ms. T. was a woman in her late forties, recently married, who came for massage because she felt tired and stressed. She was a self-employed psychotherapist, seeing about 15 to 16 clients per week. She complained of constantly feeling cold in spite of wearing several layers of clothing, warm socks, and sensible shoes. She and her husband ate a balanced whole-foods diet, took vitamin supplements, and were both regular meditators. She had consulted her primary care physician to check that the feelings of tiredness and cold were not related to any more serious ailment, but all the test results were normal.

Aromatherapy was suggested to help with the feelings of tiredness and cold, and she was also encouraged to start a fitness program to increase circulation through physical exercise. The following blend was made in a 3% dilution in 2 oz. of lotion and used in a vigorous full-body massage, with an emphasis on the feet and hands. The same oils were given to the client in a take-home blend to use in the bath:

Marjoram (*Origanum majorana*), 8 drops: relaxant, tonic

Bay laurel (*Laurus nobilis*), 10 drops: rubefacient, tonic

Black pepper (*Piper nigrum*), 10 drops: rubefacient, warming

Rosemary (*Rosmarinus officinalis*), 7 drops: rubefacient, tonic

After five massage sessions approximately 2 weeks apart, Ms. T. felt much warmer. She had continued to take baths with the blend about two or three times weekly, and felt that the exercise routine had contributed to the increased warmth and energy.

Varicose Veins

Varicose means dilated or distended. Varicose veins can occur at any age, but they are most common in women between ages 40 and 50 and generally occur in the legs. Surface veins that are varicosed are blue and bulging and should not be confused with spider veins, which are chronically dilated surface capillaries that usually produce thin red lines.

Causes and Symptoms. In some people, the valves in the veins stop working, usually because the vein has enlarged from extra pressure. The impaired valves allow blood to backflow and pool, and gravity makes the problem worse by increasing the pressure in the veins that have pooling. The main cause is unusual pressure on the veins, which slows circulation. Pressure can come from poor posture, tight clothes, obesity, constipation, or pregnancy. Standing for long periods of time may also be a factor, as a result of gravity. In some people the problem is mainly cosmetic, but for many people it is accompanied by mild to moderate pain and a feeling of fatigue or cramping in the legs. Anal varicose veins are commonly known as hemorrhoids.

Essential Oils. Generally, essential oils that are astringent and help tighten tissue have the best effects on varicose veins. Valnet indicates that cypress (*Cupressus sempervirens*) is an excellent remedy for varicosities and also suggests the very astringent lemon (*Citrus limon*).[17] Other essential oils that have beneficial effects include juniper (*Juniperus communis*), mastic (*Pistacia lentiscus*), and peppermint (*Mentha piperita*). If there is significant inflammation, essential oils such as helichrysum (*Helichrysum italicum*) and German chamomile (*Matricaria recutita*) can be added to the blend.

Methods of Application. Massage is frequently contraindicated locally over varicose veins, except for very gentle effleurage work toward the heart. Essential oils can be used in this type of massage or given to clients to apply over the area. Take-home blends are extremely important for this condition because regular daily application is required to make any change, which may take several months. Dilutions should be mild (about 2%), as application is so frequent. Blends need to be varied every few weeks to avoid allergic reactions.

Bruising

We have all had bruises. Generally not particularly serious, bruises show up as black or blue marks under the skin; they gradually fade to green and yellow and then disappear. They are discussed in the cardiovascular system because they are the result of injury to blood vessels.

Causes and Symptoms. The marks indicate areas where blood has escaped from the blood vessels and clotted in the tissue itself, usually from a direct blow of some kind. A bruise can be very small, or it can extend over large areas of the body, such as after a car accident. People who bruise unusually easily may have a vitamin C deficiency or they might suffer from hemophilia, a condition that keeps blood from clotting.

Essential Oils. Generally, bruises do not require treatment unless they are particularly painful or widespread. Oils that are anti-inflammatory and blood-moving are the most beneficial, including helichrysum (*Helichrysum italicum*), fennel (*Foeniculum vulgare*), hyssop (*Hyssopus officinalis*), rosemary (*Rosmarinus officinalis*), and sage (*Salvia officinalis*). With severe,

---

CASE STUDY 17.2

Varicose Veins

Mrs. B., age 34, had just had her second child. During her first pregnancy her legs frequently felt sore and tired, and during the second pregnancy her physician told her that she was developing varicose veins in her left lower leg. Four months after giving birth, the varicose veins showed no signs of going away. The following essential oils were blended at about a 3% dilution in a light lotion to help with the varicosities:

Blend 1

Cypress (*Cupressus sempervirens*), 40 drops: astringent, vasoconstrictor

Lemon (*Citrus limon*), 24 drops: astringent

Geranium (*Pelargonium graveolens*), 24 drops: astringent, vasoconstrictor

Peppermint (*Mentha piperita*), 4 drops: anti-inflammatory

Blend 2

Juniper (*Juniperus communis*), 20 drops: astringent

Grapefruit (*Citrus x paradisii*), 30 drops: lymphatic stimulant, astringent

Palmarosa (*Cymbopogon martinii*), 30 drops: anti-inflammatory, slightly astringent

Helichrysum (*Helichrysum italicum*), 10 drops: anti-inflammatory

Mrs. B. applied blend 1 at least once daily for about 6 weeks before switching to blend 2. She alternated the two blends every 4 to 6 weeks to avoid tolerance to the oils or the risk of allergic reaction. After 6 months of continual use, she reported that the varicose veins showed significant improvement, and her legs felt heavy and tired only rarely.

---

extensive bruising, oils such as black pepper (*Piper nigrum*), which supports the spleen (the organ that stores blood to release after a trauma), are useful.

Methods of Application. For a severe bruise with swelling and pain, essential oils in a strong dilution (10–20%), or even undiluted for smaller areas, can be used under a cold compress. The essential oils should be reapplied frequently in the first few hours to minimize the bruising. A few days later, essential oils in a milder dilution (2–3%) can be used in massage work to help move the clotted blood out of the area.

SUMMARY

- The main function of the cardiovascular system is to transport oxygen, hormones, nutrients, and wastes, such as carbon dioxide. It also regulates temperature and the pH of fluids.

- The heart beats at about 75 beats per minute. Heart rate is regulated by the autonomic nervous system, which means that it is strongly affected by physical and emotional stress.

- Blood is made up of mostly red blood cells and plasma, with white blood cells, platelets, electrolytes, and proteins.

- Arteries transport blood away from the heart and have thick, elastic walls. Veins transport blood back to the heart and have thinner walls and valves. Blood is returned to the heart by skeletal muscle contraction and the pull caused by respiration.

- Gases and nutrients are exchanged by capillaries.

- Risk factors for many problems of the cardiovascular system include lack of exercise, smoking, stress, obesity, excessive alcohol intake, and poor nutrition.

- Aromatherapy may affect the cardiovascular system by increasing parasympathetic nervous functioning or decreasing sympathetic nervous functioning; causing vasodilation and vasoconstriction; increasing local circulation; and reducing clotting.

- For high blood pressure, the hypotensive essential oils are best, used in a relaxation massage to encourage stress reduction and peripheral vasodilation.

- Angina seems to respond to essential oils that are relaxing and analgesic.

- Arrhythmia and tachycardia may be helped by essential oils that are relaxing and balancing to the cardiovascular system.

- Impaired circulation should be treated with rubefacient essential oils in a full-body massage or in baths.

- Varicose veins may be helped by the long-term application of astringent essential oils that tighten tissue.

- Bruising may be helped by the use of anti-inflammatory and circulatory-stimulating essential oils.

Review Questions

1. Match the word to the definition: (a) hypotensive, (b) rubefacient, (c) vasoconstrictor, (d) anticoagulant; (i) ginger, (ii) helichrysum, (iii) cypress, (iv) ylang ylang.
2. The regular use of spritzers or inhalers can be helpful for arrhythmia or tachycardia because they help to reduce _____ and give the client some sense of _____.
3. Which methods of application are most appropriate for a client with poor circulation?
4. Clients with diabetes are at risk of impaired circulation, leading to tissue death. To avoid this, this type of essential oil would be most beneficial: (a) astringent, (b) antispasmodic, (c) rubefacient, (d) calming.
5. Stress has been shown to be a major factor in hypertension. What types of essential oils would be beneficial?
6. Angina responds well to essential oils such as lavender and chamomile, which are both _____ and _____.
7. Should dilutions for varicose veins be strong or mild, and why?
8. Which of the following essential oils would be most appropriate for varicose veins? (a) cypress and geranium, (b) rosemary and ginger, (c) ylang ylang and jasmine, (d) sandalwood and cedarwood.
9. Name two essential oils that would be suitable for severe acute bruising with inflammation.
10. Black pepper is sometimes used when bruising is severe because it helps support the _____.

Notes

1. American Heart Association. Available at: www.americanheart.org. Accessed November 30, 2004.
2. Saeki Y. The effect of foot-bath with or without the essential oil of lavender on the autonomic nervous system: a randomized trial. Complement Ther Med 2000;8:2–7.
3. Tisserand R, Balacs T. Essential Oil Safety. London, UK: Churchill Livingstone, 1999:65.
4. Lahlou S, Figueiredo AF. Cardiovascular effects of 1,8 cineole, a terpenoid oxide present in many plant essential oils, in normotensive rats. Can J Physiol Pharmacol 2002;80(12):1125–1131.
5. Saeed SA, Gilani AH. Antithrombotic activity of clove oil. J Pak Med Assoc 1994;44(5):112–115.
6. Romine IJ, Bush, AM, Geist CR. Lavender aromatherapy in recovery from exercise. Percept Mot Skills 1999;88:756–758.
7. Ko FN, Huang TF, Teng CM. Vasodilatory action mechanisms of apigenin isolated from *Apium graveolens* in rat thoracic aorta. Biochim Biophys Acta 1999;1115(1):69–74.
8. Lahlou S, Interaminense Lde F, Leal-Cardoso JH, et al. Cardiovascular effects of the essential oil of *Ocimum gratissimum* leaves in rats: role of the autonomic nervous system. Clin Exp Pharmacol Physiol 2004; 31(4):219–225.

9. Dayawansa S, Umeno K, Takakura H, et al. Autonomic responses during inhalation of natural fragrance of Cedrol in humans. Auton Neurosci 2003;108(1–2):79–86.

10. El Tahir KEH, Ashour MMS, Al-Harbi MM. The cardiovascular actions of the volatile oil of the black seed (*Nigella sativa*) in rats: elucidation of the mechanism of action. Gen Pharm 1993;24(5): 1123–1131.

11. Saeed SA, Gilani AH. Antithrombotic activity of clove oil. J Pak Med Assoc 1994;44(5):112–115.

12. Guo S, Chen K, Weng WL, et al. Immediate effect of Kuan-xiong aerosol in the treatment of anginal attacks. Planta Med 1983;47:116.

13. Gui-Yuan Y, Wei W. Clinical studies on treatment of coronary heart disease with *Valeriana officinalis* var *latifolia*. Chung Kuo Chung Hsi I Chieh Ho Tsa Chih 1994;14(9):540–542.

14. Hong C-Z, Shellock FG, Shellock MD. Effects of a topically applied counterirritant (*Eucalyptamint*) on cutaneous blood flow and on skin and muscle temperatures. A placebo-controlled study. Am J Phys Med Rehab 1991;70:29–33.

15. Davydova OB, Turova EA, Golovach AV. The use of white and yellow turpentine baths with diabetic patients. Vopr Kurortol Fizioter Lech Fiz Kult 1998;3:3–10.

16. Nikolaevskii VV, Kononova NS, Pertsovskii AI, et al. Effect of essential oils on the course of experimental atherosclerosis. Patol Fiziol Eksp Ter 1990;5:52–53.

17. Valnet J. The Practice of Aromatherapy. Saffron Walden, UK: CW Daniel, 1992:210.

18

The Lymphatic System

The lymphatic system is the body's other circulatory mechanism, and it works together with the cardiovascular system to bring fluid to and from the tissues. Because it makes up an important part of the immune system, its efficiency is vital for our health. The lymphatic system also picks up leaked fluid from most parts of the body, and without it, the cardiovascular system could not function.

An Overview of the Lymphatic System

The lymphatic system consists of the lymphatic vessels, lymph nodes, lymphatic organs, and the lymph itself (Fig. 18.1).

Lymphatic vessels can be compared with blood vessels, in that larger and smaller ones make up a network that reaches to every cell of the body. However, unlike the cardiovascular system, the lymphatic system flows only in one direction: It sends fluid only toward the heart. From the blood capillaries, fluid is forced out at the arterial end and most of it is recaptured at the venous end. A small amount is left behind and is absorbed by the lymphatic capillaries to become lymphatic fluid, or lymph. Proteins, cell debris, viruses, and bacteria can also enter the highly permeable lymphatic capillaries. The lymph is taken through increasingly larger vessels and eventually returned to the cardiovascular system through either the right lymphatic duct or the thoracic duct, both in the thoracic region.

Lymphatic vessels have thin walls, and valves in the larger vessels prevent backflow. The lymph is circulated by pressure from movements of the skeletal muscles and from breathing, and by the contraction of smooth muscle in the larger lymphatic vessels. Figure 18.2 shows how the blood and lymph circulation interact.

The lymphatic system also consists of a network of nodes throughout the body, as well as the various glands made up of lymphatic tissue. As the lymph moves toward the heart, it is filtered through lymph nodes, small bean-shaped structures that occur in clusters along the vessels. Larger clusters are found in the inguinal, axillary, and cervical areas, and most people have experienced swollen, tender nodes during an infection in that area of the body. The nodes filter out large particles and contain white blood cells that attack pathogens such as bacteria and viruses.

The larger lymphatic organs include the spleen, the tonsils, and the thymus gland, as well as small patches of tissue (Peyer's patches) in the intestines. The spleen is a large organ with many important functions, including acting as a blood reservoir and destroying worn-out red blood cells. It also produces lymphocytes, white blood cells that are part of the immune system. The tonsils are also an important part of the immune system; located at the top of the throat, they fight pathogens that are breathed in or ingested. The thymus

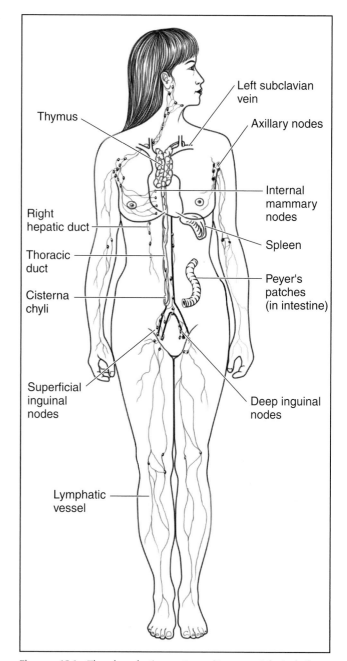

Figure 18.1 The lymphatic system. (Source: Adapted from Premkumar K. The Massage Connection Anatomy and Physiology. Baltimore: Lippincott Williams and Wilkins, 2004.)

is located just above the heart and produces hormones that help regulate certain types of lymphocytes.

The main function of the lymphatic system is to capture fluid and proteins from the interstitial spaces (spaces between cells) and transport them back to the cardiovascular system. When the system does not work efficiently, fluid collects in the tissue, making it swollen and puffy. The lymphatic system is also a key part of the immune system, filtering out and destroying pathogens before they can enter the bloodstream. Because the lymph collects waste products along with the fluid picked up from most parts of the body, it is an essential

Lymphatic system

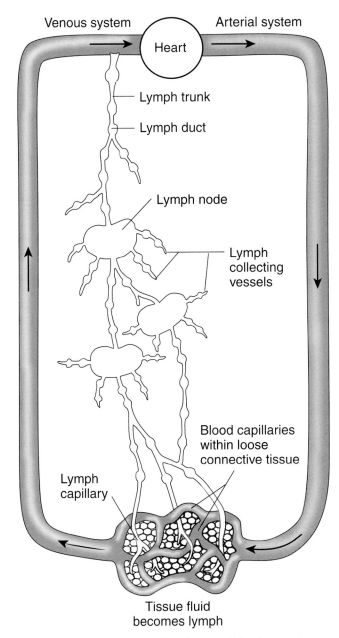

Figure 18.2 The relationship of lymphatic and blood circulation.

part of the body's detoxification process. If lymph movement is sluggish, the other channels of elimination and detoxification may become overloaded, and the person is at even more risk of a compromised immune system.

Risk Factors

Factors that have a negative effect on the lymphatic system include:

- *Lack of exercise.* Because the lymphatic system has no pump to push the lymph through the vessels, its circulation relies on movement of skeletal muscle and breathing.

- *Trauma and infection.* Lymphatic flow can be impeded by anything that blocks or damages the vessels, including injury or surgery, and infections or parasites.

How Aromatherapy Affects the Lymphatic System

There is much debate in aromatherapy circles about the extent to which essential oils can affect the lymphatic system directly. Traditionally, certain essential oils are reputed to be lymphatic stimulants, and they are often used together with lymphatic drainage techniques. However, according to Simon Mills, an experienced herbal practitioner and educator, "clinical experience suggests that this is a useful treatment, but probably not for the reasons often given."[1] He cites one study suggesting that a glass of beer actually stimulated lymph flow more effectively than any of the traditional lymphatic movers.

Most of the oils traditionally used to help move the lymph have a definite **astringent** effect, tightening tissue where they are applied, and it is possible that this firming effect helps move lymph in the superficial channels. Many of the same essential oils also have a significant effect on the organs of detoxification or elimination. In other words, they are either **hepatics,** stimulating to the liver, or **diuretics,** stimulating the kidneys to produce urine. Anything that supports detoxification in the body will have an indirect beneficial action on the lymphatic system. Increasing blood circulation will also have an effect on lymph flow, as the two are strongly connected.

Lymphatic flow stimulants: grapefruit (*Citrus x paradisii*), cypress (*Cupressus sempervirens*), lemon (*Citrus limon*), juniper (*Juniperus communis*), fennel (*Foeniculum vulgare*), geranium (*Pelargonium graveolens*)

Blood circulatory stimulants: rosemary (*Rosmarinus officinalis*), black pepper (*Piper nigrum*), cinnamon (*Cinnamomum verum*), ginger (*Zingiber officinale*), juniper (*Juniperus communis*)

Common Problems of the Lymphatic System

Because the lymphatic system is such an important part of the immune system and of the body's detoxification process, when it does not work efficiently, the most usual ailments are some kind of infection such as a cold or flu, or a worsening of a toxicity problem affecting the other systems, such as acne or dermatitis. However, only a few ailments directly show lymphatic stagnation, such as edema.

Edema

Edema is an accumulation of protein and fluid in the interstitial spaces. It can be specific to a part of the body, or it may be systemic, affecting the entire body. Over time, the trapped protein causes a thickening of connective tissue and a hardening and enlargement of the tissues in the immediate area.

Causes and Symptoms. The cause of edema is lymphostasis, a stagnation of lymph flow; the normal lymph flow is blocked in some way. Common underlying reasons include physical trauma, surgery (especially surgery removing the lymph nodes), infection, parasites, or increased capillary pressure resulting from pregnancy, heart problems, allergic response, and other factors. Gravity-induced edema results from standing or sitting for long periods of time. Edema resulting from infections or caused by trauma, such as sprains, burns, or bruises, is a normal part of the healing process and generally will resolve after some time. Edema resulting from surgery, lack of movement, or systemic ailments often needs assistance, from either manual lymphatic drainage or some form of compression.

The most common symptom is the easily observed swelling of the tissues. With edema caused by injury or infection, the tissues are often tight and hot; with edema caused by surgery or systemic conditions, the tissues are more likely to be congested and cool. With pitted edema, pressure applied to the tissues leaves an impression. Pain or discomfort caused by pressure within the tissues is common, and range of motion may be impaired.

Essential Oils. Essential oils often used in aromatherapy to move lymph and reduce swelling include grapefruit (*Citrus x paradisii*), geranium (*Pelargonium graveolens*), juniper (*Juniperus communis*), fennel (*Foeniculum vulgare*), and cypress (*Cupressus sempervirens*).

Methods of Application. The essential oils are best applied to the affected area in a moderately strong dilution (3–5%) after manual lymphatic drainage techniques, or during a superficial effleurage. Essential oils can also be applied to the skin under a cold compress, which can be particularly useful for edema resulting from trauma or surgery.

Cellulite

Cellulite is not a medical term; the word was originally used in the 1970s in spas and salons to describe the uneven, dimpled appearance of the skin found on many women's thighs and buttocks. Although cellulite is more commonly seen in women older than age 30, it can occur as early as puberty and is found in both overweight and very slim people. It is often called "orange peel skin" or "cottage cheese skin." Cellulite is not usually regarded as a health issue. It is often described as an issue of lymphatic stagnation, and certainly stimulating lymphatic circulation and blood circulation can have a temporary beneficial cosmetic effect on cellulite.

Causes and Symptoms. The causes of cellulite are not well understood. Many companies in the cosmetics industry have described cellulite as a combination of trapped fat, water, and

---

CASE STUDY 18.1

Edema

Mr. P., age 56, had multiple sclerosis and was in a wheelchair. His feet, ankles, and lower legs were greatly swollen and pitted edema was evident. The skin on the soles of his feet was dry and cracked. He had been diagnosed with multiple sclerosis about 7 years previously and the disease had progressed to the stage that he was no longer able to walk or stand. He was extremely depressed. He had requested massage mainly because of shoulder and back pain. After three sessions of shoulder and back massage, it was suggested that some drainage work with essential oils might help improve the condition of his legs. The following blend was made in a dilution of 4% in 4 oz. of lotion:

Grapefruit (*Citrus x paradisii*), 30 drops: lymphatic stimulant, antidepressant

Juniper (*Juniperus communis*), 20 drops: lymphatic stimulant

Fennel (*Foeniculum vulgare*), 18 drops: lymphatic stimulant

German chamomile (*Matricaria recutita*), 12 drops: relaxing, moisturizing for the skin

Rosemary (*Rosmarinus officinalis*), 18 drops: blood circulatory stimulant, strengthening

The blend was used in light manual lymphatic drainage on Mr. P.'s feet and legs for 10–15 minutes once a week. After several weeks, there was a noticeable difference in the swelling, especially in the feet and ankles. Mr. P. noted that his feet felt more comfortable. The cracks on the soles of the feet had almost healed and the skin was much less dry.

---

toxins that have accumulated in certain areas as a result of an unhealthy diet and lack of exercise. However, it is just as likely to be simply unevenness in the connective tissue underlying the dermis. There appear to be no symptoms other than the puckered or dimpled appearance of the skin.

There has been a lot of research on nonsurgical treatments for cellulite, including internal medications or supplements, topical creams, compression techniques, electrical stimulation, and heating pads. There is a lot of controversy regarding whether any treatments actually work at all for cellulite. Certainly, they have to be carried out regularly and consistently to have any good effects. One study stated: "At present, it can be safely stated that there is no topical medication or manipulative process to which advanced cellulite responds in a treatment period of less than 2 months."[2] Many other studies cite treatment periods of 6 months or longer. Most topical treatments consist of ingredients designed to decrease water retention and increase lymphatic and blood circulation.

Essential Oils. Essential oils used in commercial topical creams for cellulite include clove, cinnamon, ginger, peppermint, and juniper. There is no evidence to show that these have any effect on cellulite, and several of them can cause skin irritation if used in high amounts on the sensitive skin of the thighs and buttocks.

SUMMARY

- The lymphatic system consists of lymphatic vessels, nodes, organs, and lymphatic fluid (lymph). Its function is to pick up fluid at the cellular level and return it to the cardiovascular system.
- Lymph is circulated in the vessels by pressure from muscular movements, and by smooth muscle contraction in the larger lymph vessels.
- The lymphatic system is an important part of immune functioning. The lymph nodes and the tonsils trap and destroy pathogens, and the spleen and thymus help produce lymphocytes.
- If the lymphatic system is not working correctly, elimination, detoxification, and immunity may all be affected.

- Risk factors are lack of exercise and trauma or infection.
- There is some doubt as to whether essential oils traditionally used as lymphatic stimulants actually work. Astringent oils, diuretics, and circulatory stimulants may have some beneficial effect on lymph flow.
- Edema is an accumulation of blood and fluid in interstitial spaces. Manual lymphatic drainage with essential oils can be helpful.
- Cellulite is a cosmetic issue, possibly involving lymphatic stagnation. There is controversy regarding treatments, which need to be long term.

Review Questions

1. Match the word to the definition: (a) increases output of urine, (b) tightens tissue, (c) stimulates the liver; (i) astringent, (ii) diuretic, (iii) hepatic.
2. Lymphatic stagnation can lead to _____, a lowered _____ functioning, or the worsening of _____ issues, such as dermatitis.
3. Name three essential oils traditionally used to treat edema.
4. The most appropriate treatment method for edema is essential oils with: (a) deep tissue work, (b) hot compresses, (c) light effleurage or manual lymphatic techniques, (d) some form of spa therapy.
5. Cellulite is considered by some people to be trapped _____, _____, and _____ under the dermis. However, medical authorities usually consider it to be simply uneven _____.
6. Essential oils commonly used in commercial topical preparations for cellulite include: (a) rose and jasmine, (b) fennel and grapefruit, (c) lavender and rosemary, (d) cinnamon and peppermint.
7. What are the risks of essential oils commonly used in cellulite preparations, if used in high amounts on the skin?

Notes

1. Mills S. The Essential Book of Herbal Medicine. London, UK: Arkana, 1991:97.

2. Draelos ZD, Marenus KD. Cellulite. Etiology and purported treatment. Dermatol Surg 1997;23(12):1177–1181.

19

The Nervous System

For a long time the brain was regarded as the controller of the entire body. Old illustrations showed a tiny person, or homunculus, sitting inside the skull directing all the movements of the larger body. Today we know that the situation is not that simple. The nervous system, together with the endocrine system, is the master control and communication system of the body, regulating most of the complex processes that occur throughout our lives. It is also the center for learning, memory, emotion, and thought.

An Overview of the Nervous System

The nervous system has three major functions:

1. It monitors changes inside and outside the body by way of sensors.

2. It processes and interprets the information from the sensors and responds according to the body's needs.

3. It sends messages to muscles or glands to effect this response.

As the nervous system oversees so many of the checks and balances that keep the body functioning smoothly, it has to have an excellent means of communication. This is accomplished through electrical impulses that are fast, are specific, and cause an immediate response in muscles or glands.

The different parts of the nervous system are classified by either structure or function. On a structural level, there are two parts. The central nervous system (CNS), composed of the brain and the spinal cord, does most of the interpreting of data and decision making. The peripheral nervous system (PNS), made up of the spinal and cranial nerves, carries impulses to and from the CNS. Sensory (afferent) nerves carry information to the CNS, while motor (efferent) nerves carry instructions from the CNS to the various glands or muscles. Figure 19.1 shows this exchange of information and commands.

On a functional level, the efferent section of the PNS is divided into the somatic nervous system and the autonomic nervous system. The somatic nervous system allows us to voluntarily control our skeletal muscles, although some muscle reflexes are involuntary. The autonomic nervous system (ANS) is involuntary; it sends messages to glands and internal organs, which are not under our conscious control. The ANS is further divided into sympathetic and parasympathetic divisions. The sympathetic nervous system stimulates various parts of the body for action. This action is often referred to as the fight-or-flight response (see Chapter 15). The parasympathetic nervous system is often related to what is called the rest-and-repair response, and ideally the body should be in this mode for much of the time. Figure 19.2 shows a representation of these divisions.

All nervous tissue is made up of two types of cells: neurons, which transmit the electrical impulses, and neuroglia, which are supporting cells that insulate and protect the delicate neurons. Synapses are gaps between neurons, and impulses are conveyed across the synapse by neurotransmitters, chemicals manufactured by the neuron. The fatty insulating covers around some nerve fibers are called myelin sheaths, and these help nerve impulses to move faster. Neurons are unusual among the body's cells in that they do not have the ability to divide; once they die, they are not renewed (with the exception of the olfactory nerves, which are renewed about once every 60 days). As a result, there are many nervous system issues associated with aging, such as slower reaction time, loss of vision and hearing, and possibly a failing of short-term memory.

The delicate brain and spinal cord exist in a controlled environment, protected by the bony coverings of the skull and vertebrae, and are bathed in their own fluid, called the cerebrospinal fluid (CSF). Capillaries that are less permeable than usual make up the blood–brain barrier, which prevents toxins such as body wastes, proteins, and many drugs from entering the CNS.

The part of the brain that most interests aromatherapists is the limbic system, which is strongly affected by odors (see Chapter 4). This complex system regulates memory, emotions, and sexual behavior. One of the structures in the limbic brain, the hypothalamus, is the important link between the nervous system and the endocrine system, as it has nerve tissue that both conducts impulses and secretes hormones.

Risk Factors

Factors that have a negative effect on the nervous system include:

- *Trauma.* Because neurons cannot renew themselves, any damage to the nervous system is likely to be permanent. This irreversible damage can be seen in accidents that sever the spinal cord, resulting in paralysis of any muscles stimulated by nerves below the injury. The results of head injuries can be seen in many retired professional boxers who may have slurred speech, tremors, and dementia.

- *Circulatory problems.* The brain is more dependent than most tissues on oxygen carried by the blood. Health problems such as arteriosclerosis, which results in a decrease of blood and therefore oxygen to tissues, may be the cause of senility in later life.

- *Drugs and alcohol.* Drugs influence the brain mainly by altering the transmission of neurotransmitters between the synapses, and some of these changes may permanently affect the brain. For example, like boxers, chronic alcoholics tend to have symptoms of premature senility, and computed tomography scans of their brains show significant reductions in size.

- *Pain and stress.* Both of these factors appear to sensitize the nervous system, so that people with chronic pain or who have long-term stress tend to have a lower tolerance for further pain.

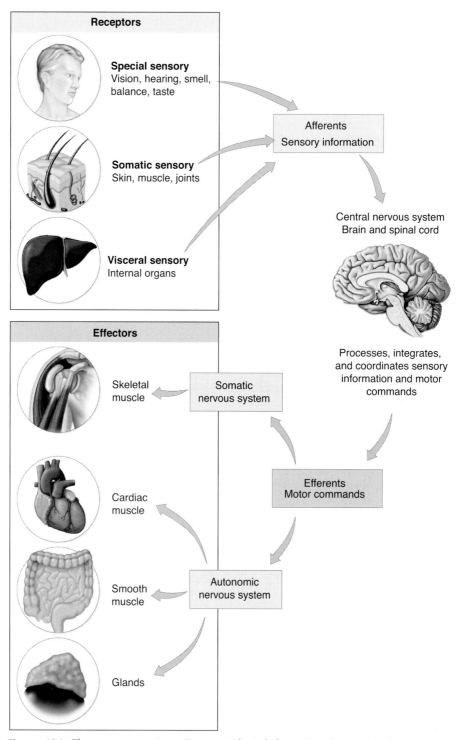

Figure 19.1 The nervous system. (Source: Adapted from Premkumar K. The Massage Connection Anatomy and Physiology. Baltimore: Lippincott, Williams and Wilkins, 2004.)

How Aromatherapy Affects the Nervous System

The olfactory system—the sense of smell—is a part of the nervous system. It is made up of nervous tissue and has the only neurons that renew themselves regularly. Chapter 4 explored the connections between the olfactory system and the limbic brain, and how odors strongly affect the working of the nervous system via the amygdala and the hypothalamus. Studies show that essential oils have a particularly strong influence on the sympathetic and parasympathetic divisions of the nervous system.[1]

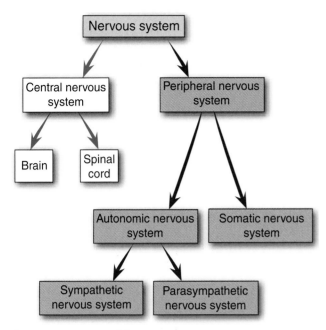

Figure 19.2 Divisions of the nervous system.

The fastest effects on the nervous system in aromatherapy are often achieved by inhalation, as the brain registers the aroma almost instantly and modulates the nervous system in response. For nerve pain, however, as in sciatica or facial neuralgia, topical application provides the most relief. Although aromatherapy is not suggested as a primary treatment for more severe diseases of the nervous system, like Parkinson's or Alzheimer's, it can help ease some of the symptoms.

Essential oils that produce the most noticeable effects are **neurodepressants,** which calm the nervous system, and **neurostimulants,** which access the sympathetic system. Some analgesic essential oils seem to be more effective for neuropathic (nerve) pain than others, and several essential oils are reputed to be **nervines,** or substances that are strengthening to the nervous system as a whole.

Neurodepressants (calming): rose (*Rosa damascena*),[2] linden blossom (*Tilia x europaea*),[3] lavender (*Lavandula angustifolia*),[4] neroli (*Citrus aurantium* var. *amara*),[5] sandalwood (*Santalum album*),[6] hops (*Humulus lupulus*),[7] Roman chamomile (*Chamaemelum nobile*),[8] bitter orange (*Citrus aurantium* var. *amara*),[9] lemongrass (*Cymbopogon citratus*),[10] valerian (*Valeriana officinalis*),[11] patchouli (*Pogostemon cablin*)[12]

Neurostimulants: black pepper (*Piper nigrum*), tarragon (*Artemisia dracunculus*), fennel (*Foeniculum vulgare*), grapefruit (*Citrus x paradisii*),[13] peppermint (*Mentha piperita*),[14] jasmine (*Jasminum grandiflorum*)[15]

Nervines: fennel (*Foeniculum vulgare*),[16] basil (*Ocimum basilicum*), clary sage (*Salvia sclarea*), rosemary (*Rosmarinus officinalis*), black spruce (*Picea mariana*), sage (*Salvia officinalis*), linden blossom (*Tilia x europaea*)

Analgesics: peppermint (*Mentha piperita*), geranium (*Pelargonium graveolens*), lavender (*Lavandula angustifolia*), nutmeg (*Myristica fragrans*), Roman chamomile (*Chamaemelum nobile*), eucalyptus (*Eucalyptus radiata*), marjoram (*Origanum majorana*)

Common Problems of the Nervous System

Many of the more emotional issues connected with the nervous system, such as anxiety and depression, were discussed in Chapter 15 under stress-related problems. In this chapter, we will focus on the more physical aspects of nervous system imbalance.

Nerve Pain

In a broad sense, all pain can be regarded as nerve pain, since we feel everything through our sensory nerves. However, we generally make distinctions between types of pain that result from different causes.[17] Many clients say they are experiencing a "muscle pain" when they feel they have damaged soft tissue in some way, and the pain tends to be more radiating and diffuse. Others refer to "nerve pain," which has a distinct character and is usually described as "sharp," "burning," "numbing," "shooting," or "knife-like." Conditions associated with nerve pain are sciatica, thoracic outlet syndrome (TOS), carpal tunnel syndrome, and trigeminal neuralgia, in which the major symptom is nerve pain, though other symptoms may also be present.

Causes and Symptoms. Nerve pain, often referred to as neuralgia, is most often caused by some kind of impingement or localized trauma to the nerve or by prolonged exposure to cold. Nerves can be impinged by a dislocated bone, a herniated disc, enlargement of the uterus during pregnancy, a tumor, or scar tissue. Other causes can be bacterial or viral infections, or diseases such as multiple sclerosis. The main symptom is the shooting pain described previously, although other problems, such as loss of motor control or weakness, may be present if there is nerve damage.

Essential Oils. Oils described as analgesic will be useful to some extent for any type of pain, and some seem to be particularly good for nerve pain. Among the essential oils listed above as analgesics, I have had particular success with nutmeg (*Myristica fragrans*), lavender (*Lavandula angustifolia*), eucalyptus (*Eucalyptus radiata*), and marjoram (*Origanum majorana*). If warmth seems to bring temporary relief from pain, some of the hotter analgesic oils, such as black pepper (*Piper nigrum*) or ginger (*Zingiber officinale*), may be used.

Methods of Application. Relaxation massage with long superficial effleurage strokes is probably most soothing for minor nerve pain, although massage is contraindicated for acute neuralgia. Compresses also may be useful. Essential oils should be used with massage or with compresses in a medium-strong dilution, such as 4–8%, depending on the size and location of the painful area.

Shingles

Shingles is an illness that affects both the skin and the nerves. The basic cause of the condition is a viral infection of the nerves.

Causes and Symptoms. When someone catches chicken-pox, the virus that causes the illness, herpes zoster, is absorbed into the nerve root where it lies dormant, possibly for decades. It may be reactivated by stress, trauma, surgery, aging, or fatigue. The first symptoms are itching or nerve pain, and a rash or blisters generally develops along the path of the affected nerve. There may also be fever and muscle pain. The rash often disappears within 3 to 4 weeks but the nerve pain can remain for several more weeks, or months.

Essential Oils. Several essential oils are reputed to be effective against the herpes zoster virus, including bergamot (*Citrus x bergamia*), tea tree (*Melaleuca alternifolia*), ravensara (*Ravensara aromatica*), and melissa (*Melissa officinalis*). Others, such as German chamomile (*Matricaria recutita*), peppermint (*Mentha piperita*), lavender (*Lavandula angustifolia*), and helichrysum (*Helichrysum italicum*), are helpful in relieving the initial itchy rash. Essential oils for nerve pain (listed previously) should be used once the skin has healed.

Methods of Application. Local massage over the shingles rash is contraindicated because of neuralgia and the possibility of infection. The essential oils should be put into a carrier for self-application by the client. During the period of the rash, I have found that cooling carriers such as aloe vera, hydrosols, or witch hazel, with essential oils in a 10% dilution, provide the most relief. Cool baths with oatmeal and 10–15 drops of essential oil are also helpful. After the skin has healed, essential oils can be applied in a 2–3% dilution, in a carrier such as oil or lotion to help with nerve pain.

Paralysis

Paralysis is the inability to contract muscles, either voluntarily or involuntarily. It may affect muscle groups in large areas of the body, leaving the person unable to walk, for example, and recovery may not be possible. On the other hand, with some types of paralysis, smaller areas of the body may be affected and recovery may be spontaneous within a matter of weeks or months. An example of the latter is Bell's palsy, which affects the muscles on one side of the face.

Causes and Symptoms. Paralysis is generally caused by a lesion (scar tissue in the CNS) or by some other kind of compression of the nerve. If there is tissue damage in the CNS, the damaged neurons often cannot repair themselves and scar tissue forms rapidly, making repair impossible. In the PNS, neurons can repair themselves when damaged,

---

CASE STUDY 19.1

Shingles

Mrs. C., age 56, had been diagnosed with shingles about 2 months previously. She had had blisters on her trunk for a few weeks, which had been itchy and painful, but these had finally disappeared after getting a topical medication from her physician. However, she had residual nerve pain, which was greatly distressing her, as it showed no signs of clearing up. She expressed feelings of depression and frustration and said that her husband had suggested a massage might help her feel better.

Aromatherapy was suggested to help with the nerve pain. Essential oils were chosen that were analgesic but also relaxing to help relieve the stress and depression. She was concerned that the essential oils might irritate the skin where the blisters had been, as it still felt slightly sensitive, so the oils were used in a 1% dilution. This was increased to 2% in later massages. The following blend was used in 2 oz. of oil:

Geranium (*Pelargonium graveolens*), 3 drops: analgesic, uplifting

Lavender (*Lavandula angustifolia*), 5 drops: analgesic, calming

Roman chamomile (*Chamaemelum nobile*), 2 drops: analgesic, calming

Nutmeg (*Myristica fragrans*), 2 drops: analgesic, antidepressant

Mrs. C. reported feeling calmer and more relaxed immediately after the massage and said that there was possibly slightly less nerve pain. However, this could have been simply a change in pain perception, since she was feeling better emotionally. The oils were given in a take-home blend to be applied when needed. She returned for two more massages, 2 weeks apart, and reported at the end of 4 weeks that the nerve pain had subsided significantly. On follow-up 1 month later, the nerve pain had disappeared completely, and Mrs. C. seemed much calmer and happier.

---

especially if the nerves are not severed, or if the cut ends are in close contact. Injury to the spinal cord or brain is a common cause of paralysis. Other causes include diseases such as multiple sclerosis or Parkinson's disease, infection, stroke, or compression on the nerve from edema, tissue swelling, or a tumor.

The major symptom is a loss of motor function, though the muscles may be slack and loose (flaccid paralysis) or tight and contracted (spastic paralysis). There may be pain, depending on the cause of the paralysis, or tremors. Secondary problems often occur as a result of the paralysis. These problems include decreased tissue and joint health from the lack of movement, postural imbalances, and emotional issues, perhaps resulting from changes in brain chemistry or the stress of the condition itself. Edema is common, resulting from the lack of movement of skeletal muscles, which help to pump lymph around the body.

Essential Oils. Since there is no cure for paralysis but spontaneous recovery occurs in a certain number of cases, aromatherapists tend to concentrate on maintaining good tissue health, using essential oils such as cypress (*Cupressus sempervirens*), grapefruit (*Citrus x paradisii*), or geranium (*Pelargonium graveolens*) to help lymphatic flow and rubefacient oils such as rosemary (*Rosmarinus officinalis*), bay laurel (*Laurus nobilis*), black pepper (*Piper nigrum*), and eucalyptus (*Eucalyptus globulus*) to encourage blood flow in the affected area. Antispasmodic oils such as petitgrain (*Citrus aurantium* var. *amara*), cardamon (*Elettaria cardamomum*), clary sage (*Salvia sclarea*), or Roman chamomile (*Chamaemelum nobile*) can be used to help avoid muscle contracture.

Methods of Application. Essential oils in a 2–3% dilution for full-body massage work well with relaxation massage to reduce spasticity and pain, or after lymphatic drainage techniques to encourage lymph flow.

Migraine Headache

More than 28 million people in the United States suffer from migraine headaches, and women are three times more likely than men to get them.[18] Migraines and migraine-type headaches are widely regarded as being a nervous system disorder with many different symptoms that can vary significantly from person to person. The symptoms have been recorded for centuries.

Causes and Symptoms. Unlike tension headaches, the causes of migraines are largely unknown, although there might be a genetic factor. Objects and situations that trigger the attacks have been closely observed and can include stress, food allergies, insomnia, aromas such as gasoline or perfumes, hunger, hormonal fluctuations, loud noises, bright lights, and medications.

The list of symptoms is equally long and includes throbbing pain in the head, often on one side only; visual disturbances; hypersensitivity to light, sounds, and smells; nausea; and muscle achiness. Sufferers often need to lie down in a quiet, dark room for several hours until the migraine dies down. The chronic pain, as well as the unpredictability of attacks, which can mean time lost from work, is stressful. Some people can accurately predict when they will get a migraine

several hours in advance because of unusual physical symptoms, such as excessive yawning. Many will know up to an hour in advance because of visual disturbances.

Essential Oils. For some people in the middle of a migraine, the very thought of a smell can make them sick. This is not the time to try to treat a migraine with aromatherapy! For those people who are able to predict their migraines, essential oils such as peppermint (*Mentha piperita*),

---

CASE STUDY 19.2

Bell's Palsy

Mr. R., age 33, had Bell's palsy, a type of facial paralysis, probably caused by exposure to a chill while camping. The muscles on the left side of his face were completely flaccid, and the left eye and left side of the face sagged slightly. He was unable to close his left eye. His physician had given him an eye patch and antibiotic drops to help prevent infection of the left eye, but otherwise no medication was prescribed. His doctor was optimistic, as spontaneous recovery occurs in about 70% of cases, and had recommended that Mr. R. have facial and neck massage to maintain tissue health and circulation. Although he was experiencing no pain, he was embarrassed by the fact that his facial expressions were distorted because he worked as a salesman and could not smile without grimacing.

Bay laurel and rosemary were used as rubefacient oils to help with blood circulation, as they are warming without being too harsh on the sensitive skin of the face. A blend of the following oils was made at a 2% dilution:

Bay laurel (*Laurus nobilis*), 8 drops: warming and soothing

Rosemary (*Rosmarinus officinalis*), 8 drops: rubefacient, stimulating to circulation

Cypress (*Cupressus sempervirens*), 8 drops: lymph stimulant

The massage and the oil blend produced a feeling of relaxation in the facial muscles, which had felt tense to Mr. R. The remainder of the oil was sent home with him to apply once daily. He returned for weekly facial massage sessions, showing a gradual increase in facial movement on the left side between weeks 5 and 7. He continued to use the oil blend at home because he enjoyed the sensation of warmth from it. He made a complete recovery within 8 weeks.

lemon (*Citrus limon*), lavender (*Lavandula angustifolia*), or basil (*Ocimum basilicum*) can sometimes avert an attack. Peppermint, with its beneficial effect on pain and nausea and its sharp, fresh smell, would be the only oil I would recommend trying during a migraine-type headache.

Between episodes, essential oils can be used to lower stress levels, improve sleep, relax muscles, and work on any other issue that may be a trigger for the migraines. Geranium (*Pelargonium graveolens*) used regularly seems to work particularly well for women who suffer from hormonally triggered migraines. Marjoram (*Origanum majorana*) and rosemary (*Rosmarinus officinalis*) are useful to help reduce hypertonicity.

Methods of Application. During a migraine, peppermint can be used undiluted on the head, if the smell can be tolerated. Often a couple of drops of the oil on the temples will bring some people almost instant relief, or 2–3 drops on the occiput with a cold compress on top can be helpful. The same techniques, or gentle aromatherapy massage to the neck and shoulder muscles, can help avoid a migraine. Between headaches, massage and essential oils can be used to reduce hypertonicity and trigger points.

Epilepsy

Epilepsy is the tendency to have repeated seizures caused by unusual activity in the brain. The typical preconception of an epileptic fit is that of the person falling to the floor and writhing. In fact, this type of seizure, called grand mal, is not commonly seen, particularly since about 75% of people control their epilepsy with medications.

Causes and Symptoms. The seizures that occur are a symptom that normal brain functioning has been disrupted in some way, and often the underlying causes are not known. Epilepsy can also be the result of scarring, caused by trauma to the head, a stroke, or an infection or disease affecting the brain. Seizures can be triggered by many factors, especially emotional stress, flashing lights, alcohol, lack of sleep, and food allergies. As with migraines, sufferers can sometimes predict seizures in advance because of unusual physical sensations, and they occasionally find ways to avert them. When one of my clients with epilepsy felt these warning signs, he would try to resolve any emotional stress, especially ongoing disagreements with other people, and was often successful in avoiding a seizure.

Symptoms can be mild, such as a brief loss of consciousness and a blank stare for several seconds to a minute. Other symptoms include muscle spasms, to greater or lesser degrees.

Essential Oils. Many essential oils have been contraindicated for use with people who have epilepsy, for fear of triggering an attack. However, according to Tisserand and Balacs, "the only recorded cases where seizures have been induced by essential oils, the oils were taken orally."[19] With clients whose epileptic seizures are triggered by strong smells, the therapist should use only the mildest smelling oils in a very mild dilution. For others, research shows that aromatherapy can actually be helpful, especially when used for stress reduction. One report from the seizure clinic of a hospital in England stated that of 100 patients treated with aromatherapy, a third were seizure-free for at least a year.[20] Essential oils that would be particularly beneficial include bergamot (*Citrus x bergamia*), bitter orange (*Citrus aurantium* var. *amara*), lavender (*Lavandula angustifolia*), Roman chamomile (*Chamaemelum nobile*), ylang ylang (*Cananga odorata*), clary sage (*Salvia sclarea*), and marjoram (*Origanum majorana*).

Methods of Application. Full-body relaxation massage with essential oils in a fairly mild dilution of 1–2% will be most helpful. Clients can also use the essential oils at home in vaporizers, spritzers, or baths as part of a stress-reduction program.

Parkinson's Disease

Causes and Symptoms. The cause of Parkinson's disease is unknown. The disease involves degeneration of the neurons of the basal ganglia, a part of the brain's cerebral cortex that helps govern movement. The neurons secrete the neurotransmitter dopamine. Drugs that depress dopamine activity, such as tranquilizers, can trigger Parkinson's-type syndrome, as can street drugs and other toxins, or repeated head trauma (e.g., from boxing). The main symptoms are tremors, rigidity of muscles and joints, difficulty in balancing, and bradykinesia, a difficulty in initiating and carrying out voluntary movements. There may be many other symptoms as the disease progresses. It may progress slowly or rapidly.

Essential Oils. As there is no cure for Parkinson's, the approach is to try to lessen the symptoms by decreasing sympathetic nervous system activity. Stress appears to worsen symptoms, and calming essential oils, such as Roman chamomile (*Chamaemelum nobile*), bitter orange (*Citrus aurantium* var. *amara*), neroli (*Citrus aurantium* var. *amara*), linden blossom (*Tilia vulgaris*), and rose (*Rosa damascena*), help the client enter parasympathetic functioning.[21] Nervines such as basil (*Ocimum basilicum*) and black spruce (*Picea mariana*) may be useful late in the disease, as clients tend to fatigue easily. I have found that using antispasmodic oils such as basil (*Ocimum basilicum*) or petitgrain (*Citrus aurantium* var. *amara*) while giving massage tends to decrease spastic movements.

Methods of Application. Essential oils to reduce sympathetic nervous system activity can be used in a relaxation massage (1–2%), or by the client at home in a vaporizer.

Alzheimer's Disease

Alzheimer's disease (AD) is a progressive degenerative disease of the brain that eventually causes dementia. About 5–15% of people older than age 65 develop the disease.

Causes and Symptoms. The exact cause of AD is unknown, but it involves a reduction in acetylcholine, a neurotransmitter that stimulates skeletal muscle cells, as well as structural changes in the brain, resembling twists and tangles. Symptoms are often mild at the outset and may be overlooked, but they get progressively more serious. They include short-term memory loss, mood swings, a short attention span, and confusion, eventually leading to dementia and hallucinations.

Essential Oils. Medical treatment for AD has concentrated on developing drugs that inhibit the breakdown of acetylcholine, and various studies have investigated essential oils that may have the same effect. None of these studies has been on live subjects, so their findings are only suggestive as far as aromatherapeutic topical applications are concerned. One study stated that sage (*Salvia officinalis*), clary sage (*Salvia sclarea*), Spanish sage (*Salvia lavandulaefolia*), melissa (*Melissa officinalis*), and lime (*Citrus aurantifolia*) reduced the enzyme that breaks down acetylcholine.[21]

Other studies have been directed toward helping patients deal with the dementia that is a feature of late Alzheimer's. Several of these have shown lavender to be useful in calming patients and improving sleep, and one showed that Roman chamomile had the same effects.[22] Other calming oils would also presumably work well for the restlessness and anxiety of late Alzheimer's, such as sweet orange (*Citrus sinensis*), rose (*Rosa damascena*), sandalwood (*Santalum album*), and ylang ylang (*Cananga odorata*).

Methods of Application. Vaporizers used by care providers are probably the easiest way to introduce aromatherapy to Alzheimer's patients in the late stage, although baths and footbaths have also been used in hospitals. For those with mild Alzheimer's symptoms, relaxation massage is probably most helpful, to promote parasympathetic functioning, which may help reduce overall symptoms slightly.

Multiple Sclerosis

Multiple sclerosis (MS) is a difficult disease to diagnose because early symptoms are often mild and remissions are frequent, especially at the beginning. MS often affects younger people, typically between ages 20 and 40. The disease is extremely unpredictable on a day-to-day basis, making prognoses almost impossible. This means that someone who has MS is likely to experience depression.

Causes and Symptoms. Multiple sclerosis is caused by a breakdown of the myelin sheaths around nerves in the central nervous system, resulting in scar tissue, or scleroses. This leads to a short-circuiting of nerve impulses, and muscle control becomes increasingly difficult. As the scleroses increase, symptoms become more severe. MS is thought to be an autoimmune disease, but other factors seem to be important. There may be a genetic component, a virus may trigger the autoimmune response, and climate seems to play a role because the disease primarily affects people living in temperate areas. Stress, food allergies, and some toxins also seem to worsen symptoms.

The most common symptom is spasticity, with tremors, muscle weakness, and problems with balance. Paralysis especially in the legs can be seen in late MS, often with resulting edema. Fatigue, speech problems, and pain are also common, as well as a long list of other symptoms. The progression of the disease is unpredictable, with frequent remissions. One person may have only mild symptoms that do not worsen throughout her life, while another may rapidly decline, with less frequent remissions and more severe symptoms.

Essential Oils. There is no typical client with MS, as the level and number of symptoms vary enormously. This means that treatment has to be individually based and that issues such as edema and pain will have to be addressed. However, it is always helpful to decrease sympathetic nervous system activity, by using calming oils such as neroli (*Citrus aurantium* var. *amara*), rose (*Rosa damascena*), lavender (*Lavandula angustifolia*), sandalwood (*Santalum album*), or sweet orange (*Citrus sinensis*). These will also address the anxiety and depression that affect many clients with MS. Because fatigue is a common factor, essential oils that boost energy can be useful. These include black spruce (*Picea mariana*), pine (*Pinus sylvestris*), ginger (*Zingiber officinale*), rosemary (*Rosmarinus officinalis*), and cardamon (*Elettaria cardamomum*).

Methods of Application. Essential oils in a 1–3% dilution can be used in a relaxation massage to reduce spasticity, increase tissue health, and decrease sympathetic nervous system activity. Oils can be used in a 3–5% dilution on areas that have been treated with lymphatic drainage techniques. Essential oils can also be vaporized, used in baths, foot baths, and spritzers by the client to reduce stress.

SUMMARY

- The function of the nervous system is to monitor changes inside and outside the body, process this information, and send messages to muscles or glands to make a response to the change.

- Communication within the nervous system is by electrical impulses between neurons.

- Risk factors include trauma to neurons, circulatory problems leading to a lack of oxygen to the brain, drugs and alcohol, and pain and stress.

- Essential oils have a strong effect on the parasympathetic and sympathetic divisions of the autonomic nervous system. Inhalation produces the fastest effects because of its direct effect on the hypothalamus, but nerve pain may require topical application for most relief.

- Essential oils that influence the nervous system are categorized as neurodepressants, neurostimulants, those that help nerve pain, and nervines.

- Analgesic essential oils are most effective for neuralgia and for the later stages of shingles, in which nerve pain may last for months.

- With paralysis, essential oils are used mostly to encourage circulation and maintain tissue health.

- Migraine headaches, multiple sclerosis, epilepsy, and Parkinson's disease are treated mostly with calming essential oils to reduce stress. They can also be treated symptomatically, which will vary from individual to individual.

- With Alzheimer's disease, essential oils are used mostly in the later stages to reduce the agitation common in dementia.

Review Questions

1. What parts of the brain are most strongly affected by aromatherapy? (a) medulla oblongata and brain stem, (b) hypothalamus and limbic brain, (c) cerebellum, (d) cerebrum.
2. Match the definitions with the words: (a) calming to the sympathetic nervous system, (b) stimulating to the nervous system, (c) pain relieving, good for neuralgia, (d) strengthening to the nervous system; (i) analgesic, (ii) nervine, (iii) neurostimulant, (iv) neurodepressant.
3. Why is local massage contraindicated in the early stages of shingles? What treatment methods would be more appropriate?
4. Name three carriers that would be suitable for the inflammation found in early shingles.
5. Essential oils are used in paralysis to encourage the flow of _____ and _____, as this will help maintain healthy tissue.
6. The following essential oils may be helpful in preventing a migraine as it is just starting: (a) vetiver and ginger, (b) rose and jasmine, (c) peppermint and lemon, (d) cinnamon and clove.
7. The method of application that affects both the parasympathetic and sympathetic nervous system most quickly is _____.
8. Name two essential oils that have successfully been used to calm the dementia of late Alzheimer's disease.
9. Parkinson's disease and multiple sclerosis both require essential oils that help reduce spasm. Examples of these include: (a) basil and petitgrain, (b) helichrysum and fir needle, (c) myrrh and frankincense, (d) lemon and grapefruit.
10. Aromatherapy seems to be most helpful for epilepsy when used to reduce _____.

Notes

1. Haze S, Sakai K, Gozu Y. Effects of fragrance inhalation on sympathetic activity in normal adults. Jpn J Pharmacol 2002;90(3):247–253.
2. Kirov M, Bainova A, Spasovski M. Rose oil. Acute and subacute oral toxicity. Med Biol Info 1988;3:8–14.
3. Buchbauer G, Jirovetz L, Jager W. Passiflora and lime-blossoms: motility effects after inhalation of the essential oils and of some of the main constituents in animal experiment. Arch Pharm 1992;325(4):247–248.
4. Guillemain J, Rousseau A, Delaveau P. Neurodepressive effects of the essential oil of *Lavandula angustifolia* Mill. Ann Pharm Fr 1989;47(6):337–343.
5. Jager W, Buchbauer G, Jirovetz L, et al. Evidence of the sedative effects of neroli oil, citronellal and phenylethyl acetate on mice. J Essent Oil Res 1992; 4:387–394.
6. Okugawa H, Ueda R, Matsumoto K, et al. Effect of a-santalol and b-santalol from sandalwood on the central nervous system in mice. Phytomedicine 1995;2(2):119–126.
7. Hansel R, Wohlfart R, Coper H. Sedative-hypnotic compounds in the exhalation of hops (I). Z Naturforsch 1980;35(11–12):1096–1097.
8. Rossi T, Melegari M, Bianchi A, et al. Sedative, anti-inflammatory and anti-diuretic effects induced in rats by essential oils of varieties of Anthemis nobilis: a comparative study. Pharmacol Res Comm 1988;20 (Suppl. 5):71–74.
9. Carvalho-Freitas MI, Costa M. Anxiolytic and sedative effects of extracts and essential oil from Citrus aurantium L. Biol Pharm Bull 2002;25(12):1629–1633.
10. Seth G, Kokate CK, Varma KC. Effect of essential oil of *Cymbopogon citratus* Stapf. on the central nervous system. Ind J Exp Biol 1976;14 (3):370–371.
11. Hendriks H, Bos R, Woerdenbag HJ, et al. Central nervous depressant activity of valerianic acid in the mouse. Planta Med 1985;51:28–31.
12. Haze S, Sakai K, Gozu Y. Effects of fragrance inhalation on sympathetic activity in normal adults. Jpn J Pharmacol 2002;90(3):247–253.
13. Ibid.
14. Warm JS, Dember WN. Effects of fragrances on vigilance performance and stress. Perfumer Flavorist 1990;15:15–18.

15. Karamat E, Imberger J, Buchbauer G, et al. Excitatory and sedative effects of essential oils on human reaction time performance. Chem Senses 1992;17:847.

16. Nagai H, Nakagawa M, Fujii W, et al. Effects of odors on humans (ii). Reducing effects of mental stress and fatigue. Chem Senses 1991; 16:198.

17. Premkumar K. The Massage Connection. Baltimore: Lippincott Williams and Wilkins, 2004:345.

18. The National Headache Foundation. Available at: www.headaches.org. Accessed November 30, 2004.

19. Tisserand R, Balacs T. Essential Oil Safety. London, UK: Churchill Livingstone, 1999:68.

20. Betts T. Use of aromatherapy (with or without hypnosis) in the treatment of intractable epilepsy—a two-year follow-up study. Seizure 2003;12(18):534–538.

21. Perry N, Court G, Bidet N, et al. European herbs with cholinergic activities: potential in dementia therapy. Int J Geriatr Psychol 1996;11: 1063–1069.

22. Wolfe A, Herzeberg J. Can aromatherapy oils promote sleep in severely demented patients? Int J Geriatr Psychol 1996;11:926–927.

20

The Immune System

The immune system can also be thought of as the immune function, because it is more the interrelated mechanisms of various systems and body parts than an individual system in itself. The activities of the immune system range throughout the lymphatic, endocrine, integumentary, and cardiovascular systems, and even the digestive system. Many parts of the body play a role in protecting the body against the threat of infection and illness, or in repairing any damage.

An Overview of the Immune System

The body has many forms of defense against infection. The herbalist Simon Mills vividly described these different mechanisms as being like a walled castle; the outer walls block external invaders (nonspecific immunity), and the internal defenses (specific immunity) are increasingly sophisticated. "The further in the trouble penetrates, the more involved and specific the defences and the more complex the issues for the body."[1] Figure 20.1 shows the various parts of the body involved in the immune system.

In **nonspecific immunity,** the skin and mucous membranes form the first level of defense. Not only physical barriers that are difficult for pathogens to penetrate, they also contain various acids and enzymes that kill invaders. Friendly bacteria on the skin crowd out less innocent pathogens, mucus in respiratory passages traps bacteria and viruses, and stomach acids and enzymes kill them.

If pathogens manage to get past the physical barriers, the next level of nonspecific response is activated. This level of defense consists of white blood cells circulating through the body's tissues. The two main types are phagocytes, which surround and digest foreign or dead matter, and natural killer cells, which recognize and destroy foreign cells. Chemicals released by various cells are also important parts of nonspecific immunity, and these include complement, cytokines, prostaglandins, kinins, pyrogens, and histamine, all of which have different roles either in the destruction of invading cells or in increasing inflammation. Inflammation itself is part of the immune response, as the increased heat helps kill pathogens, speed up metabolism, and switch on other parts of the immune system.

In **specific immunity,** lymphocytes, cells of the lymphatic system, play a key role. T cells recognize antigens (substances that the immune system regards as a threat to the body) and either destroy them directly or activate other parts of the specific immune response. B cells differentiate into two types. Plasma cells produce antibodies, also called immunoglobulins, which destroy antigens in various ways, and memory cells store data about the antigens for future recognition. This means that if the same virus or bacterium invades our cells in the future, the specific immune response is so swift and overwhelming that symptoms of the illness do not even occur. This process is known as **acquired immunity.** Humans also have **innate immunity,** a type of specific immunity that is genetically determined and prevents certain viruses and bacteria that infect animals from affecting humans. Figure 20.2 shows the different levels of immunity.

Risk Factors

Because immune functioning relies on so many different systems and body parts, it can be adversely affected by many factors. However, certain situations seem to affect immunity more strongly than others, including:

* *Stress.* Stress suppresses the immune response, as many people with chronic health issues have noticed. It is generally recognized that asthmatic attacks, herpes lesions, migraine headaches, and dermatitis rashes can all be triggered by emotional or physical stress.

* *Poor nutrition.* A lack of the appropriate vitamins and minerals can lead to a depletion of the whole system and lowered immunity. Excessive sugar consumption and being significantly overweight or underweight are factors in lowered immunity.

* *Difficult emotional states.* Many mental and emotional states can be factors, although depression seems to lower immunity the most.

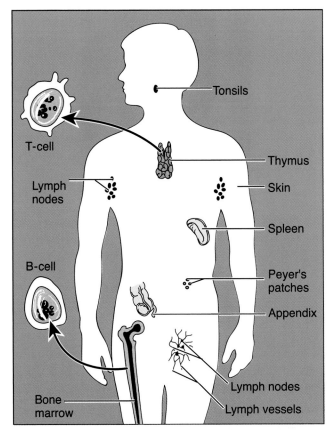

Figure 20.1 The immune system.

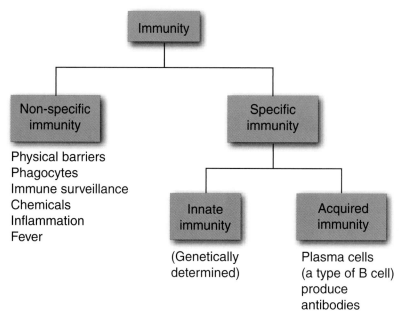

Figure 20.2 Levels of immunity.

- *Poor self-care.* In addition to poor nutrition, lack of regular sleep and exercise can contribute to lowered immunity.
- *Illness.* The physical and emotional stress of being ill lowers the immune defenses, thereby making a recurrence of illness more likely.

How Aromatherapy Affects the Immune System

Aromatherapy aids immunity in two main ways. First, essential oils can attack pathogens directly. Research has shown many essential oils to be antibacterial, antiviral, or antifungal.[2] (Some are also antiparasitic, but they probably have to be taken internally to be effective, which is outside the scope of practice of massage therapy.) Being lipophilic, essential oils can probably penetrate the walls of cells, with the result that they can target pathogens in a very specific way. In French aromatic medicine, the **aromatogram** has been used for several decades. This is a laboratory technique designed to test various essential oils against a bacterial culture taken from a patient, to see which oil has greatest activity against that bacterial strain. Using this test, physicians can determine which essential oils are most effective for the patient. Two patients with the same type of infection may need different essential oils in their treatment protocols because of the different strains of bacteria present or because of their overall health patterns.

Second, various essential oils are considered in aromatherapy circles to be immune-boosting. This is an interesting concept, and its underlying premise is that aromatherapy can be effective in increasing the body's own defenses against disease. Known in French medicine as terrain support, it has parallels in the medical field of psychoneuroimmunology.

The French concept of **terrain support** is that a person's health needs to be supported during the long term, rather than simply fighting disease in the short term. The "terrain" idea originated as a counterbalance to the concept of illness caused by invading "germs." The word terrain literally means "soil," which is a metaphor for an environment in which things grow. As in gardening, if the soil is kept healthy and balanced, the plants have a better chance of survival. If the body and mind are healthy and balanced, the likelihood that the person will get sick is much lower. The proponents of terrain support point to the fact that if 10 people are exposed to an infection, only one or two will catch it. Look after a person's general well-being, and infections will cease to be a problem.

The other aspect of terrain support is that individual clients will need different remedies depending on their underlying strengths and weaknesses. According to Kenner and Requena, "Implicit in the idea of the terrain, likewise, is that even if we assume a specific external disease pathogen, an individual living organism's response is so complex that there is no predictable outcome of the disease or its treatment."[3] This means that the therapist needs a good understanding of the essential oils used when selecting a remedy. A client who is overweight, has high blood pressure, and feels constantly anxious will need a different blend for an infection than a client who is underweight, feels fatigued, and craves sugar.

Holistic aromatherapy, with its use of lower doses of essential oils in mild forms of application, tends to have a strengthening and balancing effect on the terrain, and certain essential oils are recognized in aromatherapy as being particularly appropriate in long-term use to support healthy immune functioning. These are not necessarily the oils that are used to combat infection during acute illnesses but are often included in remedies during these illnesses to strengthen the client and are used when the client is not ill to maintain homeostasis. Essential oils high in alcohols, or alcohols and esters, are often considered to be good terrain supports.

Emotional and mental stress and its effects on the immune system, such as the decrease in white blood cells, have been mentioned in Chapter 15. This is the subject of **psychoneuroimmunology (PNI),** a branch of medicine that explores how the mind can affect immunological processes via the nervous system. In *Molecules of Emotion,* Candace Pert explains how these systems are intimately linked by neurochemicals. For example, cells of the immune system have been found to produce endorphins—brain chemicals that promote well-being, happiness, and lack of pain. According to Pert, "the immune cells are making the same chemicals that we conceive of as controlling mood in the brain."[4] She goes on to show how the mind and body have a two-way connection, with particular implications for the immune system.

Aromas can play a large role in mediating this communication. As we have seen, the olfactory bulb is an extension of the limbic brain—a part of the brain that regulates the nervous system and emotion—and studies show that removing the olfactory bulb in animals will lower T cell count, negatively affecting the immune system.[5] Studies also show that immune system functioning can be improved by inhaling aromas,[6] possibly by lowering the amount of stress hormones in the body and increasing our feelings of well-being.

Antibacterials: As most essential oils have antibacterial qualities to some degree, only the ones with the strongest effect on the largest variety of bacteria are included here: cinnamon bark (*Cinnamomum zeylanicum*),[7] clove bud (*Syzygium aromaticum*),[8] basil (*Ocimum gratissimum*),[9] lemongrass (*Cymbopogon citratus*),[10] oregano (*Origanum vulgare*),[11] tea tree (*Melaleuca alternifolia*),[12] thyme (*Thymus vulgaris* all chemotypes, but especially CT thymol)[13]

Antivirals: cinnamon bark (*Cinnamomum zeylanicum*), tea tree (*Melaleuca alternifolia*), marjoram (*Origanum majorana*),[14] eucalyptus (*Eucalyptus* spp; all species with a high percentage of 1,8 cineole, e.g., *E. globulus* or *E. radiata*),[15] ravensara (*Ravensara aromatica*), peppermint (*Mentha piperita*),[16] clove (*Syzygium aromaticum*),[17] lemongrass (*Cymbopogon citratus*),[18] sandalwood (*Santalum album*)[19]

Antifungals: Essential oils high in aldehydes are generally strong antifungals. These include melissa (*Melissa officinale*), lemongrass (*Cymbopogon citratus*), may chang (*Litsea cubeba*),[20] *Eucalyptus citriodora*, and many more. Other strong antifungal oils include those that are high in

alcohols or phenols: geranium (*Pelargonium graveolens*), palmarosa (*Cymbopogon martinii*),[21] patchouli (*Pogostemon cablin*),[22] clove (*Syzygium aromaticum*), petitgrain (*Citrus aurantium* var. *amara*), and spearmint (*Mentha spicata*).[23]

Terrain (immune) supports: bay laurel (*Laurus nobilis*), frankincense (*Boswellia carteri*), lavender (*Lavandula angustifolia*), petitgrain (*Citrus aurantium* var. *amara*), geranium (*Pelargonium graveolens*), marjoram (*Origanum majorana*), myrrh (*Commiphora myrrha*), thyme (*Thymus vulgaris* CT geraniol or linalool), palmarosa (*Cymbopogon martinii*), lemon (*Citrus limon*).[24] Tea tree (*Melaleuca alternifolia*) is also a good terrain support, but I try to avoid it in blends designed for long-term use, as it tends to be overused in commercial products and as a result clients have generally been exposed to it a lot, with the resulting risk of allergic reaction.

Common Problems of the Immune System

Many common illnesses, such as bacterial, viral, or fungal infections, are considered to be outside the massage therapist's scope of practice. Certainly, massage is contraindicated for clients who have an acute infection with a fever, and few clients would expect their massage therapist to help them treat any kind of infection. However, many massage therapists have clients with chronic diseases involving the immune system, for whom aromatherapy treatment in conjunction with their regular massage work could be helpful. Massage is well documented as strengthening immune functioning, and many clients with chronic illnesses derive benefit from it on this level. Using aromatherapy can increase this benefit. Also, massage therapists are in physical contact with many people daily. It makes sense for them to learn how to boost their own immune system and to treat infections as soon as they appear.

Depressed Immunity

A depressed immune system is one that is not working efficiently. Clients range from those who catch colds too often during the winter to those with severely compromised immune systems, such as clients with HIV/AIDS. Although these are very different problems, massage and aromatherapy treatment is aimed at strengthening the immune system as well as easing symptoms.

Causes and Symptoms. Any of the risk factors mentioned, such as poor nutrition, stress, lack of sleep, or depression, can result in lowered immune function. Chronic illnesses, such as rheumatoid arthritis, chronic fatigue syndrome, or type 2 diabetes, often include depressed immunity as part of the condition. The main symptom of a depressed immune system is the frequency of infections these clients catch. They often have a cold, a sore throat, an infected cut or sore, an abscessed tooth, and so on. Some may have mild infections, such as athlete's foot, which can last for months or even years. Every infection they get further weakens the immune system.

Essential Oils. It is very important for the therapist to try to establish the underlying factors associated with a client's lowered immunity, as this will determine the choice of essential oils to use and make treatment significantly more effective. The terrain support oils listed above should always be used, but they can be combined with antidepressant oils, detoxifying oils, adrenal supports, or soothing sedative oils, depending on the issues involved. For example, if dealing with a client who has been working very long hours, is exhausted, worries constantly, and has depressed immunity, a good blend might include:

Black spruce (*Picea mariana*), for exhaustion, adrenal support

Frankincense (*Boswellia carteri*), to help with worry, terrain support

Petitgrain (*Citrus aurantium* var. *amara*), to help with worry, terrain support

Rosemary (*Rosmarinus officinalis*), to help with tiredness, stimulating to all systems

Methods of Application. Almost any method of application can be used in these cases, the important factor being regular use over a period of time. Since massage has been shown to be stimulating to the immune system, using essential oils in regular massage will possibly be the most beneficial form of treatment. However, aromatherapy should also be used between sessions. Because effective treatment may take a considerable time, blends should be changed every 4 to 6 weeks to avoid the risk of allergic reaction and in case the client becomes tolerant to the essential oils. Most aromatherapists agree that dilutions should be fairly mild, probably 1–2% in a massage. This formula seems to be more strengthening, and many of the more severely affected clients may not be able to tolerate higher doses.

Autoimmune Diseases

Autoimmune diseases include a large number of chronic illnesses, such as rheumatoid arthritis (RA), systemic lupus erythematosus (SLE), type 1 diabetes, multiple sclerosis (MS), and Crohn's disease. Many of these illnesses are discussed in other chapters, as their primary symptoms fall within a particular system. Authorities often disagree over which illnesses can be classified as autoimmune diseases. These diseases develop when the immune system loses its ability to distinguish between invading pathogens and the body's own cells. As a result, it produces antigens and T cells that attack and damage the tissues of the body. About 5% of adults (two-thirds of them women) in the United States have autoimmune diseases.

CASE STUDY 20.1

Depressed Immunity

Mr. F., age 28, came for massage sessions to help with tight shoulders, high stress, and feelings of anxiety. During his intake interview, he reported that he had a tendency to catch frequent colds. He also had athlete's foot, which had persisted off and on for over a year in spite of over-the-counter topical medications. He had a high-stress job with long hours and swam in a public pool several times weekly to help reduce stress.

Aromatherapy was incorporated into his massage sessions to help with stress relief and to boost overall immune functioning. He also expressed interest in using essential oils to try to resolve the athlete's foot. The following blend was used at a 2% dilution during the massage:

Bay laurel (*Laurus nobilis*), 4 drops: terrain support, warming for muscles

Frankincense (*Boswellia carteri*), 3 drops: terrain support, calming, stress relief

Marjoram (*Origanum majorana*), 3 drops: terrain support, calming, relaxing to muscles

Lemon (*Citrus limon*), 2 drops: terrain support, antidepressant

A take-home remedy for the athlete's foot contained essential oils that were both terrain supports and antifungals, at a 5% dilution:

Palmarosa (*Cymbopogon martinii*), 18 drops: antifungal, terrain support

Lemongrass (*Cymbopogon citratus*), 6 drops: antifungal

Geranium (*Pelargonium graveolens*), 24 drops: antifungal, terrain support

Patchouli (*Pogostemon patchouli*), 12 drops: antifungal

Mr. F. also started wearing natural fiber socks to reduce moisture around the feet, which could be contributing to the fungal infection, and took up a different form of exercise temporarily, as swimming pools and communal changing areas often harbor fungal infections. Massage sessions were continued on a weekly basis for stress reduction and to relieve tight muscles. The athlete's foot resolved completely within 6 weeks, and Mr. F. reported feeling generally more energetic. Over the following winter, he only caught one cold, which was a great improvement in his immune functioning compared with the previous winter.

Causes and Symptoms. The immediate cause is the confusion in the immune system that identifies the body's own cells as a threat. The reasons some people develop autoimmune diseases and others do not are unclear, but there may be a genetic factor, as some families seem prone to autoimmune diseases, even though different family members may have different types of autoimmune illnesses. Other possible factors are viral and bacterial infections, which might cause the immune system to start reacting in an abnormal way as a side-effect. Symptoms vary enormously, depending on the illness involved, but all autoimmune diseases show damage to body tissue and some kind of inflammation.

Essential Oils. The main medical treatments for autoimmune diseases are anti-inflammatory drugs and immunosuppressive drugs. Studies show that essential oils can be used as **immunosuppressives,** to reduce immune responses that are overactive. Michael Alexander, an aromatherapy researcher, suggests that essential oils can be used to not only suppress the immune response but also "retrain" the immune system to react normally, using the learned odor response.[25] In other words, after a certain period, even the smell of the oils should "remind" the body to reduce the overactive response (see Chapter 4). This idea is supported by a case study on a patient with lupus erythematosus who was given standard medication together with a strong taste (cod liver oil) and smell (rose). After some sessions in which medication was paired with the cod liver oil and the rose oil, the smell and taste alone were given between the standard medication treatments, and as a result, the patient was able to continue improvement on only half the usual dose of medications. Five years after the study, the patient was still doing well.[26]

Essential oils that suppress the immune/inflammatory process work by inhibiting certain chemicals in the body, such as arachidonic acid, a precursor of many inflammatory substances. These essential oils include cardamon (*Elettaria cardamomum*), Himalayan cedar (*Cedrus deodara*),[27] cinnamon leaf (*Cinnamomum zeylanicum*), clove (*Syzygium aromaticum*), ginger (*Zingiber officinale*), nutmeg (*Myristica fragrans*), palmarosa (*Cymbopogon martinii*), and turmeric (*Curcuma longa*). These oils should be combined with essential oils that work on symptom relief for the various diseases. (Symptoms are discussed in the other body systems chapters.)

Methods of Application. Application methods will depend on the illness involved and the body system most affected. Refer to the specific autoimmune diseases discussed in other chapters.

Chronic Fatigue Syndrome

Chronic fatigue syndrome (CFS) is an illness that is widely misunderstood and not well documented. Patients have often been told that they are imagining their symptoms or that they are simply lazy. However, it is estimated that between 75 and 265 people out of every 100,000 suffer from CFS.

Causes and Symptoms. The exact cause of CFS is not known. Immunological dysfunction might be a factor because nonself antibodies are often found in the bloodstream, and some researchers have found lower numbers of natural killer cells or activity. However, the inflammation and tissue damage associated with autoimmune disease is not present. Other possible factors include viral or bacterial infections, allergies, and food intolerances—all of which point to some kind of immune imbalance. The National Center for Infectious Diseases suggests that there may be multiple causes all leading to a common end point.[28]

The major symptom is extreme fatigue, which is not improved by rest and is worsened by any physical or mental activity. Sufferers describe it as debilitating, to the extent that they may find it difficult to get out of bed, or even read. Other symptoms include muscle aches, severe pain and fatigue after exertion that can last longer than 24 hours, impaired memory and concentration, and insomnia. There may be many other symptoms, which vary from person to person. The condition can last for years and is very unpredictable. Some people recover completely, some recover to a certain extent, and some get worse. There is no known cure.

Essential Oils. The most important are oils to improve stamina and decrease tiredness. Adrenal supports and stimulating tonics are most suitable. These include black spruce (*Picea mariana*), pine (*Pinus sylvestris*), ginger (*Zingiber officinale*), rosemary (*Rosmarinus officinalis*), and cardamon (*Elettaria cardamomum*).

As the condition can last for an extremely long time, terrain supports are also essential (see list above). Other essential oils should be chosen for symptomatic relief, such as oils for muscular pain or for digestive problems. Frankincense (*Boswellia carteri*) seems to be a particularly effective oil for many symptoms, especially insomnia and difficulty concentrating, as well as being a good terrain support.

Methods of Application. Aromatherapy massage can be helpful in reducing muscular pain, although cool compresses with essential oils may be preferable for the severe pain experienced after exertion. Vaporized blends to help with insomnia are also frequently useful, because this common symptom tends to make all other symptoms of the condition more severe and difficult to manage. A useful treatment regimen is a sedating blend for late evening and a stimulating, strengthening blend for self-application in the mornings and early afternoons. Terrain supports should be a feature of all of these blends.

Allergies

Allergies are the sixth leading cause of chronic disease in the United States. More than 50 million people suffer from allergies, costing the healthcare system $18 billion per year. Allergic diseases can affect many systems of the body, most commonly the skin, digestive system, and respiratory system.

Specific allergic illnesses are discussed in the relevant chapters for the body systems.

Causes and Symptoms. Symptoms vary widely, depending on the system most affected by the allergy. However, all of them have in common the inflammation that leads to the red eyes, swollen respiratory passages, and skin rashes that commonly characterize allergies. In some ways similar to autoimmune diseases, people with allergies have a hyperactive immune system, although in this case it reacts to harmless substances such as pollen, or everyday foods, rather than attacking the body's own tissues. However, tissue damage can still result as a side-effect of the war waged on other substances. The main chemical involved in allergic response is histamine, which causes blood vessels to dilate and become leaky. This produces edema, large amounts of mucus, and smooth muscle contractions (which affect the respiratory and digestive systems).

Essential Oils. Essential oils need to be chosen to deal symptomatically with the allergic response, depending on the body system involved. However, essential oils that both suppress the release of histamine and help control inflammation are always needed. These include German chamomile (*Matricaria recutita*),[29] Roman chamomile (*Chamaemelum nobile*), Himalayan cedar (*Cedrus deodara*), turmeric (*Curcuma longa*), lavender (*Lavandula angustifolia*),[30] and tea tree (*Melaleuca alternifolia*).[31]

Methods of Application. These will vary, depending on the system most affected by the allergic reaction. The most important thing to remember when working with clients with allergies is that less is always better. Dilutions should be very mild, partly because treatment is often long-term, but also because the system has the potential to overreact to any substance. There is a huge literature of case studies of clients developing allergies to essential oils, even the ones listed above. To avoid this, it is essential to use mild dilutions (probably 1–1.5% in massage), change oil blends frequently (about every 4 weeks at least), and use only the freshest essential oils, as studies show that allergic reactions are more common when oxidized oils are used.[32]

Candidiasis

Candidiasis is the most common fungal infection in humans. It usually produces superficial, annoying symptoms, but in someone who is severely immune-compromised, it may become a systemic illness, with serious implications for health. Even in its milder, superficial form, many naturopathic doctors suggest that it can lead to a wide range of other problems.

Causes and Symptoms. *Candida albicans* is a yeast that normally lives in the intestinal tract. The infection, candidiasis, can spread to various other parts of the body, causing a variety of symptoms. The reasons for the spread include internal antibiotic treatment, chemotherapy, immunosuppres-

sive treatment, vitamin C deficiency, and impaired immunity. Candidiasis is more common in pregnant women, newborn babies, the elderly, and people with diabetes. The areas usually affected are moist regions of the skin, such as the groin, the mouth, and the vagina. General symptoms are itching and irritation, and, in the case of vaginal candidiasis, a thick discharge. Urinary tract infections are also commonly experienced by a person with candidiasis. It has also been suggested that candidiasis can lead to a wide range of debilitating symptoms, such as depression, mood swings, PMS, an inability to concentrate, tiredness, digestive problems, allergies, and migraines.

Essential Oils. The most beneficial effects seem to be caused by the antifungal oils. The alcohol-rich antifungals, such as geranium (*Pelargonium graveolens*), palmarosa (*Cymbopogon martinii*), and patchouli (*Pogostemon cablin*),[33] will probably be easiest to use for candidiasis, as the infection tends to spread in mucous membranes and other sensitive areas. Potentially irritating oils such as lemongrass (*Cymbopogon citratus*) and melissa (*Melissa officinalis*) can be used as part of the blend, making up perhaps about 10% of the total essential oil content.

Methods of Application. The oils can be used in full-body relaxation massage, as stress tends to trigger some of the symptoms of candidiasis. However, they should also be used between massage sessions and can be given in take-home blends to be used in the bath.

Viral Infections

Massage therapists are not called upon to treat viral infections, but it is important for any person who is in frequent physical contact with many other people to know how to treat themselves if they get sick. Many massage therapists are self-employed, often without health insurance themselves, and cannot easily afford to take time off work. The most common viral infections, colds and flus, can mean several days, or even weeks, of missed work.

The easiest and most effective way to treat a viral infection is to deal with it as soon as it appears. At the first sign of a ticklish throat, a slight fever, or simply a feeling that something is not right, it is best to use essential oils in fairly high doses (depending on your sensitivity) to get rid of the virus quickly.

Causes and Symptoms. Viruses are parasites that take over the living cells of plants or animals. Once a virus gets inside the cell it uses the cell's own enzymes to reproduce and make large numbers of viral particles, which are released to infect other cells. Different viruses can cause illnesses in any of the systems of the human body. However, the most common are viruses that affect the respiratory system, resulting in sore throats, coughing and sneezing, and congestion in the respiratory tract.

Essential Oils. Antiviral oils, such as eucalyptus (*Eucalyptus radiata*), marjoram (*Origanum majorana*), ravensara (*Ravensara aromatica*), or tea tree (*Melaleuca alternifolia*), can be used with most otherwise healthy adults at high doses for short periods of time. Ginger (*Zingiber officinale*) and cardamon (*Elettaria cardamomum*) seem to be particularly helpful for the type of viral infection that is characterized by chills and shivering.

Methods of Application. From personal experience, I have found baths and foot baths to be most effective when trying to head off a viral infection. Therapists with little previous exposure to essential oils should try moderate amounts (10–15 drops in a full bath), while those with more experience with essential oils may want to try higher amounts (20–25 drops). (Ginger should be used in much lower amounts in both cases, or blended with the other oils mentioned.) Essential oils should be diluted in honey or milk before being used, to reduce the likelihood of skin irritation with these higher amounts.

SUMMARY

- Immune functioning includes many body systems, including the lymphatic, endocrine, digestive, integumentary, and cardiovascular systems.

- Nonspecific immunity defends against all pathogens and includes the skin and mucous membranes, phagocytes, natural killer cells, and certain chemicals.

- Specific immunity targets individual pathogens and includes T cells, which kill specific antigens, and B cells, which produce antibodies and store memory of specific antigens (acquired immunity). Innate immunity is a type of specific immunity that is genetically determined.

- Risk factors include stress, poor nutrition, emotional states (especially depression), lack of sleep or exercise, and illness.

- Essential oils help the immune system either by attacking pathogens directly or by boosting immunity, partly through their effects on the nervous system and stress.

- In autoimmune diseases and in allergies, essential oils can be used to calm a hyperfunctioning immune system and to lower inflammation.

- In chronic fatigue syndrome, essential oils are used symptomatically, often to reduce fatigue and muscular pain.

- Antifungal essential oils are most beneficial for candidiasis.

- It may be possible to shorten the course of a viral illness by using high amounts of essential oils for a very short period of time.

Review Questions

1. With regard to pathogens, most essential oils are anti-_____, many are anti-_____, and only some are strongly anti-_____.
2. How can essential oils penetrate cell walls to attack pathogens?
3. What is an aromatogram used for?
4. In treating allergies, essential oils that help suppress the release of histamine include: (a) bergamot and grapefruit, (b) fennel and aniseed, (c) chamomile and Himalayan cedar, (d) peppermint and spearmint.
5. Essential oils high in these chemical groups are good antifungals: (a) aldehydes, (b) ketones, (c) monoterpenes, (d) esters.
6. Anti-_____ oils are important when treating autoimmune diseases and allergies.
7. Why should dilutions be mild when treating allergies?
8. Name three essential oils that are useful for treating the fatigue that is a symptom of chronic fatigue syndrome.
9. The mildest essential oils are most appropriate for treating candidiasis because: (a) the yeast tends to grow in sensitive areas of the body, (b) people with this infection tend to become hypersensitive to all substances, (c) only babies and older adults typically have candidiasis, (d) the infection is never severe.
10. Essential oils high in this chemical group are usually regarded as good terrain-support oils, suitable for long-term use to boost overall health: (a) phenols, (b) aldehydes, (c) ketones, (d) alcohols.

Notes

1. Mills S. The Essential Book of Herbal Medicine. London, UK: Arkana, 1991:67.
2. Farag RS, Shalaby RS, El-Baroty GA, et al. Chemical and biological evaluation of the essential oils of different *Melaleuca* species. Phytother Res 2004;18(1):30–35.
3. Kenner D, Requena Y. Botanical Medicine. Brookline, MA: Paradigm Publications, 2001:21.
4. Pert C. Molecules of Emotion. New York: Scribner, 1997:183.
5. Komori T, Yamamoto M, Matsumoto T, et al. Effects of imipramine on T cell subsets in olfactory bulbectomized mice. Neuropsychobiology 2002;46(4):194–196.
6. Moynihan JA, Karp JD, Cohen N, et al. Immune deviation following stress odor exposure: role of endogenous opioids. J Neuroimmunol 2000;102(2):145–153.
7. Deans SG, Ritchie G. Antibacterial properties of plant essential oils. Int J Food Microbiol 1987;5:165–180.
8. Singh BS, Singh G. Antibacterial activity of the essential oils of three medicinal plants. Ind Drugs 1978;15(11):227–229.
9. Ramaoelina AR, Terrom GP, Bianchini JP, et al. Antibacterial action of essential oils extracted from Madagascar plants. Arch L'Institute Pasteur Madagasc 1987;53(1):217–226.
10. Onawunmi GO, Ogunlana EO. A study of the antibacterial activity of the essential oil of lemongrass (*Cymbopogon citratus* (DC.) Stapf). Int J Crude Drug Res 1986;24(2):64–68.
11. Sivropoulou A, Papanikolaou E, Nikolaou C, et al. Antimicrobial and cytotoxic activities of *Origanum* essential oils. J Agricult Food Chem 1996;44(5):1202–1205.
12. Nelson RRS. *In vitro* activities of five plant essential oils against methicillin-resistant *Staphylococcus aureus* and vancomycin-resistant *Enterococcus faecium*. J Antimicrob Chemother 1997;40:305–306.
13. Svoboda KP, Deans SG. Biological activities of essential oils from selected aromatic plants. Acta Horticult 1995;390:203–209.
14. Bourne KZ, Bourne N, Reising SF, et al. Plant products as topical microbicide candidates: assessment of *in vitro* and *in vivo* activity against *Herpes simplex* virus type 2. Antiviral Res 1999;42:219–226.
15. Penoel D. *Eucalyptus smithii* essential oil and its use in aromatic medicine. Br J Phytother 1992;2(4):154–159.
16. Schumacher A, Reichling J, Schnitzler P. Virucidal effect of peppermint oil on the enveloped viruses herpes simplex virus type 1 and type 2 in vitro. Phytomedicine 2003;10(6–7):504–510.
17. Benencia F, Courreges MC. *In vitro* and *in vivo* activity of eugenol on human herpes virus. Phytother Res 2000;14:495–500.
18. Minami M, Kita M, Nakaya T, et al. The inhibitory effect of essential oils on herpes simplex virus type-1 replication in vitro. Microbiol Immunol 2003;47(9):681–684.
19. Benencia F, Courreges MC. Antiviral activity of sandalwood oil against *Herpes simplex* viruses -1 and -2. Phytomedicine 1999;6(2):119–123.
20. Gogoi P, Baruah P, Nath SC. Antifungal activity of the essential oil of *Litsea cubeba* Pers. J Essent Oil Res 1997;9:213–215.
21. Singatwadia A, Katewa SS. *In vitro* studies on antifungal activity of essential oil of *Cymbopogon martinii* and *Cymbopogon citratus*. Ind Perfumer 2001;45(1):53–55.
22. Yang D, Michel D, Mandin D, et al. Antifungal and antibacterial properties, *in vitro*, of three Patchouli essential oils of different origins. Acta Botanica Galla 1996;143(1):29–35.
23. Galal EE, Adel MS, El-Sherif S, et al. Evaluation of certain volatile oils for their antifungal properties. J Drug Res 1973;5(2):235–245.
24. Komori T, Fujiwara R, Nomura J, et al. Effects of citrus fragrance on immune function and depressive states. Neuroimmunomodulation 1995;2:174–180.
25. Alexander M. Aromatherapy and immunity: how the use of essential oils aids immune potentiality. Int J Aromather 2002;12(1):49–56.
26. Olness K, Ader R. Conditioning as an adjunct in the pharmacotherapy of lupus erythematosus. J Dev Behav Pediatr 1992;13(2):124–125.
27. Shinde UA, Phadke AS, Nair AM, et al. Preliminary studies on the immunomodulatory activity of *Cedrus deodara* wood oil. Fitoterapia 1999;70:333–339.
28. National Center for Infectious Diseases. Available at: www.cdc.gov/ncidod/diseases/cfs. Accessed November 28, 2004.
29. Patzelt-Wenczler R, Ponce-Poschl E. Proof of efficacy of Kamillosan (R) cream in atopic eczema. Eur J Med Res 2000;5(4):171–175.
30. Kim HM, Cho SH. Lavender oil inhibits immediate-type allergic reaction in mice and rats. J Pharm Pharmacol 1999;51(2):221–226.
31. Koh EJ, Pearce AL, Marshman G, et al. Tea tree oil reduces histamine-induced skin inflammation. Br J Dermatol 2002;147(6):1212–1217.
32. Khanna M, Qasem K, Sasseville D. Allergic contact dermatitis to tea tree oil with erythema multiforme-like id reaction. Am J Contact Dermat 2000;11(4):238–242.
33. Harris R. Progress with superficial mycoses, using essential oils. Int J Aromather 2002;12(2):83–91.

21

The Integumentary System

Although massage and aromatherapy affect many body systems, the one that all massage therapists must work with constantly is the integumentary system. In holistic aromatherapy, treatments are most often given by applying the essential oils to the skin. The texture, age, and sensitivity of the skin must all be taken into account when assessing a client for aromatherapy massage, and sensitivities to essential oils are generally manifested as skin problems—rashes, itching, and eruptions. The skin can also inform aromatherapists about the health or emotional state of their clients because many internal diseases are manifested as skin disorders, and people will often become red or pale in response to emotional disturbance.

An Overview of the Integumentary System

The most obvious function of the skin is to protect the underlying tissues from abrasion, heat, ultraviolet (UV) light, and dehydration. It also protects the body from pathogens, partly because of its slightly acidic nature and partly because of various enzymes and biochemicals present on the skin surface. It regulates body heat by sweating; excretes salt, water, and wastes; and synthesizes vitamin D from sunlight.

The skin has various layers, of which the most superficial is the epidermis. The epidermis contains cells that produce keratin, a tough protective protein, and melanin, a pigment that protects the skin from UV rays. The stratum corneum is the most superficial layer of the epidermis, mostly consisting of keratin and dead cells. The cells of the stratum corneum are shed continually.

Under the epidermis is a layer of connective tissue called the **dermis,** which contains sebaceous glands, sweat glands, nerve endings, blood capillaries, lymphatic vessels, and hair follicles. The connective tissue contains collagen and elastin fibers that are flexible and allow the skin to stretch and recoil to its original size. Stretch marks occur when the skin is stretched beyond its capacity and the elastin and collagen are damaged.

Beneath the dermis is a layer of subcutaneous tissue, which consists of adipose (fat) and connective tissue. Although this is not strictly part of the skin, it provides stability and connects the skin to underlying structures. The adipose tissue helps retain heat, and it acts as a shock absorber and an energy reservoir. Essential oils tend to be attracted to this layer of fatty tissue, and the amount of adipose tissue will determine how quickly essential oils enter the bloodstream and therefore how quickly they are used and excreted by the body. Individuals who are very overweight, with a large amount of fatty tissue, will have slower absorption of essential oils. Athletes, with a very thin adipose layer, may actually require milder dilutions. Figure 21.1 shows the primary integumentary structures.

Risk Factors

Factors that have a negative effect on the integumentary system include:

- *Trauma.* Physical trauma, such as cutting or burning the skin, leads to local tissue damage, which often heals completely without outside help because skin cells have the capacity to regenerate quickly. However, larger wounds may lead to scarring. Any rupture of the protective layers of skin also leaves the body more vulnerable to infection, and in the case of burns, to dehydration.

- *Overexposure to sunlight.* The dangers of sunburn have been well documented, and although a certain amount of exposure to sunlight is necessary for the body, larger amounts of UV radiation may cause genetic alterations in cells, increasing the risk of skin cancer.

- *Overexposure to cold.* Severe cold may damage the skin and external body tissues as a result of a disruption in the blood supply. This is commonly known as frostbite.

- *Inadequate hydration.* Dehydration adversely affects the entire body but may have permanent effects on the skin.

- *Stress.* Stress usually aggravates already existing skin conditions, and most people with eczema and psoriasis experience flare-ups in stressful situations.

How Aromatherapy Affects the Integumentary System

Aromatherapy has a very direct influence on the skin, and essential oils are often applied topically in holistic treatments. As we saw in Chapter 4, certain constituents of essential oils penetrate the stratum corneum relatively easily because they have a small molecular size and are lipophilic. They also use hair follicles and sebaceous glands to bypass the stratum corneum, so that areas of skin dense in glands and follicles have a higher rate of absorption. The quality of the client's skin is also important in assessing absorption; the skin of young children and older people is much thinner and absorbs substances more quickly.

Essential oils can be classified according to their actions on the integumentary system. Aromatherapy is a good remedy for skin inflammation, but not all anti-inflammatory oils can be used to relieve inflammation. Ginger, for example, is often used to counter the inflammation found in arthritis, as it suppresses certain chemicals produced by the body. However, it is also directly heating to the skin, making it contraindicated in cases of skin

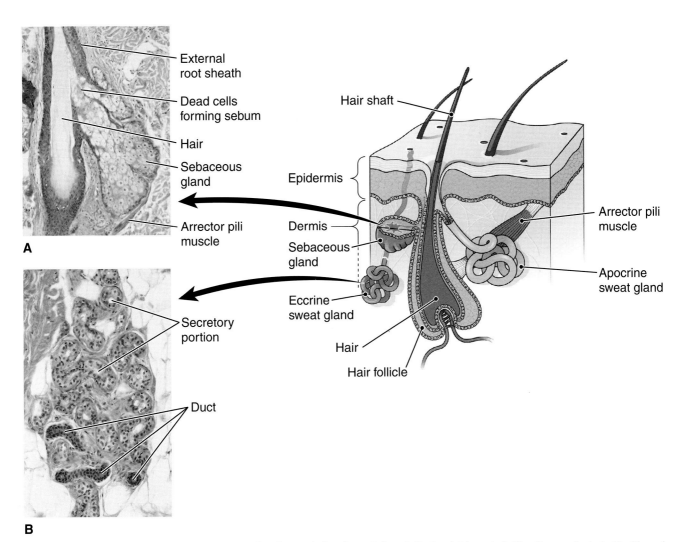

Figure 21.1 The integumentary system. (Reprinted with permission from Cohen B, Taylor J. Memmler's The Human Body in Health and Disease, 10th ed. Baltimore: Lippincott Williams & Wilkins, 2005.)

irritation. The cooling anti-inflammatories only are used for skin inflammation.

Other essential oils are considered **cicatrizant,** or wound healing. These oils are frequently used to encourage cell regeneration in situations in which the skin and underlying tissue have been damaged. **Antipruritic** essential oils reduce or prevent itching. Most essential oils are drying to the skin, especially if used in large amounts, as they are such concentrated substances, but some oils are considered moisturizing when used in mild or moderate dilutions.

Anti-inflammatories: lavender (*Lavandula angustifolia*),[1] German chamomile (*Matricaria recutita*),[2] yarrow (*Achillea millefolium*), tea tree (*Melaleuca alternifolia*),[3] rose (*Rosa damascena* or *centifolia*)[4]

Cicatrizants: rose (*Rosa damascena* or *centifolia*),[5] lavender (*Lavandula angustifolia*),[6] German chamomile (*Matricaria recutita*),[7] frankincense (*Boswellia carteri*), myrrh (*Commiphora myrrha*), helichrysum (*Helichrysum italicum*), neroli (*Citrus aurantium* var. *amara*). The infused oils of St. John's wort (*Hypericum perforatum*) and calendula (*Calendula arvensis*)[8] are also cicatrizant and can be used as carriers for the essential oils.

Anti-pruritics: lavender (*Lavandula angustifolia*), tea tree (*Melaleuca alternifolia*),[9] peppermint (*Mentha piperita*)

Moisturizers: German chamomile (*Matricaria recutita*), mandarin (*Citrus reticulata*),[10] sweet orange (*Citrus sinensis*), rose (*Rosa damascena* or *centifolia*), geranium (*Pelargonium graveolens*), palmarosa (*Cymbopogon martinii*)

Common Problems of the Integumentary System

Clients generally do not see massage therapists about skin problems. They are more inclined to consult an esthetician or a dermatologist. However, massage therapists spend most of their working time applying substances to their clients' skin, and it would be at least useful to know what essential oils may be beneficial for certain issues, even if that is not the main focus of the massage. Also, recovery from extensive burns or wounds often requires physical rehabilitation, which may include massage therapy to reduce adhesions and increase range of motion. Patience is necessary when dealing with skin problems, as they are often long-standing issues and rarely improve quickly. Therapists may also need to try several essential oils in the relevant categories before finding which oils a particular client responds to best.

Scars

Massage therapists frequently encounter scar tissue, which generally affects much more than just the skin.

Causes and Symptoms. We often think of scars as being visible reminders on the skin of a wound or surgery. However, scar tissue can be the result of *any* injury or activity that causes inflammation in the connective tissue, and may not be visible on the skin. Healing of tissue after injury depends on the extent of the injury and on the area of the body involved. Minor injuries to the skin often heal extremely fast, leaving very little trace after a few days, as epidermal cells have the capacity to regenerate very quickly. Cells of the nervous system and skeletal muscular system are often replaced instead by fibrous tissue, which may cause adhesions that can restrict range of motion and cause pain. And trauma to larger areas of the skin, deep burns, and delayed healing can produce visible scars that do not disappear.

Essential Oils. For minor wounds and scrapes, very mild antiseptic essential oils can be useful in cleansing the wound and ensuring rapid healing by preventing infection. The best oils for this in my experience are lavender (*Lavandula angustifolia*), lavandin (*Lavandula x intermedia*), and tea tree (*Melaleuca alternifolia*) because of their combination of strong antibacterial properties and extreme gentleness on the skin. Essential oils in water can be used to clean the wound initially and can then be applied in a moderate dilution (4–6%) in aloe vera gel to avoid infection.

Cicatrizant oils are also important because they encourage rapid cell regeneration, thereby counteracting the slow growth that can result in excessive scarring. With larger scars, such as scars from surgery, it is important to remember that even after the wound has closed over, the surface tissue is much more sensitive than normal skin and cannot be treated in the same way. Undiluted lavender oil is often recommended for the treatment of scars, and for mature scars this may be a good option. However, undiluted essential oils on new scars will often cause rashes and

skin irritation. The infused oils of calendula and St. John's wort are much gentler on this fragile tissue and have shown excellent healing properties. Other carrier oils often used by aromatherapists for scar healing are rose hip seed oil (*Rosa rubiginosa*) and callophyllum (*Calophyllum inophyllum*). After about a month, mild dilutions of the cicatrizant essential oils can be added (up to 1%), and the amount of essential oils in the blend can be increased as the scar matures.

For scar tissue that shows no visible scarring on the skin, the anti-inflammatory oils will be useful for more recent injury or illness, as inflammation sets the stage for the buildup of fibrotic tissue and adhesions. With mature scar tissue, the rubefacient essential oils, such as rosemary (*Rosmarinus officinalis*), ginger (*Zingiber officinale*), juniper (*Juniperus communis*), and black pepper (*Piper nigrum*), will help soften rigid tissue and bring blood and nutrients to the area to help with remodeling.

Methods of Application. For skin scarring, essential oils can be applied in appropriate dilutions directly to the site of the scar. As frequent application is ideal, blends should be given to clients to apply at home at least once a day. Essential oils can also be used with any massage techniques, such as skin rolling, fascial spreading, and cross-fiber friction, the massage therapist normally uses to treat underlying scar tissue and adhesions. Dilutions will depend on the size of the area involved; they can range from 2–3% for larger areas to 10% for very small areas.

Burns

Burns are a type of injury to the skin, frequently resulting in scarring that can be treated using the oils and techniques described previously. However, clients will sometimes arrive with a relatively new smaller burn, or even with extensive sunburn, which contraindicates massage locally but can be treated with aromatherapy to make the client more comfortable.

Causes and Symptoms. Burns are caused by intense heat such as from flames or hot liquids, by chemical substances such as acids, by UV light, and by electrical sources. Burns may range in severity from a reddening of the skin surface to the destruction of the epidermis, dermis, and the underlying tissues.

Essential Oils. Burns that have caused damage beyond the epidermis should not be treated by the aromatherapist because broken skin absorbs essential oil much more rapidly and unpredictably. The client should be encouraged to seek medical attention if the burn is widespread. For superficial burns, I prefer essential oils that are both anti-inflammatory and cicatrizant, such as lavender (*Lavandula angustifolia*) and German chamomile (*Matricaria recutita*), to reduce the heat

Mature Scar Tissue

Mr. R was a bank clerk in his early thirties. He had undergone a surgical operation on his hip as a 2-year-old and the surgical scar had elongated as he had grown. At this point, the scar was about 12 inches long and very noticeable. There seemed to be no particular underlying adhesions, and range of motion was not restricted. As the scar had existed for over 30 years, I was not particularly optimistic that there would be any benefit, but the client expressed interest in using essential oils on the scar mostly for cosmetic reasons. A blend was made with lavender (*Lavandula angustifolia*) essential oil at a 25% dilution in jojoba oil, and this was applied by the client twice daily. After several months of application, he reported that the scar tissue felt softer and more pliable, and that it appeared to have narrowed slightly.

from the burn and promote rapid healing of skin cells. Tiny amounts of peppermint (*Mentha piperita*) can be added for its cooling effect.

With widespread burns, for which the client has been hospitalized and is in the later stages of healing, the essential oils mentioned above for scar healing will be most appropriate. Extensive burns are extremely traumatic, as the client must come to terms with the stress of the incident itself, a very painful rehabilitation process, and possibly permanent changes in movement and appearance. The section on emotional issues in Chapter 15 will be helpful in choosing essential oils to help with the posttraumatic stress.

Methods of Application. For superficial burns in the acute and early subacute stages, essential oils can be applied to the skin in a mild dilution (1–3% depending on the size of the area) in aloe vera gel, which is cooling and soothing. For very large areas, such as a sunburnt back, the essential oils can be used in a spritzer and sprayed over the area. The preparations should be given to the client to apply at home, as frequent application will lead to more rapid healing.

Dermatitis/Eczema

The terms "dermatitis" and "eczema" are used interchangeably, and the problem affects about one in five people at some point in their lives.

Causes and Symptoms. Dermatitis literally means inflammation ("itis") of the skin ("derma") and is usually characterized by red inflamed skin, sometimes accompanied by flaking, pustules, or itching. It may be acute or chronic. Most forms of dermatitis are noncontagious.

There are various types of dermatitis, the most common being atopic, contact, and seborrheic. Atopic dermatitis is particularly prevalent in children, and genetic factors are suspected as a cause because there is often a family history of either dermatitis or asthma. Contact dermatitis may be either *irritant,* which is provoked by harsh chemicals, friction, detergents, etc., or it may be *allergic,* in which case the irritant is a substance such as rubber or perfume that most people do not react to. Seborrheic dermatitis commonly causes dry, flaky, irritated skin on the scalp, face, and possibly chest. The causes are unknown, but it may be related to a yeast infection. All types of dermatitis are aggravated by stress, harsh soaps, and other irritants, such as extreme temperatures or pollution.

Essential Oils. All types of dermatitis are characterized by inflammation, so the cooling anti-inflammatory essential oils listed previously are always helpful. As dry skin is often a feature, moisturizing oils such as rose (*Rosa damascena*), mandarin (*Citrus reticulata*), geranium (*Pelargonium graveolens*), and palmarosa (*Cymbopogon martinii*) are also used in treatment. The infused oil of calendula (*Calendula officinalis*) in my experience is extremely healing and moisturizing, and I use it as a carrier for treating dermatitis.

Seborrheic dermatitis may need a slightly different treatment, as there is some evidence to suggest that it may be related to a yeast infection, and antifungal essential oils may be particularly indicated. One study reported that a long-term case of seborrheic dermatitis that only responded temporarily to steroid treatment was completely resolved by using a combination of geranium (*Pelargonium graveolens*), palmarosa (*Cymbopogon martinii*), bay laurel (*Laurus nobilis*), tansy (*Tanacetum annuum*), and spike lavender (*Lavandula latifolia*) essential oils.[11]

Methods of Application. Essential oils should be applied to the affected area in a light, easily absorbed carrier, in a mild dilution (1–2%). Frequent applications will increase the rate of healing, so take-home blends are helpful.

Psoriasis

More than 4.5 million people in the United States are affected by either psoriasis or psoriatic arthritis.

Causes and Symptoms. Psoriasis is a chronic noncontagious disease that manifests in the skin and occasionally in the joints. It is a genetic disease, probably caused by the immune system sending faulty signals that accelerate the growth of skin cells. Skin cells usually grow, mature, and are shed within about 28 days, but for people with psoriasis this process can accelerate to about 3 to 6 days. This typically results in patches of inflamed skin covered with white, flaky scales. Psoriasis may affect only small areas of the body, commonly the scalp, elbows, knees, or trunk, although a small percentage of people have much larger areas affected. Many people carry the gene for psoriasis but never develop skin lesions, and it is believed that the symptoms are triggered by emotional stress, injury, infection, or reaction to drugs.[12] There is no known cure for psoriasis, and treatments concentrate on managing symptoms.

Essential Oils. Psoriasis is notoriously difficult to treat with either conventional or complementary therapies. According to one study, aromatherapy does not seem to alleviate symptoms significantly but is probably best used to help clients deal with stress as one way to avoid flareups.[13] However, in my experience some clients with psoriasis may experience quite a dramatic improvement in symptoms after using essential oils, while others show no change at all. Any of the essential oils that help decrease sympathetic nervous system activity and are also anti-inflammatory, such as lavender (*Lavandula angustifolia*), German chamomile (*Matricaria recutita*), and rose (*Rosa damascena*), will be helpful, as there is a significant amount of inflammation with psoriasis. Also useful are essential oils or carrier oils that soften the skin, such as mandarin (*Citrus reticulata*), rose (*Rosa damascena* or *centifolia*), geranium (*Pelargonium graveolens*), palmarosa (*Cymbopogon martinii*), and calendula (*Calendula officinalis*) infused oil.

Methods of Application. A mild dilution (about 2%) applied daily directly to the affected area will produce the best results. Improvement can be seen in as little as a week, or may take several months.

CASE STUDY 21.2

Psoriasis

Mr. K was a 46-year-old man with psoriasis. He initially came for aromatherapy massage for stress relief. He had raised, white flaking patches on his elbows, knees, and a large patch on his lower back. There was no cracked skin but a significant amount of inflammation under the flaking, and slight itching. There seemed to be no history of allergies or particular skin sensitivity. The blend used for the aromatherapy massage was given as a take-home remedy to be applied directly twice daily to the areas affected by psoriasis, and a spritzer was also made for stress relief to be used as needed.

Massage/take-home blend

Lavender (*Lavandula angustifolia*), 18 drops: anti-inflammatory, calming

Helichrysum (*Helichrysum italicum*), 6 drops: anti-inflammatory, calming

Spritzer

Neroli (*Citrus aurantium* var. *amara*), 3 drops: calming

Grapefruit (*Citrus x paradisii*), 7 drops: antidepressant, emotional balancer

Blue cypress (*Callitris intratropica*), 2 drops: calming, grounding

The client reported that the itching disappeared after 2 days and the size and redness of the lesions decreased slowly. There was significant improvement after 2 weeks of use, especially on the low back. The client continued to use the blend occasionally if the areas flared up.

SUMMARY

- The main function of the integumentary system is to protect the body against abrasion, heat, UV light, dehydration, and pathogens. The skin also helps regulate body heat, excrete wastes, and synthesize vitamin D.

- The skin is made up of the epidermis, with the outer layer being the stratum corneum, which sheds cells continually, and the dermis, which contains glands, nerves, blood and lymphatic vessels, and hair follicles. Below this is a layer of fatty tissue that helps retain heat and absorbs shocks.

- Risk factors include trauma, UV light, extreme cold, dehydration, and stress.

- Essential oils have small molecules and are lipophilic, enabling certain constituents to pass through the epidermis and dermis. Those with an influence on the skin are classi-

fied as anti-inflammatory, cicatrizant, antipruritic, and moisturizing.

- New scars are very sensitive tissue and should be treated at first with infused oils and carrier oils. Cicatrizant essential oils can be added in increasing amounts as the scar ages.

- Rubefacient oils can be used for underlying mature scar tissue to bring blood to the area and soften tissue.

- Burns are best treated with anti-inflammatory and cicatrizant essential oils.

- Dermatitis/eczema responds best to anti-inflammatory and moisturizing essential oils and carrier oils.

- Psoriasis does not seem to respond well to aromatherapy treatment, except for the use of essential oils in stress relief.

Review Questions

1. Areas of the skin high in this have higher rates of absorption: (a) nerve endings and fat cells, (b) collagen and elastin, (c) blood and lymph vessels, (d) glands and hair follicles.
2. Babies and the elderly have higher rates of skin absorption. (T / F) Why? Why not?
3. Match the term with its definition: (a) increases hydration, (b) promotes rapid cell regeneration, (c) brings blood to the area, (d) helps stop itching; (i) cicatrizant, (ii) moisturizing, (iii) antipruritic, (iv) rubefacient.
4. Why is ginger (*Zingiber officinale*), which is anti-inflammatory, not used to treat skin inflammation?
5. Name two infused oils and two carrier oils that are used in aromatherapy to treat scarring.
6. For burns, essential oils are chosen to reduce _____ and promote rapid _____.
7. A cooling carrier for recent superficial burns would be: (a) a light lotion, (b) aloe vera gel, (c) cocoa butter, (d) sesame oil.
8. Seborrheic dermatitis is best treated with antifungal oils because it is possibly caused by a(n) _____ infection.
9. Athletes, who tend to have a thinner layer of subcutaneous fat, probably need: (a) rubefacient essential oils, (b) stronger dilutions of essential oils, (c) milder dilutions of essential oils, (d) anti-inflammatory essential oils.
10. Rubefacient essential oils are used for old scar tissue because they help to _____ tissue.

Notes

1. Kim HM, Cho SH. Lavender oil inhibits immediate-type allergic reaction in mice and rats. J Pharm Pharmacol 1999;51(2):221–226.
2. Safayhi H, Sabieraj J, Sailer ER, et al. Chamazulene: an antioxidant-type inhibitor of leukotriene B4 formation. Planta Med 1994; 60(5):410–413.
3. Koh KJ, Pearce AL, Marshman G, et al. Tea tree oil reduces histamine-induced skin inflammation. Br J Dermatol 2002;147(6):1212–1217.
4. Kirov M, Vankov S. Rose oil and girosital. Med Biol Info 1988;3:3–7.
5. Kirov M, Vankov S. Rose oil and girosital. Med Biol Info 1988;3:3–7.
6. Hartman D, Coetzee JC. Two US practitioners' experience of using essential oils for wound care. J Wound Care 2002;11(8):317–320.
7. Glowania HJ, Raulin C, Swoboda M. Effect of chamomile on wound healing—a clinical double-blind study. Z Hautkrankheiten (Berlin) 1987;62(17):1267–1271.
8. Lavagna SM, Secci D. Efficacy of hypericum and calendula oils in the epithelial reconstruction of surgical wounds in childbirth with caesarean section. Il Farmaco 2001;56:451–453.
9. Ro YJ, Ha HC, Kim CG, et al. The effects of aromatherapy on pruritus in patients undergoing hemodialysis. Dermatol Nurs 2002;14(4): 231–256.
10. Monges P, Joachim G, Bohor M, et al. Comparative *in vivo* study of the moisturizing properties of three gels containing essential oils: mandarin, German chamomile, orange. Nouveau Dermatol 1994;13:470–475.
11. Allan R. Case study: seborrhoeic dermatitis. Int J Aromather 2003; 13(1):47–48.
12. The National Psoriasis Foundation. Available at: www.psoriasis.org. Accessed November 28, 2004.
13. Harrison PV, Weaver J. Aromatherapy and psoriasis. J Dermatol Treat 1993;4(3):163.

22

The Female Reproductive System

The reproductive system is unique in that it is the only system without which the body can continue to survive, and in fact it does not become very obvious until puberty. However, it has enormous impact on both physical and emotional functioning. Both my own experience and research studies show that problems associated with the female reproductive system respond favorably to complementary therapies, including aromatherapy and massage. At present there is little evidence that complementary therapies provide effective options for the male reproductive system.

An Overview of the Female Reproductive System

The function of the female reproductive system is to produce ova (eggs) for fertilization by sperm produced by the male reproductive system, and to provide a safe and nurturing environment for the developing fetus during pregnancy. The entire process is regulated by the endocrine system. The internal structures of the female reproductive system are the ovaries, the fallopian tubes, the uterus, the cervix, and the vagina (Fig. 22.1).

The ovaries are a pair of organs that produce oocytes (developing eggs), which are released about once every 28 days in the process of ovulation. The maturation and release of the oocyte are stimulated by hormones produced by the pituitary gland, in response to hormones from the hypothalamus. When an oocyte is released, it travels down the fallopian tubes, where fertilization by a sperm cell might take place. The ovaries also produce hormones, such as estrogen and progesterone, that regulate the various stages of the menstrual cycle, and relaxin, which relaxes the pubic symphysis and pelvic joints during pregnancy.

If fertilization occurs, the fertilized egg implants itself in the wall of the uterus and begins to develop. If the egg is not fertilized it is expelled. Hormones cause the endometrium, the

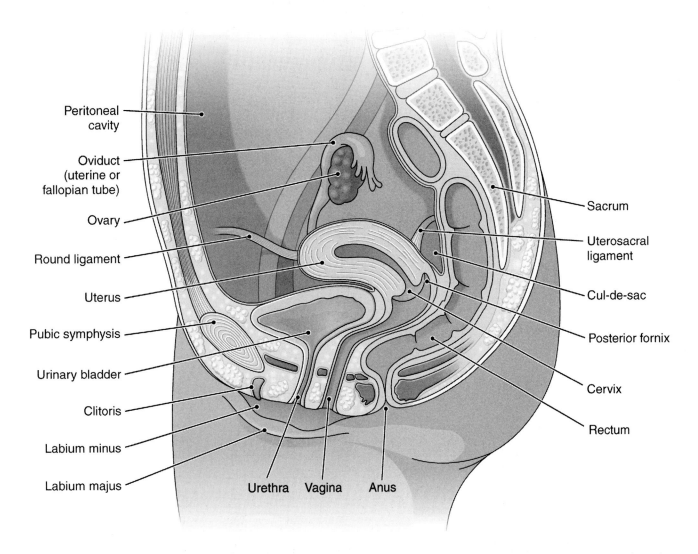

Figure 22.1 Internal structures of the female reproductive system. (Reprinted with permission from Cohen B, Taylor J. Memmler's The Human Body in Health and Disease, 10th ed. Baltimore: Lippincott Williams & Wilkins, 2005.)

inner lining of the uterus, to become thinner and start to break down. The endometrium is shed as menstrual flow.

Puberty usually occurs between the ages of 10 and 15, when rising hormone levels lead to many changes in the body, especially in the reproductive system. Estrogen causes the breasts to grow in females, and menarche (first menstrual period) usually occurs about 2 years later. The menstrual cycle often takes some time to regularize, and ovulation and fertility may not become dependable for another 2 years.

Many changes happen to the mother's entire body throughout pregnancy. The hormones that are released during pregnancy cause weight gain from fluid retention. The volume of blood increases by up to a liter and the heart must work harder to pump it around the body. Oxygen and nutrients are required by the growing fetus, so the rate of respiration increases, as do thirst and appetite. The breasts largely consist of fat and connective tissue in nonpregnant women, but during pregnancy, hormones cause the milk-producing glands to enlarge and occupy most of the breast.

Menopause is a gradual phase culminating in the cessation of the menstrual cycle. As a result of the decrease in estrogen production by the ovaries, ovulation and menstruation become irregular and finally stop, signaling the end of reproductive capability. Menopause usually occurs between the ages of 45 and 55, and what is known as perimenopause, the transition period to menopause, may last for several years. Fluctuating hormone levels during perimenopause can lead to uncomfortable physical symptoms, and lower hormone levels during menopause have effects on the entire body, not just on the reproductive system. The risk of both osteoporosis and atherosclerosis increases significantly after menopause, largely because of the lower levels of estrogen.

Risk Factors

Factors that have a negative effect on the reproductive system include:

- *Stress.* Sympathetic nervous system activity disrupts the regular functioning of the reproductive system. Because many reproductive functions are controlled by the hypothalamus, which is a regulator of the autonomic nervous system, it is easy to see how emotions and stress can affect the reproductive system. Many women experience a cessation of menstruation when they are under unusual stress, and others find that stress can affect fertility, making it more difficult to get pregnant.

- *Poor nutrition.* If a woman is not getting adequate nutrition, menstrual periods may cease and pregnancy will be more difficult to achieve. A high sugar or caffeine intake seems to intensify the symptoms of PMS.

- *Alcohol.* Alcohol consumption is a risk factor for breast cancer, as alcohol seems to change how the body metabolizes estrogen.[1]

- *Environmental estrogens.* Pesticides, plastics, and other human-made products contain estrogen-like compounds. It has been suggested that they have some role in causing various cancers of the reproductive system, but their actions on the body are not yet well understood.

How Aromatherapy Affects the Female Reproductive System

Odors have a strong influence on the limbic system, including the hypothalamus, which regulates the female reproductive system via the pituitary. Many experiments to show the effects of aromas on the body, such as those by the researcher Martha McClintock, have focused on charting the response of the menstrual cycle to odors.[2] This is presumably partly because menstruation is a very obvious endocrine marker, but also because the reproductive system is especially sensitive to influence from the limbic brain. Many women using aromatherapy find that symptoms of PMS, menstruation, and menopause may be alleviated by inhaling essential oils. Essential oils that are calming are likely to have a beneficial effect on the reproductive system, through their influence on the hypothalamus and the autonomic nervous system.

Certain essential oils have been traditionally regarded in aromatherapy as having **estrogenic** properties, and some of them have been proven in scientific studies to have compounds that bind to estrogen receptors in the body.[3] They may have a mild regulatory effect on the female reproductive system.

Aside from these oils, which have a general balancing influence, many essential oils have a direct effect on various symptoms experienced before and during menstruation, pregnancy, and menopause. The most important of these are the antispasmodic oils, which can help provide relief from cramping. Essential oils that are classified as **emmenagogues,** substances that promote menstrual flow, can also be helpful for cramping and menstrual pain. Contrary to what is written in many texts, there is no evidence that emmenagogues pose a risk during pregnancy, as they only encourage menstruation when the menstrual cycle actually occurs.

Calming: rose (*Rosa damascena*), linden blossom (*Tilia x europaea*), lavender (*Lavandula angustifolia*), neroli (*Citrus aurantium* var. *amara*), sandalwood (*Santalum album*), Roman chamomile (*Chamaemelum nobile*), bitter orange (*Citrus aurantium* var. *amara*), patchouli (*Pogostemon cablin*)

Estrogenics: aniseed (*Pimpinella anisum*), fennel (*Foeniculum vulgare*),[4] geranium (*Pelargonium graveolens*),[5] sage (*Salvia officinalis*), and essential oils high in citral, such as lemongrass (*Cymbopogon citratus*) and melissa (*Melissa officinalis*)[6]

Antispasmodics: basil (*Ocimum basilicum*), black pepper (*Piper nigrum*), cardamon (*Elettaria cardamomum*), clove (*Syzygium aromaticum*), ginger (*Zingiber officinale*), marjoram (*Origanum majorana*), rosemary (*Rosmarinus officinalis*),[7] fennel (*Foeniculum vulgare*),[8] clary sage (*Salvia sclarea*), Roman chamomile (*Chamaemelum nobile*)

Emmenagogues: basil (*Ocimum basilicum*), fennel (*Foeniculum vulgare*), juniper (*Juniperus communis*), peppermint (*Mentha piperita*), rosemary (*Rosmarinus officinalis*), sage (*Salvia officinalis*), thyme (*Thymus vulgaris* CT thymol)

Common Problems of the Female Reproductive System

A significant number of issues affecting the female reproductive system appear to respond well to aromatherapy and massage therapy. Even if underlying issues cannot be resolved, symptomatic relief is often possible.

Dysmenorrhea

Dysmenorrhea, or painful menstruation, is a common condition. It probably affects most women at some point in their lives. Chronic severe dysmenorrhea can be disabling for some women for several days each month.

Causes and Symptoms. The main symptom is a cramping pain in the low abdomen and/or low back, which usually starts at the onset of menstruation but can also occur premenstrually. If the pain is severe, nausea and a slight fever may also be present. Most menstrual pain is caused by powerful contractions of the uterine muscle. For most women there is no known underlying cause. However, for a certain percentage of women with severe chronic dysmenorrhea, the pain may be the result of pelvic infection, cysts or fibroids, or **endometriosis,** a disease in which the lining of the uterus (the endometrium) migrates outside the uterus and causes growths, internal bleeding, and scar tissue formation.

Essential Oils. The most effective oils are the emmenagogues and antispasmodics (see lists previously). Several of these, such as Roman chamomile (*Chamaemelum nobile*), black pepper (*Piper nigrum*), ginger (*Zingiber officinale*), and peppermint (*Mentha piperita*), are also analgesic, making them particularly helpful.

If endometriosis is known to be the cause, adding essential oils that are vasoconstrictors and anti-inflammatories to the blend may provide some relief over the long term. According to the Endometriosis Association, internal bleeding and inflammation are common with this problem.[9] Essential oils that are both vasoconstricting and anti-inflammatory include cypress (*Cupressus sempervirens*), geranium (*Pelargonium graveolens*), and lemon (*Citrus limon*).

Methods of Application. For women who find some relief from the pain in warmth directly over the lower abdomen, essential oils can be used in a moderate dilution of about 5–7% under a warm compress, either on the abdomen or low back. Massage with essential oils on the low back and gluteal area can also bring some relief.

Premenstrual Syndrome

Most women experience PMS, a range of uncomfortable symptoms in the week before their menstrual periods. According to the Mayo Clinic, as many as 70–90% of menstruating women experience at least one premenstrual symptom.[10]

Causes and Symptoms. The cause of PMS is unknown, although it obviously has to do with hormonal fluctuations, as symptoms generally disappear after menopause or during pregnancy. The large range of symptoms are both psychological (irritability, anxiety, mood swings, food cravings, depression, insomnia) and physical (water retention, fatigue, breast tenderness, acne, migraine). Of these symptoms, women may experience only one or two, or they may experience many.

Essential Oils. Oils that are thought to be estrogenic and/or generally balancing to hormones can be used throughout the month to prevent symptoms. These oils include geranium (*Pelargonium graveolens*), aniseed (*Pimpinella anisum*), fennel (*Foeniculum vulgare*), sage (*Salvia officinalis*), and melissa (*Melissa officinalis*).

Other oils can be used symptomatically, for example, grapefruit (*Citrus x paradisi*) or juniper (*Juniperus communis*) for water retention, black spruce (*Picea mariana*) for fatigue, and frankincense (*Boswellia carteri*) or grapefruit (*Citrus x paradisi*) for food cravings. Geranium (*Pelargonium graveolens*) tends to work well for the acne that appears during PMS, and most of the citrus oils, especially bergamot (*Citrus x bergamia*), are useful for mood swings. Jasmine (*Jasminum grandiflorum*) seems to be very effective for any depression associated with PMS.

Methods of Application. Application methods will depend on the symptoms being treated. Full-body massage with essential oils in a mild dilution (2–3%) is very helpful for psychological symptoms, insomnia, water retention, and fatigue. Spritzers, diffusers, or stick inhalers used throughout the month seem to help prevent many of the symptoms of PMS, although blends should be changed at least every 2 months to avoid allergic reaction or tolerance to the blend.

Issues During Pregnancy

Pregnancy massage is a growing industry, with specialized props, body cushions, and tables being produced to ensure client comfort and safety. There are many misconceptions about the use of aromatherapy during massage, but it is clear that holistic aromatherapy, using essential oils topically and in inhalations in low to moderate doses, is a safe option for treating some of the problems associated with pregnancy. Certain essential oils should be avoided during pregnancy (see Chapter 10), but Tisserand and Balacs draw a clear distinction between those that should not be used at all and those that are safe topically, but not internally.[11] Many essential oils

PMS

Ms. C. was a woman in her early thirties who came for aromatherapy massage sessions for stress relief. She was a nurse in a nursing home for the elderly and her work was reasonably stressful, but she commented that it only overwhelmed her during the week before her menstrual period. She frequently felt weepy and unable to cope with the normal work routine at this time and had strong cravings for chocolate. Other symptoms included being more tired premenstrually, having difficulty concentrating on forms and charts, and feeling slightly depressed.

She agreed to use a take-home aromatherapy blend, as well as having regular massage sessions twice a month. The same blend was used in the massage and in a take-home spritzer, to make use of the learned odor response. The following oils were used in a 2% blend:

Geranium (*Pelargonium graveolens*), 8 drops: hormone balancer

Fennel (Foeniculum vulgare), 6 drops: estrogenic, tonic

Sandalwood (*Santalum album*), 4 drops: centering, calming, antidepressant

Grapefruit (*Citrus x paradisi*), 3 drops: antidepressant, appetite balancer

Frankincense (*Boswellia carteri*), 3 drops: calming, appetite balancer

After 1 month, melissa (*Melissa officinalis*) was substituted for the fennel, because Ms. C. commented that she did not particularly like the "liquorice" smell. After 2 months, she reported that she felt more balanced and less overwhelmed at work. The chocolate cravings were more manageable, particularly if she used the spritzer immediately when she experienced them. She purchased some of the essential oils because she wanted to use them in different ways, such as in baths and diffusers. At a 6-month follow-up she said that many of the premenstrual symptoms had either disappeared or felt more within her control.

currently contraindicated for pregnancy in aromatherapy texts, such as fennel (*Foeniculum vulgare*) or rosemary (*Rosmarinus officinalis*), are safe for external use in all trimesters.

Pregnancy is in no way an illness, and most women feel extremely healthy throughout their term. However, there are a number of issues ranging from inconvenient to painful that can easily be resolved with the use of aromatherapy and massage.

Morning Sickness. Affecting at least 50% of women, typically in early morning for the first trimester, morning sickness can occur at any time of day and sometimes for the entire 9 months. An inhaler or spritzer with peppermint oil (*Mentha piperita*) at about a 1% dilution can be helpful. Ginger (*Zingiber officinale*) is also frequently recommended, but in my experience, it is more effective as a tea made from the root or as a crystallized candy.

Low-Back Pain. Pain in the lower back area usually is most noticeable in the last trimester, when the weight of the abdomen causes the pelvis to tilt forward, constricting the low back. Local massage with essential oils to relax muscles, such as black pepper (*Piper nigrum*), cardamon (*Elettaria cardamomum*), ginger (*Zingiber officinale*), and lavender (*Lavandula angustifolia*), in a 3% dilution seems to relieve aches in this area.

Constipation. Fairly common especially in later pregnancy, constipation results from the pressure of the fetus on the intestines and the lack of tone in the intestinal muscles because of the influence of the hormone relaxin. Very gentle abdominal massage with essential oils such as black pepper (*Piper nigrum*), ginger (*Zingiber officinale*), rosemary (*Rosmarinus officinalis*), sweet orange (*Citrus sinensis*), or fennel (*Foeniculum vulgare*) in a 2–3% dilution is useful.

Varicose Veins. Even women with no other risk factors for varicose veins frequently develop them during later pregnancy, as a result of the pressure on veins running through the pelvic area. Cypress (*Cupressus sempervirens*), lemon (*Citrus limon*), and geranium (*Pelargonium graveolens*) are often beneficial and should be given as a 2% dilution in lotion or oil to be used by the client over the area every day.

Urinary Tract Infections. Infection of the urinary tract is common in late pregnancy when the head of the fetus descends into the pelvis, often irritating the bladder. Essential oils that are antibacterial, yet mild on mucous membranes, can be used in an abdominal and low-back massage and given in a take-home blend to be used in baths. These oils include lavender (*Lavandula angustifolia*), geranium (*Pelargonium graveolens*), sandalwood (*Santalum album*), and tea tree (*Melaleuca alternifolia*).

Leg Cramps. Cramping of the legs is more common in later pregnancy, and it can interfere with sleep. Useful essential oils are black pepper (*Piper nigrum*), clary sage (*Salvia sclarea*), marjoram (*Origanum majorana*), lavender (*Lavandula angustifolia*), and petitgrain (*Citrus aurantium* var. *amara*). These can be applied in a 2% dilution during a massage or given as a take-home blend to be applied as needed.

Edema. Caused by the various hormones produced during pregnancy, edema is most noticeable as puffy ankles, swollen feet, and sometimes swollen hands. Localized lymphatic drainage work with essential oils in a 3% dilution, or a foot bath with 4–6 drops of essential oils, will be helpful. Essential oils to help move lymph include cypress (*Cupressus sempervirens*), geranium (*Pelargonium graveolens*), grapefruit (*Citrus x paradisi*), and lemon (*Citrus limon*).

Stretch Marks. Stretch marks are caused when the body grows more quickly than the skin can stretch to accommodate it. They are typically seen across the abdomen during pregnancy. They can also occur across the chest, abdomen, thighs, or buttocks after growing spurts in adolescence, as a result of rapid weight gain, or from a rapid increase in muscle size because of working out intensively. Essential oils such as lavender (*Lavandula angustifolia*), neroli (*Citrus aurantium* var. *amara*), mandarin (*Citrus reticulata*), or helichrysum (*Helichrysum italicum*) can be added in a 1–2% dilution to a heavy lotion made with rich, nourishing carrier oils such as avocado oil, vitamin E oil, wheat germ oil, cocoa butter, and Shea butter. This blend should be used daily in early pregnancy to avoid stretch marks, as they do not respond to treatment after they appear.

Postnatal Depression. Affecting up to 10% of women who have given birth recently, postnatal depression can range from mild cases of weepiness to severe cases that might need medical treatment. The main cause seems to be the strong hormonal fluctuations that occur when a woman gives birth, aggravated by common feelings of being overwhelmed by responsibility, increased demands, and lack of sleep.

Studies show that essential oils can be extremely effective in helping with depression, especially citrus oils,[12] such as lemon (*Citrus limon*) or grapefruit (*Citrus x paradisi*). Fennel essential oil (*Foeniculum vulgare*) has been shown to reduce depression, mental stress, and fatigue,[13] and other essential oils such as rose (*Rosa damascena*), geranium (*Pelargonium graveolens*), marjoram (*Origanum majorana*), and ylang ylang (*Cananga odorata*) are traditionally used in aromatherapy to help with depression. Jasmine (*Jasminum grandiflorum*) is frequently recommended for postnatal depression; however, it is an antigalactagogue, reducing breast milk production even by its smell, and its use is not advised in any form for breast-feeding women. Full-body aromatherapy massage is one of the best treatments for any form of depression, but this may be impractical for a mother with a newborn. Essential oils should be given as any take-home treatment that the mother is likely to use frequently.

Issues During Menopause

Like pregnancy, menopause is part of a healthy woman's life, yet it can have uncomfortable side effects. Although several essential oils have been identified as containing **phytoestrogens,** which are plant compounds resembling human estrogen that may bind with estrogen receptors in the body, there is no scientific evidence to suggest that they have strong effects during perimenopause or menopause. However, they may have a general balancing effect, and aromatherapy can certainly be used to help with many of the inconvenient or distressing sensations experienced at this time.

Chaste berry (*Vitex agnus castus*) is a relatively new essential oil, although the fruits have traditionally been used in herbal medicine. Some recent studies have been conducted on the effects of the oil on menopausal symptoms. Aromatherapy researcher and author Janina Maria Sørenson describes the pharmacological action as "mainly hormonal, balancing the female endocrine system and counteracting oestrogen dominance through a dopaminergic principle."[14] Barbara Lucks reports on a study in which many of the 23 women using the oil commented that it alleviated both physiological and emotional symptoms of perimenopause.[15] The participants in the study could inhale the oil or apply it topically. This result is certainly encouraging, but chaste berry is new as an essential oil, rather than an herb, and long-term use of any essential oil that has not had either scientific testing for safety or a recorded history of safe use is always dubious.

Hot Flashes. Although they can occur at any time, night sweats, or hot flashes, can disturb sleep. Essential oils can be given for home use in the form of a spritzer, which can be sprayed directly onto the skin when needed to cool and calm. Cooling essential oils include blue cypress (*Callitris intratropica*), German chamomile (*Chamaemelum nobile*),[16] clary sage (*Salvia sclarea*), geranium (*Pelargonium graveolens*), lavender (*Lavandula angustifolia*),[17] palmarosa (*Cymbopogon martinii*), rose (*Rosa damascena*), and the citrus oils.

Increased Perspiration. Excessive perspiring often accompanies hot flashes, and a spritzer can be made for both, using the essential oils listed above combined with oils that are slightly astringent, helping to close pores and slow down perspiration. These oils include cypress (*Cupressus sempervirens*), juniper (*Juniperus communis*), lemon (*Citrus limon*), and grapefruit (*Citrus x paradisi*).

Emotional Changes. Because of the strong hormonal changes during this period of life, many women experience depression, anxiety, irritability, or mood swings. Good mood balancers include the citrus oils, especially bergamot (*Citrus x bergamia*),[18] cardamon (*Elettaria cardamomum*), clary sage (*Salvia sclarea*), jasmine (*Jasminum grandiflorum*), rose (*Rosa damascena*),[19] and ylang ylang (*Cananga odorata*).

Difficulty Concentrating. Although not typically documented as a symptom of menopause, many women going through perimenopause experience a mild loss of short-term memory, difficulty concentrating, or general fuzzy-headedness. Essential oils that are traditionally used in aromatherapy to stimulate the brain and help with concentration and memory include basil (*Ocimum basilicum*),[20] frankincense (*Boswellia carteri*), lemon (*Citrus limon*), peppermint (*Mentha piperita*), and rosemary (*Rosmarinus officinalis*).

SUMMARY

- The function of the female reproductive system is to produce eggs for fertilization by sperm and to provide an environment for the growth of the fetus during pregnancy. Menstruation starts during puberty and ends at menopause.

- The reproductive system is regulated by hormones, principally estrogen and progesterone, that control the menstrual cycle. The release of these hormones is triggered by the hypothalamus via the pituitary gland. The ovaries also secrete the hormone relaxin during pregnancy.

- The ovaries produce oocytes, which travel down the fallopian tubes to the uterus. If fertilized, the egg will implant in the wall of the uterus and begin to develop. If unfertilized, the egg will be expelled and the endometrium (inner lining of the uterus) will be shed as the monthly menstrual flow.

- Risk factors include stress, poor nutrition, alcohol, and environmental estrogens.

- Aromatherapy affects the reproductive system mainly through the effects of essential oils on the hypothalamus.

Estrogenic oils that bind to estrogen receptors in the body may have a regulatory effect. Essential oils also provide symptomatic relief before and during menstruation, pregnancy, and menopause.

- Antispasmodic essential oils and emmenagogues are helpful for dysmenorrhea.

- Vasoconstrictors and anti-inflammatory oils may be useful for clients with endometriosis.

- PMS should be treated symptomatically, although estrogenic/hormone balancing essential oils may be useful to help prevent symptoms.

- See Chapter 10 for specific contraindications for pregnancy. Most essential oils classified as emmenagogues do not pose a risk during pregnancy.

- During perimenopause, estrogen-balancing essential oils may be helpful. Essential oils can also be used for symptomatic relief.

Review Questions

1. Because the reproductive system is regulated by hormones released by the _____, which is part of the limbic brain, odors have a strong effect on this system.
2. Some essential oils have compounds that are similar to this human hormone: (a) progesterone, (b) testosterone, (c) adrenaline, (d) estrogen.
3. Do essential oils that are emmenagogues present a risk during pregnancy? Why or why not?
4. Dysmenorrhea is best treated with anti-_____ and _____ essential oils.
5. Inhalation of essential oils can be an effective treatment for PMS. (T / F)
6. Name two essential oils that are generally considered to be helpful in preventing the symptoms of PMS.
7. Which of the following guidelines should be followed during pregnancy? (a) All essential oils should be avoided completely during pregnancy, (b) most oils are safe in mild to moderate dilutions, (c) essential oils must be avoided in the first trimester but are safe thereafter, (d) essential oils can only be used in inhalations, except for the last trimester.
8. Which essential oil is recommended in inhalation for morning sickness?
9. Describe a typical treatment for constipation during pregnancy.
10. To avoid stretch marks during pregnancy, essential oils should be applied topically in a: (a) light carrier oil, (b) gel base, (c) heavy rich carrier, (d) spritzer.
11. Jasmine should not be used for postnatal depression. (T / F) Why or why not?
12. Phytoestrogenic essential oils may be useful during menopause for _____.
13. Cooling essential oils such as _____ or _____ may be helpful for hot flashes.
14. Cypress and lemon may help with excessive perspiration because they are: (a) phytoestrogenic, (b) phototoxic, (c) detoxifying, (d) astringent.

Notes

1. Weil A. From a lecture on breast cancer, Integrative Medicine Retreat, Hollyhock, BC, Canada, August 2004.

2. Stern K, McClintock MK. Regulation of ovulation by human pheromones. Nature 1998;392(6672):177–179.

3. Howes MJ, Houghton PJ, Barlow DJ, et al. Assessment of estrogenic activity in some common essential oil constituents. J Pharm Pharmacol 2002;54(11):1521–1528.

4. Albert-Puleo M. Fennel and anise as estrogenic agents. J Ethnopharmacol 1980;2(4):337–344.

5. Geldof AA, Engel C, Rao BR. Estrogenic action of commonly used fragrant agent citral induces prostatic hyperplasia. Urol Res 1992;20: 139–144.

6. Howes MJ, Houghton PJ, Barlow DJ, et al. Assessment of estrogenic activity in some common essential oil constituents. J Pharm Pharmacol 2002;54(11):1521–1528.

7. Ramadan A, Afifi NA, Fathy MM, et al. Some pharmacodynamic effects and antimicrobial activity of essential oils of certain plants used in Egyptian folk medicine. Vet Med J Giza 1994;42(1):263–270.

8. Ostad SN, Soodi M, Shariffzadeh M, et al. The effect of fennel essential oil on uterine contraction as a model for dysmenorrhea, pharmacology and toxicology study. J Ethnopharmacol 2001;76(3):299–304.

9. The Endometriosis Association. Available at: www.endometriosisassn .org. Accessed October 14, 2004.

10. The Mayo Clinic. Available at: www.mayoclinic.com. Accessed October 14, 2004.

11. Tisserand R, Balacs T. Essential Oil Safety. London, UK: Churchill Livingstone, 1999:111.

12. Komori T, Fujiwara R, Tanida M, et al. Effects of citrus fragrance on immune function and depressive states. Neuroimmunomodulation. 1995;2:174–180.

13. Nagai H, Nakagawa M, Nakamura M, et al. Effects of odors on humans (II). Reducing effects of mental stress and fatigue. Chem Senses 1991;16:198.

14. Sørenson JM. A natural female hormone balancer. In Essence 2002;1 (1):14–19.

15. Lucks B. *Vitex Agnus-Castus* essential oil and menopausal balance: a self-care survey. Int J Aromather 2003;13(2):161–168.

16. Tubaro A, Zilli C, Redaelli C, et al. Evaluation of anti-inflammatory activity of a chamomile extract topical application. Planta Med 1984; 50(4):359.

17. Kim H-M, Cho S-H. Lavender oil inhibits immediate-type allergic reaction in mice and rats. J Pharm Pharmacol 1999;51:221–226.

18. Komori T, Fujiwara R, Tanida M, et al. Effects of citrus fragrance on immune function and depressive states. Neuroimmunomodulation 1995;2:174–180.

19. Umezu T. Anticonflict effects of plant-derived essential oils. Pharmacol Biochem Behav 1999;64(1):35–40.

20. Manley CH. Psychophysiological effect of odor. Crit Rev Food Sci Nutr 1993;33(1):57–62.

23

The Respiratory System

The respiratory system is unique among the systems of the body in that it has both a voluntary and an involuntary action. Every day we breathe thousands of times, quite unconsciously, not needing to think to inflate or deflate our lungs. Yet if we want to, at any point we can choose to change our breathing pattern. If we are angry or nervous we might breathe slowly and deeply to try to control our feelings. Women in labor are taught to pant shallowly. And we will sometimes take in a deep breath and heave a sigh to express boredom or disgust. We use our breathing deliberately to calm down from strong emotional states, ease pain or discomfort, express our feelings, and help us to concentrate. Conversely, pain and strong emotions can upset our normal regular breathing patterns. The nervous system and the respiratory system have strong influences on each other.

An Overview of the Respiratory System

Cells need energy to carry out their basic functions, to make repairs, and to divide and grow. This energy is provided by nutrients, but most cells need oxygen to metabolize the nutrients. In this process oxygen is used up and carbon dioxide is released. The cardiovascular system collects the carbon dioxide and transports it to the lungs, where it is expelled from the body by breathing out. Fresh oxygen is breathed in and is carried by the blood to all the tissues of the body. The respiratory system has specialized structures and tissues to facilitate this exchange of oxygen and carbon dioxide. The other functions of the system are to produce sound, to help with venous return through the change in thoracic pressure, and as part of the olfactory system. Figure 23.1 shows the upper and lower tracts of the respiratory system.

The upper respiratory tract is of obvious importance to aromatherapists because it contains the olfactory receptors at the top of the nasal cavity (see Chapter 4). In breathing, the air enters the nose, which acts as a filter, trapping dust and other particles with hairs and mucus. The nasal cavity and the sinuses warm and moisten the air before it enters the pharynx, or throat, which is the common passageway for both air and food. The auditory tubes that drain the middle ear also open into the upper pharynx, with the result that ear infections are often linked to sore throats and tonsillitis. The tonsils are clusters of lymphatic tissue around the top of the throat that trap bacteria and other pathogens and prevent them from penetrating any deeper into the body.

The lower respiratory tract starts with the larynx, also called the voice box. The larynx houses the vocal cords, ligaments that are expanded and contracted by the laryngeal muscles; they vibrate to produce sound as air moves past them. Sensitive nerves in the larynx trigger a cough reflex if food enters the area. The trachea, or windpipe, is a tube largely made of cartilage that leads from the larynx to the lungs. It branches into the two bronchi, which in turn divide many times into smaller passageways called bronchioles. These lead to alveolar ducts, which in turn lead to air-filled sacs called alveoli. The alveoli are separated from an extensive network of tiny blood capillaries by a membrane only one cell thick. This facilitates the exchange of oxygen and carbon dioxide from the capillaries to the lungs and back again.

The lungs consist of the bronchi, bronchioles, alveoli, blood vessels, and other connective tissue. They lie in the rib cage, resting on the diaphragm, the large muscle that contracts, together with the external intercostal muscles, to increase the size of the thoracic cavity and draw air into the lungs. Exhalation is mostly passive, relying on the elastic recoil of the lungs as the muscles of inhalation relax. Forced exhalation is the expulsion of air from the lungs by the internal intercostals and the abdominal muscles.

Risk Factors

Factors that have a negative effect on the respiratory system include:

- *Smoking.* Smoking and secondhand smoke are the biggest risk factors for many kinds of respiratory diseases, including lung cancer and emphysema, and they can trigger or exacerbate others, such as asthma. Smoking also lowers the amount of oxygen available to the body, making tissue healing slower and causing many other health problems.

- *Industrial fumes or dust.* These factors have been shown to cause chronic obstructive pulmonary disease and asthma. Many of the most extreme case studies of people developing allergic reactions to essential oils have been from the industrial processing of plant material.

- *Stress.* Stressful situations tend to make people breathe quickly and shallowly. If this becomes a chronic breathing pattern, there is a risk that the person may not be taking in enough oxygen, thereby starving cells and tissues.

How Aromatherapy Affects the Respiratory System

Unlike most other systems of the body that are affected by the absorption of essential oil components into the blood, or affected indirectly via the brain, the respiratory system is directly influenced by essential oils. Most essential oils are extremely volatile, which means that they are easily inhaled in various treatment modalities, reaching the tissues of both the upper and lower respiratory tracts virtually intact. As a result, aromatherapy has a very strong effect on the system, and essential oils have been extensively used in scientific and medical studies to alleviate respiratory problems. Inhalation is by far the safest method of application for essential oils and also the most effective as far as the respiratory system is concerned.

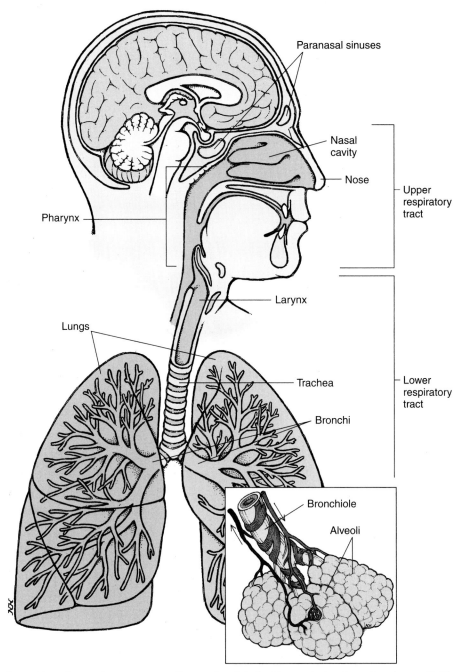

Figure 23.1 The respiratory system. (Source: Reprinted with permission from Premkumar K. The Massage Connection Anatomy and Physiology. Baltimore: Lippincott Williams & Wilkins, 2004.)

Essential oils can be classified according to their actions on the respiratory system. Some are **expectorant,** meaning loosening of mucus in the lungs, making it easier to cough up. Others are more suitable for the thick, sticky mucus that is almost impossible to cough up, as they are **mucolytics,** substances that break down mucus and make it more liquid. Some are useful as **antitussives** to stop coughing, or antispasmodics, for the type of spasmodic cough found in asthma or whooping cough. Some oils

work as **decongestants** for clearing the sinuses, while many are effective against viral or bacterial infections of the sinuses or lungs. Most essential oils traditionally used in aromatherapy to treat respiratory issues are highly immunostimulating.

Steam inhalation is popular for many respiratory ailments, especially when there is mucus involved. It is important to emphasize that smaller amounts of essential oils appear to work better as expectorants than larger amounts. One study stated that the expectorant action declined progressively as the concentration of the volatile oils increased.[1] Using 2–3 drops in personal steam inhalation devices is recommended, and even this may be too strong for some people.

Many oils are ideally suited to treat respiratory symptoms because of their volatile and antibacterial nature. A few oils are very useful in blends, including eucalyptus (*Eucalyptus radiata*), frankincense (*Boswellia carteri*), peppermint (*Mentha piperita*), and spike lavender (*Lavandula latifolia*).

Essential oils used with small children for respiratory disorders should be especially mild in both action and dose because stronger components, such as menthol (found in peppermint essential oil), have been suspected to cause respiratory distress or collapse.[2]

Antibacterials: peppermint (*Mentha piperita*),[3] cinnamon bark (*Cinnamomum zeylanicum*), lemongrass (*Cymbopogon citratus*), thyme (*Thymus vulgaris* CT thymol),[4] spike lavender (*Lavandula latifolia*)[5] (Note: Cinnamon bark, lemongrass, and thyme CT thymol should be used only in diffusion or steam inhalation when blended with other less irritating oils. They should make up no more than 10% of the essential oil blend.)

Antivirals: eucalyptus (*Eucalyptus radiata, E. globulus, E. smithii*),[6] ginger (*Zingiber officinale*), pine (*Pinus sylvestris*), cardamon (*Elettaria cardamomum*), tea tree (*Melaleuca alternifolia*), niaouli (*Melaleuca quinquinervia* CT cineole), cajeput (*Melaleuca cajeputi*), ravensara (*Ravensara aromatica*), spike lavender (*Lavandula latifolia*), black pepper (*Piper nigrum*)

Expectorants: turmeric (*Curcuma longa*),[7] nutmeg (*Myristica fragrans*),[8] eucalyptus (*Eucalyptus radiata*), black spruce (*Picea mariana*), ginger (*Zingiber officinale*), rosemary (*Rosmarinus officinalis*)

Mucolytics: inula (*Inula graveolens*), helichrysum (*Helichrysum italicum*)

Antispasmodics: clary sage (*Salvia sclarea*), petitgrain (*Citrus aurantium* var. *amara*), marjoram (*Origanum majorana*), basil (*Ocimum basilicum*), tarragon (*Artemesia dracunculus*), fennel (*Foeniculum vulgare*), frankincense (*Boswellia carteri*)

Antitussives: peppermint (*Mentha piperita*),[9] cypress (*Cupressus sempervirens*), black spruce (*Picea mariana*), sage (*Salvia officinalis*)

Decongestants: eucalyptus (*Eucalyptus radiata*), cardamon (*Elettaria cardamomum*), rosemary (*Rosmarinus officinalis*), spike lavender (*Lavandula latifolia*), bay laurel (*Laurus nobilis*)

Safe essential oils for children's respiratory problems: eucalyptus (*Eucalyptus smithii*), rosalina (*Melaleuca ericifolia*), green myrtle (*Myrtus communis*), palmarosa (*Cymbopogon martinii*), frankincense (*Boswellia carteri*)

Common Problems of the Respiratory System

Although many respiratory issues can be effectively treated with aromatherapy, massage therapists do not often see acute problems, such as pneumonia. They are more likely to be asked to help relieve the symptoms of chronic issues, such as sinusitis or asthma.

Sinusitis

Sinusitis is an inflammation of one or several of the sinus cavities, usually as a result of an infection. It may be acute or chronic.

Causes and Symptoms. Because the mucous membrane in the sinuses is continuous with the throat and nasal passages, infections can spread easily throughout these areas. These infections may be either viral, from a cold virus, or bacterial, such as from a tooth abscess. Food sensitivities or changes in pressure during a flight can trigger symptoms. Depending on which sinus is inflamed, symptoms range from toothache to headache, pain above or below the eyes, to earache. Other symptoms include fever, nasal discharge, and a feeling of stuffiness or pressure behind the nose. The person will often have difficulty breathing.

Essential Oils. Decongestants, such as eucalyptus (*Eucalyptus radiata*), rosemary (*Rosmarinus officinalis*), or spike lavender (*Lavandula latifolia*), often work well for blocked sinuses. Peppermint (*Mentha piperita*) is often added to blends, not because it clears the sinuses but because it stimulates the cold receptors in the nose, giving the sensation of being able to breathe more easily.[10] It is also an effective analgesic for sinus headaches. If the mucus seems to be particularly thick and difficult to clear, inula (*Inula graveolens*) or helichrysum (*Helichrysum italicum*) should be used with the decongestant blend, to break down the mucus.

Methods of Application. Massage is contraindicated with fever, but otherwise a short facial massage, including drainage techniques, with essential oils in a 5% dilution (lower with sensitive skin) can be extremely effective. Doing a steam inhalation before the massage will help drain the sinuses, and essential oils seem to be most effective in clearing air passages when they are used in small amounts. With a commercial steam inhaler, about 5–10 drops will be sufficient for one session. Tissues should be available for the client, as drainage can be quite significant.

Respiratory Allergies (Hay Fever)

Respiratory allergies are commonly known as hay fever, although few of them are actually grass allergies. Other terms include seasonal allergic rhinitis. It is estimated that more than 26 million people in the United States have hay fever symptoms every year.

Causes and Symptoms. Any allergic reaction shows an underlying dysfunction of the immune system (see Chapter 20). There are various triggers for respiratory reactions, including plant pollens, mold, dust mites, and animal dander. Many people also have similar symptoms when exposed to chemicals such as paints, plastics, and cigarette smoke. These are not true allergic reactions, but are classified as chemical sensitivities. Symptoms of respiratory allergies include congested nasal and sinus passages, mucus in the lungs, red weepy eyes, sneezing, and feeling tired and generally slightly ill.

Essential Oils. As with any allergic reaction, essential oils that both suppress the release of histamine and help reduce inflammation are useful. These oils include German chamomile (*Matricaria recutita*), Roman chamomile (*Chamaemelum nobile*), Himalayan cedar (*Cedrus deodara*), turmeric (*Curcuma longa*), lavender (*Lavandula angustifolia*), and tea tree (*Melaleuca alternifolia*). Other essential oils can be blended with the anti-inflammatories to help alleviate symptoms. Eucalyptus (*Eucalyptus radiata*), spike lavender (*Lavandula latifolia*), and rosemary (*Rosmarinus officinalis*) will help decongest nasal passages, while black spruce (*Picea mariana*) and pine (*Pinus sylvestris*) are both good expectorants and adrenal supports for fatigue.

Methods of Application. Inhalation is always effective for respiratory disorders. Steam inhalation is recommended for both upper and lower respiratory congestion. Essential oils can also be used in a spritzer to try to avoid symptoms. Dilutions should be very mild because treatment is often long term and also to avoid the risk of allergic reactions to the essential oils from a hypersensitive immune system. Blends should be changed about every 4 weeks if they are to be used regularly, and oils should be fresh.

Asthma

Asthma is a chronic inflammatory condition that can be life-threatening if it is not properly managed. According to the American Lung Association, it was estimated that 20 million people in the United States had asthma in 2002, and the number of emergency room visits for the problem was close to 1.9 million.[11]

Causes and Symptoms. The underlying issue with asthma is a chronic inflammation and hypersensitivity of the bronchial tubes. There is often a genetic predisposition, but environmental pollution or food allergies also may be causes. Attacks may be triggered by allergic reactions, exercise, respiratory infections, cigarette smoke, sudden temperature change, or stress. Any of these may cause a narrowing of the bronchi, resulting in coughing, wheezing, and shortness of breath. Symptoms are often worse at night, as lying down narrows the airways. Episodes may be frequent or uncommon, severe or mild, and people may be asymptomatic between attacks.

CASE STUDY 23.1

Hay Fever

Mrs. L., age 49, had seasonal respiratory allergies. She had experienced the allergies since about the age of 15 and had been taking prescription medications for the problem since her mid-twenties. The symptoms were only present in spring and occasionally early summer, and if she started taking the medication in late February through May, she could avoid most of the symptoms. Without the medications, she had nasal congestion, frequent sneezing, red irritated eyes, and a slightly puffy face, especially around the eyes. She came for an aromatherapy consultation in late January, as she was interested in seeing if a more natural remedy could help with her symptoms.

A blend was made for her to use in a spritzer several times during the day, and also to massage into her hands or feet once daily. The spritzer was at a 2% dilution, while the massage blend was at a 4% dilution:

Blend 1:

Himalayan cedar (*Cedrus deodora*), 8 drops: anti-inflammatory, suppresses histamine production

Roman chamomile (*Chamaemelum nobile*), 4 drops: anti-inflammatory, suppresses histamine production

Lavender (*Lavandula angustifolia*), 12 drops: anti-inflammatory, suppresses histamine production

A second blend was made so that she could alternate these every few weeks to avoid tolerance or allergic reaction:

Blend 2:

Turmeric (*Curcuma longa*), 6 drops: anti-inflammatory, suppresses histamine production

German chamomile (*Matricaria recutita*), 8 drops: anti-inflammatory, suppresses histamine production

Tea tree (*Melaleuca alternifolia*), 10 drops: anti-inflammatory, suppresses histamine production

Mrs. L. continued to use these two blends throughout the next few months. By June she reported that she had had much fewer symptoms, although she sneezed slightly more than previous years when she had taken medication. Overall she was very pleased with the results and planned to use aromatherapy the following year.

Essential Oils. The anti-inflammatory oils are useful on a long-term basis to calm any underlying allergic reaction. These include German chamomile (*Matricaria recutita*), Roman chamomile (*Chamaemelum nobile*), Himalayan cedar (*Cedrus deodara*), turmeric (*Curcuma longa*), lavender (*Lavandula angustifolia*), and tea tree (*Melaleuca alternifolia*). Other oils may be chosen on the basis of symptoms. Eucalyptus (*Eucalyptus radiata*) and rosemary (*Rosmarinus officinalis*) are excellent expectorants and decongestants, while the antispasmodic and antitussive oils, such as peppermint (*Mentha piperita*), clary sage (*Salvia sclarea*), tarragon (*Artemesia dracunculus*), or fennel (*Foeniculum vulgare*), help with the tiring spasmodic cough that accompanies asthma.

Because stress seems to be a frequent trigger, calming essential oils such as lavender (*Lavandula angustifolia*) or mandarin (*Citrus reticulata*) may be helpful, especially in take-home blends. I almost always include frankincense (*Boswellia carteri*) in blends for clients who have asthma because it is antispasmodic and calming, as well as being a mild expectorant and anti-inflammatory.

Methods of Application. Massage is frequently used to treat the fascial restrictions around the chest and back that are common with asthma and the muscular tightness frequently found in the back, neck, and shoulders. Essential oils can be used with this massage in dilutions of 1–5%, depending on the age of the client and the size of the area being treated. Using strong dilutions around the face and neck area is not recommended because the bronchial hypersensitivity could trigger coughing. Spritzers and other take-home blends with essential oils to relax sympathetic nervous system activity can be helpful in preventing symptoms.

Steam inhalation is commonly contraindicated in aromatherapy texts for clients with asthma, in case it provokes an attack. However, a quick survey of my clients and students with asthma showed that while several of them could not tolerate steam even in a sauna, for example, others felt it helped their symptoms and had even been recommended by their doctors to do steam inhalations regularly. If therapists wish to try steam inhalation with an asthmatic client, they should check first with the client's physician, and even then use aromatic steam inhalation for only short periods of time (no longer than 1–2 minutes).

Chronic Obstructive Pulmonary Disease

Chronic obstructive pulmonary disease (COPD) includes chronic bronchitis and emphysema, which often coexist and have many similar symptoms. They are both diseases in which the airflow to or from the lungs is obstructed.

Causes and Symptoms. In chronic bronchitis, the airways become inflamed from long-term irritation, in 80–90% of cases from cigarette smoking. Exposure to industrial dust or fumes may also cause the problem. There is a chronic cough, increased mucus, and shortness of breath. The chest may lose

---

CASE STUDY 23.2

Asthma

B. was a 9-year-old boy who had been diagnosed with asthma at around age 4. He had wheezing and shortness of breath, especially during physical exercise, if he was in a stressful situation, or with sudden temperature changes. He did not seem to have allergic reactions to substances, although he was definitely sensitive to cigarette smoke and dust. The family owned a dog and often went for walks in the woods and neither the dog nor the woods seemed to cause B. any problems. He was slightly overweight, which his physician felt might contribute to his symptoms. He frequently had respiratory infections during the winter months. His parents were interested in using aromatherapy at home, but did not think B. would appreciate a massage session.

Two blends were made as an upper back and/or chest rub at a 2% dilution, to be applied by the parents. Each blend was used for several weeks and then alternated with the other blend to avoid tolerance and allergic reaction. His parents also decided to use rosalina (*Melaleuca ericifolia*) in a room humidifier when B. had a respiratory infection, as this oil helps both upper and lower respiratory infections, is milder for use with children, and is sedative for use at night.

Blend 1:

Eucalyptus (*Eucalyptus smithii*), 8 drops: antiviral, antitussive, expectorant

Palmarosa (*Cymbopogon martinii*), 8 drops: antiviral, antibacterial, stress reduction

Pine (*Pinus sylvestris*), 8 drops: expectorant, immune stimulant

Blend 2:

Cardamon (*Elettaria cardamomum*), 8 drops: expectorant, antispasmodic

Black spruce (*Picea mariana*), 10 drops: expectorant, immune stimulant

Frankincense (*Boswellia carteri*), 6 drops: antispasmodic, stress reduction

At a 3-month follow-up (in February), his parents reported that B. had had far fewer infections than usual during the winter. The infections that he did have were of shorter duration. He also seemed to have more stamina for physical exercise.

mobility, there is an increased risk of respiratory infections, and over time **hypoxemia** (oxygen deprivation) may occur.

Emphysema is characterized by irreversible lung damage. The connective tissue in the lungs loses its elasticity and eventually breaks down, resulting in impaired gas exchange in the alveoli. The bronchioles may also start to collapse, leading to obstruction. Symptoms include coughing and shortness of breath. As in chronic bronchitis, this often leads to hypoxemia. As the disease progresses, there may be pulmonary hypertension, leading to heart failure. Like chronic bronchitis, emphysema is caused by chronic irritation, most often by cigarette smoke, although a small number of people have a genetic tendency to get the disease.

Essential Oils. In treating the symptoms of COPD, one of the aims is to reduce the fascial restrictions that often occur, which restrict the free movement of the chest and upper back. Massage with essential oils that help hypertonicities can be very useful. Marjoram (*Origanum majorana*) and clary sage (*Salvia sclarea*) are both oils that help relax tight muscles and are also antispasmodic, useful for the coughing of COPD. The antitussive and antibacterial properties of peppermint (*Mentha piperita*) can be helpful, as can its property of making clients feel that they are breathing more easily, due to its stimulation of cold receptors in the respiratory tract. Any of the antispasmodic and antitussive oils will be of use generally. The all-round respiratory properties of frankincense (*Boswellia carteri*), together with its ability to decrease sympathetic nervous system activity, make it ideal for most blends.

For the heavy mucous production of chronic bronchitis, the expectorant oils are indicated. Eucalyptus (*Eucalyptus radiata*), black spruce (*Picea mariana*), and rosemary (*Rosmarinus officinalis*) are probably the oils that are most effective and least likely to further irritate the bronchi.

Methods of Application. Because of the coughing and the irritation of the airways found in bronchitis and emphysema, steam inhalation with essential oils is not advisable. Massage to reduce the fascial adhesions in the chest and

upper back is useful with essential oils in a 2–4% dilution. Chest rubs in a 2–4% dilution can be made to help with coughing and shortness of breath.

Cystic Fibrosis

Cystic fibrosis (CF) is the most common fatal genetic disease among Caucasians. About 30,000 people in the United States have CF, and it is most prevalent among those of northern European origin.

Causes and Symptoms. The cause is genetic, and both parents must carry the defective gene for it to be passed on. CF affects the respiratory tract, and frequent wheezing, pneumonia, and a chronic cough with thick mucus are common. Other symptoms include a weakened immune system and digestive system. Cystic fibrosis is a progressive disease with no current cure, and the most common cause of death is infection with the *Pseudomonas aeruginosa* bacterium. However, because of antibiotics and other treatments to help with breathing, life expectancies have increased to about 30 years.

Essential Oils. The most useful essential oils are the mucolytics, inula (*Inula graveolens*) and helichrysum (*Helichrysum italicum*), which help thin the mucus to expel it from the lungs. Clients with CF are often on mucus-thinning medications, but essential oils will also help this persistent problem. The expectorant oils also may be helpful. The *Pseudomonas* bacteria are notoriously resistant to antibiotics, and the use of certain essential oils may help avoid infection. Studies show that basil (*Ocimum basilicum*),[12] clove (*Syzygium aromaticum*),[13] cumin (*Cuminum cyminum*),[14] oregano (*Origanum vulgare*),[15] and lemon myrtle (*Backhousia citriodora*)[16] are effective against *Pseudomonas*.

Methods of Application. Physical therapy for the chest, including tapotement and postural drainage, is frequently used on a daily basis with people who have CF. Essential oils can be added to this treatment to help expel phlegm from the lungs. Steam inhalation can also be used to help break up mucus and to prevent bacterial infections in the lower respiratory tract.

SUMMARY

- Respiration can be both a voluntary and an involuntary action. It can be used to help control physical and psychological states.

- The main function of the respiratory system is to provide oxygen needed for the metabolism of nutrients. It also expels carbon dioxide produced by this process.

- The nose and sinuses filter, warm, and moisten air. The olfactory receptors are located in the nasal passages.

- The air goes next to the larynx (voice box), the trachea, and then the bronchi. These divide into many smaller bronchi-

oles, leading to alveoli—air-filled sacs with an abundant capillary blood supply for the exchange of gases.

- Risk factors for respiratory infection and disease include smoking, industrial fumes or dust, and stress.

- The tissues of the respiratory system can be directly exposed to essential oils, which are volatile and easily inhaled. Inhalation is both safe and effective.

- Essential oils for respiratory use are classified as expectorant, mucolytic, antitussive, antispasmodic, and decongestant. They may also attack respiratory pathogens directly.

- Essential oils that are high in menthol (e.g., peppermint) should not be used with young children.

- Sinusitis responds well to decongestants and mucolytics, especially in steam inhalations and facial massage.

- For asthma and hay fever, oils to reduce histamine production may be helpful. Other essential oils may be used symptomatically.

- Steam inhalations may produce an asthmatic attack and should not be used without a doctor's release for clients who have asthma.

- COPD, which includes emphysema and chronic bronchitis, responds well to essential oils that are antispasmodic and relaxing to muscles. Expectorant oils will probably be necessary with chronic bronchitis.

- Mucolytic and expectorant essential oils are helpful for the heavy mucus caused by cystic fibrosis. Essential oils can also be used to help prevent bacterial infections in the lungs.

Review Questions

1. What is the safest and most effective form of treatment for most respiratory problems?
2. Match the word with the definition: (a) breaks up mucus and makes it liquid, (b) helps decrease coughing, (c) clears sinus passages, (d) loosens mucus, making it easier to cough up; (i) expectorant, (ii) antitussive, (iii) mucolytic, (iv) decongestant.
3. Which essential oil should be avoided with small children? Which of these components is responsible? (a) methyl chavicol, (b) menthone, (c) menthol, (d) methyl salicylate
4. Some oils, such as cinnamon, may be irritating to mucous membranes when inhaled. What percentage of the essential oil blend should they be, at most?
5. List two treatment methods used with essential oils for sinusitis.
6. With an allergic reaction, such as hay fever, essential oils are used to suppress the release of _____ by the body.
7. Match the essential oils with their properties: (a) mucolytic, (b) expectorant, (c) antitussive, (d) decongestant; (i) peppermint, (ii) inula, (iii) spike lavender, (iv) ginger.
8. There is disagreement over whether _____ is contraindicated as a treatment method for asthmatic clients.
9. The most useful types of essential oil for cystic fibrosis are the _____ and the _____.
10. Chronic bronchitis and emphysema are both examples of chronic obstructive pulmonary disorder, but only one has pronounced mucus. Which one? Give an example of an essential oil that would be beneficial.

Notes

1. Boyd EM, Sheppard EP. The effect of inhalation of citral and geraniol on the output and composition of respiratory tract fluid. Arch Int Pharmacodyn 1970;188:5–13.
2. Davis S, Livingstone A. Respiratory collapse and *Karvol* capsules. Aust J Hosp Pharm 1986;16(4):273–274.
3. Shkurupii VA, Kazarinova NV, Ogirenko AP, et al. Efficiency of the use of peppermint (Mentha piperita L) essential oil inhalations in the combined multi-drug therapy for pulmonary tuberculosis. Probl Tuberk 2002;4:36–39.
4. Inouye S, Takizawa T, Yamaguchi H. Antibacterial activity of essential oils and their major constituents against respiratory tract pathogens by gaseous contact. J Antimicrob Chemother 2001;47(5):565–573.
5. Von Frohlich E. A review of clinical, pharmacological and bacteriological research into *Oleum spicae*. Weiner Medizinische Wochenschrift 1968;15:345–350.
6. Penoel D. *Eucalyptus smithii* essential oil and its use in aromatic medicine. Br J Phytother 1992;2(4):154–159.
7. Li C, Li L, Luo J, et al. Effect of turmeric volatile oil on the respiratory tract. Zhongguo Zhong Yao Za Zhi 1998;23(10):625–625.
8. Boyd EM, Sheppard P. Nutmeg oil and camphene as inhaled expectorants. Arch Otolaryngol (Chicago) 1970;92(4):372–378.
9. Schafer D, Schafer W. Pharmacological studies with an ointment containing menthol, camphene and essential oils for bronchiolitic and secretolytic effects. Arzneimittel-forschung 1981;31(1):82–86.
10. Burrow A, Eccles R, Jones AS. The effects of camphor, eucalyptus and menthol vapour on nasal resistance to airflow and nasal sensation. Acta Otolaryngol 1983;96:157–161.
11. American Lung Association. Available at: www.lungusa.org. Accessed November 5, 2005.
12. Opalchenova G, Obreshkova D. Comparative studies on the activity of basil—an essential oil from Ocimum basilicum L—against multidrug resistant clinical isolates of the genera Staphylococcus, Enterococcus and Pseudomonas using different test methods. J Microbiol Methods 2003;54(1):105–110.
13. Briozzo J, Nunez L, Chirife J, et al. Antimicrobial activity of clove oil dispersed in a concentrated sugar solution. J Appl Bacteriol 1989;66 (1):69–75.
14. Menghini A, Savino A, Lollini MN, et al. The antimicrobial activity by direct contact and microatmosphere of certain essential oils. Plantes Medicinales Phytotherapie 1987;21(1):36–42.
15. Lambert RJ, Skandamis PN, Coote PJ, et al. A study of the minimum inhibitory concentration and mode of action of oregano essential oil, thymol and carvacrol. J Appl Microbiol 2001;91(3):453–462.
16. Hayes AJ, Markovic B. Toxicity of Australian essential oil Backhousia citriodora (Lemon myrtle). Part 1. Antimicrobial activity and in vitro cytotoxicity. Food Chem Toxicol 2002;40(2):535–543.

24

The Digestive System

Kew Gardens, the large botanical gardens in the sub-urbs of London, has a motto: "All life depends on plants." We are totally dependent on green plants for our daily nutrition, whether we eat them directly or absorb their nutrients via meat from an animal. Food molecules from plants and animals are broken down into their component chemicals and absorbed and used for energy. These processes are the function of the digestive system. The digestive tract extends from the mouth to the anus.

An Overview of the Digestive System

Taste (gustation) and smell (olfaction) are the body's chemical senses, and both of them play an important role in digestion. Smells prepare the digestive system for food, triggering brain impulses that stimulate the production of saliva and digestive enzymes. There are four true tastes: sweet, salty, bitter, and sour. All other flavors are odors that reach the olfactory system through the back of the mouth. People who lose their sense of smell complain that food no longer has any flavor. They may lose weight along with their interest in food, or they may gain weight as they eat more in an attempt to regain some satisfaction with food.

Figure 24.1 shows the main digestive structures and organs, starting with the mouth. Food is mechanically broken down by the teeth and softened and moistened by saliva. Some enzymes in the saliva begin the chemical breakdown of carbohydrates, and others kill bacteria. When the food is swallowed, it goes down the esophagus, through the pharynx, to the stomach. *Peristalsis,* or rhythmic movements of the smooth muscle, propels the food downwards.

Food stays in the stomach for 30 minutes to 4 hours and is mixed with gastric acids and enzymes to break it down further and to kill bacteria. The stomach absorbs some salts, some drugs such as aspirin, and alcohol, which is why some medications work within 20–30 minutes and why it is easy to get drunk on an empty stomach. The semi-liquid chyme is then sent to the small intestine.

The small intestine, the body's major digestive organ, consists of three parts: the duodenum, where most of the breakdown of food takes place, and the jejunum and the ileum, both of which function in absorption. Movement here is slower, with food taking about 5 hours to move through. The length (about 20 feet) and the structure of the small intestine, with numerous projections increasing the surface area, make it well suited to absorption. The small intestine also secretes various substances, such as intestinal juices and hormones, which help with breakdown and absorption. Blood that contains the substances absorbed from food gets sent immediately to the liver.

The liver has many effects on the digestive system. It produces bile, the substance vital for the digestion and absorption of fats. Bile is sent to the gallbladder, where it is stored and

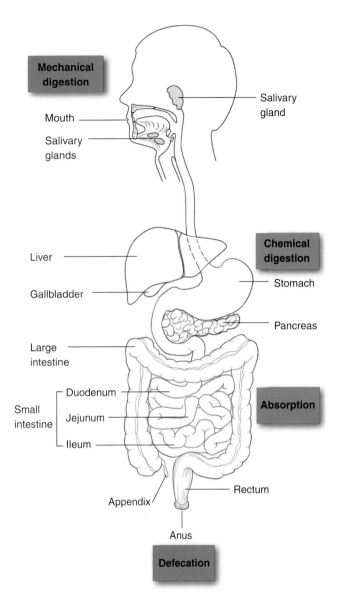

Figure 24.1 The digestive system. (Source: Adapted from Premkumar K. The Massage Connection Anatomy and Physiology. Baltimore: Lippincott Williams and Wilkins, 2004.)

concentrated, before going to the small intestine. The liver also helps maintain blood glucose levels by storing and releasing glycogen and removes toxins, drugs, pathogens, and hormones from the blood it receives from the small intestine, before circulating it to the rest of the body.

The pancreas produces pancreatic enzymes that are sent to the small intestine to help break down proteins, carbohydrates, and fats. The pancreas also helps regulate blood glucose levels by producing the hormone insulin.

The main function of the large intestine is to expel the undigested parts of the food we eat. Most water is reabsorbed by the small intestine, but the large intestine also absorbs some water, sodium, and some minerals. It also absorbs vitamins, such as K and B complex, that are produced by intestinal bacteria.

Risk Factors

Factors that have a negative effect on the digestive system include:

- *Stress.* Stress is probably the factor with the highest impact on the digestive system, which is directly influenced by the sympathetic and parasympathetic divisions of the nervous system. It has been proven that digestion effectively stops when the sympathetic system is active, with the result that chronic stress can lead to many forms of digestive dysfunction. Stress often makes people eat too fast, and this too can cause digestive disorders.

- *Poor nutrition.* A diet that is low in fiber can slow down elimination, and fatty or greasy foods may lead to indigestion. Many people, especially of Asian or Native American origin, are lactose-intolerant, and eating dairy products can upset their digestion. Many people have intolerances to certain foods, which may cause diarrhea or digestive pain. Diets high in sugar and refined carbohydrates lead to many problems, especially to type 2 diabetes.

- *Lack of exercise.* Peristalsis seems to be more effective with regular exercise, and a lack of muscle tone, especially in abdominal and pelvic floor muscles, can cause problems in elimination.

- *Postural imbalance.* Poor posture can prevent the muscles of the abdomen and low back from contracting, leading to digestive difficulties.

How Aromatherapy Affects the Digestive System

Many essential oils are derived from spices and herbs that are frequently used in cooking, such as cinnamon, ginger, rosemary, and bay laurel. These are used in cuisines around the world, not just as flavorings but because they affect the digestion, encouraging peristalsis, calming spasms, stimulating the production of bile to digest fats, or even killing harmful bacteria. However, most scientific studies have been on the effects of essential oils when they are taken internally. The results of these studies do not necessarily mean that the oils will have the same effects when used topically. However, some essential oil components do absorb into the bloodstream, so there may be a correlation.

Because the digestive system is governed by the nervous system, the most effective use of essential oils may be to calm and soothe the client, reducing sympathetic tone and increasing parasympathetic activity. For this reason, essential oils that are **neurodepressant,** or calming to the nervous system, are often used in blends for digestive disorders. Digestion is also strongly affected by secretions from the liver, and the use of essential oils that are **hepatic,** or strengthening to the liver, is often beneficial.

Neurodepressants (calming): rose (*Rosa damascena*), linden blossom (*Tilia x europaea*), lavender (*Lavandula angustifolia*), neroli (*Citrus aurantium* var. *amara*), Roman chamomile (*Chamaemelum nobile*), bitter orange (*Citrus aurantium* var. *amara*)

Antispasmodics: peppermint (*Mentha piperita*),[1] tarragon (*Artemesia dracunculus*), nutmeg (*Myristica fragrans*),[2] lavender (*Lavandula angustifolia*),[3] cardamon (*Elettaria cardamomum*),[4] melissa (*Melissa officinale*),[5] basil (*Ocimum basilicum*), rose (*Rosa damascena*),[6] sweet orange (*Citrus sinensis*), Roman chamomile (*Chamaemelum nobile*)

Digestive stimulants: sage (*Salvia officinalis*), fennel (*Foeniculum vulgare*), rosemary (*Rosmarinus officinalis*)

Appetite stimulants: cardamon (*Elettaria cardamomum*), lemon (*Citrus limon*), peppermint (*Mentha piperita*), bergamot (*Citrus bergamia*), fennel (*Foeniculum vulgare*), tarragon (*Artemesia dracunculus*)

Hepatics: helichrysum (*Helichrysum italicum*), fennel (*Foeniculum vulgare*),[7] carrot (*Daucus carota*), basil (*Ocimum basilicum*), peppermint (*Mentha piperita*),[8] rosemary (*Rosmarinus officinalis*), lemon (*Citrus limon*)

Common Problems of the Digestive System

Massage therapists do not address the symptoms of acute digestive disorders in their practices and only chronic issues are discussed here. However, many clients with chronic ailments, such as irritable bowel syndrome, have discovered that they can greatly alleviate their symptoms with aromatherapy massage.

Irritable Bowel Syndrome

Irritable bowel syndrome (IBS) is the most common problem of the digestive system in Western countries. It affects 10–20% of adults in the United States,[9] and a majority of sufferers are women. IBS is also known as nervous indigestion, irritable colon, spastic colon, spastic colitis, or mucous colitis.

Causes and Symptoms. IBS is characterized by spasms in the large intestine, with no apparent physical defect in the digestive tract. Often starting during childhood or early adulthood, attacks usually are triggered by stressful situations and/or food intolerances. The most common foods that start or aggravate symptoms include wheat products, dairy foods, citrus fruits, fruits or vegetables that are very high in fiber, greasy or fatty foods, and alcohol. Chocolate, caffeine, and carbonated drinks and simply overeating can also trigger symptoms.

The most common symptoms are alternating constipation and sudden diarrhea; clients might experience one of

CASE STUDY 24.1

Irritable Bowel Syndrome

Ms. S., age 52, came for aromatherapy massage sessions because of irritable bowel syndrome. Her physician had recommended various forms of stress reduction, including bodywork. She looked pale, exhausted, and slightly overweight. She said that her job was fairly stressful, but that she probably took it too seriously. Her partner was currently working in another part of the country and she was trying to decide whether or not to join him. The decision making was causing her extra stress. Her main symptoms were short periods of constipation, followed by sudden acute diarrhea, stomach cramps made worse by certain foods, bloating, and a general feeling of dragging tiredness. She was aware that sugary foods made her irritable bowel syndrome worse in general, but felt addicted to them for emotional comfort and to help with the tiredness.

She agreed to have weekly aromatherapy massage sessions for stress reduction, and she was interested in using the essential oils at home. The following blend was made in a 2% dilution for use in the massage session, and was given in a 4% dilution for self-massage of the abdomen:

Roman chamomile (*Chamaemelum nobile*), 3 drops: antispasmodic, calming

Tarragon (*Artemesia dracunculus*), 5 drops: antispasmodic

Lavender (*Lavandula angustifolia*), 6 drops: antispasmodic, calming

Cardamon (*Elettaria cardamomum*), 6 drops: antispasmodic, antidepressant

Sweet orange (*Citrus sinensis*), 4 drops: antispasmodic, calming

A second blend was given for home use, to help increase energy and stamina. This was a neat blend, 4 drops to be put on a washcloth and used on the body in the morning shower:

Black spruce (*Picea mariana*), 40 drops: adrenal support

Peppermint (*Mentha piperita*), 8 drops: stimulating, antispasmodic

Rosemary (*Rosmarinus officinalis*), 20 drops: stimulating, tonic, strengthening

The blends were used at home and in weekly massages for 6 weeks, during which time Ms. S. seemed to become increasingly relaxed and cheerful. She reported that she had had fewer episodes of sudden diarrhea, and that she seemed to be able to think more clearly at work and about her personal situation. She looked more energetic and talked about her future more. At the end of this time, she decided that she could not afford further massages but wanted to continue using aromatherapy at home. In a follow-up 3 months later she said that the improvements in energy and bowel function were continuing.

these more than the other. Lower abdominal pain and cramping are other major symptoms. Additional symptoms include bloating, gas, nausea, and halitosis. People with IBS often find their lives greatly restricted, as they have to stay within range of a restroom because of the unpredictable attacks of diarrhea.

Essential Oils. Stress is by far the most significant trigger with IBS, and essential oils that calm the client and restore parasympathetic functioning are the most important treatment. Any of the neurodepressant oils listed previously will be helpful, combined with any of the antispasmodic oils, as the major symptoms are caused by intestinal spasm. Peppermint (*Mentha piperita*) has been successfully used internally in conventional allopathic medications to relieve IBS symptoms.[10] In my experience of treating clients with IBS, peppermint also has good effects on spasm and pain when used topically. Basil (*Ocimum basilicum*) is useful, both for its strengthening effects on the nervous system and as an antispasmodic. Tarragon (*Artemesia dracunculus*) is an underused oil in aromatherapy that has significant antispasmodic effects, and Roman chamomile (*Chamaemelum nobile*) is frequently used for IBS with good results.

Methods of Application. Essential oils used in a moderate dilution (up to 5%) in an abdominal massage can be very helpful during the constipation stage of IBS, and can also help to relieve the bloating and pain that accompany this phase. Diarrhea is a contraindication to abdominal massage. Use of the calming essential oils in a milder dilution (1–3%) in a full-body massage, or in take-home blends such as spritzers, can be helpful in reducing the effects of stress on the intestines.

Inflammatory Bowel Disease

Inflammatory bowel disease (IBD) refers to both ulcerative colitis and Crohn's disease.

Causes and Symptoms. Ulcerative colitis causes inflammation in the lining of the large intestine, while Crohn's disease causes inflammation in the lining and wall of the large intestine and/or the small intestine. Not much is known about the causes of IBD, although there may be a possibility of a genetic factor. Changes in the immune system have been observed with IBD, although whether it is an autoimmune disease remains unclear.

Ulcerative colitis and Crohn's disease have similar symptoms, with abdominal pain, diarrhea, rectal bleeding, and weight loss commonly reported. Both diseases have periods of remission and relapse.

Essential Oils. According to the American Gastroenterological Association, stress is probably not a cause of IBD, but it might aggravate the symptoms.[11] Essential oils that calm the autonomic nervous system will be helpful (see list of neurodepressants previously). Since IBD is an inflammatory problem, essential oils such as German chamomile (*Matricaria recutita*), yarrow (*Achillea millefolium*), helichrysum (*Helichrysum italicum*), lavender (*Lavandula angustifolia*), and turmeric (*Curcuma longa*), which are both calming and anti-inflammatory, may be useful.

Methods of Application. The focus of the treatment is on stress reduction, with essential oils used in a mild dilution (1–3%) in a full-body relaxation massage. Gentle abdominal massage can be used if the client is not experiencing a flare-up of symptoms. Take-home blends of calming essential oils in any form that the client is likely to use regularly can be helpful in reducing stress.

Constipation

Constipation is a symptom, rather than an illness, although it can create other health problems. Many people have chronic, intermittent, or temporary constipation.

Causes and Symptoms. Constipation may be a symptom of many other illnesses, such as IBS, IBD, multiple sclerosis, Parkinson's disease, and diabetes. It can also be a side-effect of pregnancy, surgery of any kind, or certain medications. Lifestyle factors include a diet low in fiber, inadequate water intake, stress, poor muscle tone, and a lack of exercise. Pain or discomfort may be experienced when passing stools, and bowel movements are infrequent. Other results of constipation include abdominal pain and cramping, low-back pain, bloating and gas, nausea, lack of appetite, headaches, and halitosis.

Essential Oils. Traditional remedies for constipation in aromatherapy include fennel (*Foeniculum vulgare*), rosemary (*Rosmarinus officinalis*), black pepper (*Piper nigrum*), ginger (*Zingiber officinale*), marjoram (*Origanum majorana*), and sweet orange (*Citrus sinensis*).

Methods of Application. The most common treatment is abdominal and low-back massage with essential oils in a moderate dilution of 3–5%. Full-body relaxation massage is also helpful if constipation is stress-related. Abdominal massage can be taught to clients to perform at home if the problem is chronic, and aromatherapy blends can be sent with them for this purpose.

SUMMARY

- The function of the digestive system is to provide nutrients for conversion into energy to meet the body's needs.

- Taste and smell are both important for digestion.

- Food is broken down in the mouth by the teeth and salivary enzymes, in the stomach by gastric enzymes and mechanical churning, and in the small intestine by enzymes from the pancreas and bile from the liver and gallbladder.

- Most absorption takes place in the small intestine. Nutrient-rich blood is sent immediately to the liver for processing.

- Expulsion of undigested food parts is carried out by the large intestine, which also absorbs some water, minerals, and vitamins.

- Risk factors for digestive disorders include stress, poor diet, lack of exercise, and postural imbalances.

- Essential oils that influence the digestive system are classified as calming, antispasmodic, digestive stimulants, appetite stimulants, and hepatics.

- Irritable bowel syndrome is best treated with antispasmodic and destressing essential oils.

- Inflammatory bowel disease may respond to anti-inflammatory and destressing essential oils.

- Constipation may be helped by essential oils in an abdominal and low-back massage.

Review Questions

1. The effects of holistic aromatherapy on the digestive system have not been scientifically proven, as most studies are on essential oils used _____.

2. Name two essential oils that are traditionally used to stimulate appetite.

3. _____ is the most significant trigger for irritable bowel syndrome, so _____ essential oils are often used in treatments.

4. Inflammatory bowel disease is best treated with essential oils in a: (a) deep tissue massage on the low back, (b) relaxation massage, (c) deep abdominal massage, (d) inhalation.

5. Many essential oils that are traditionally used to treat the digestive system are also found as food flavorings. (T / F)

6. Basil and tarragon are examples of essential oils that are _____ for the digestive system.

7. Name two essential oils that are both calming and anti-inflammatory.

8. Match the essential oil with its property: (a) antispasmodic, (b) appetite stimulating, (c) stimulating to peristalsis, (d) calming; (i) rose, (ii) cardamon, (iii) sweet orange, (iv) fennel.

9. Essential oils in an abdominal massage for constipation should be used in a dilution of: (a) 1%, (b) 3–5%, (c) 5–8%, (d) 10–15%.

Notes

1. Taylor BA, Luscombe DK, Duthie HL. Inhibitory effect of peppermint oil on gastrointestinal smooth muscle. Gut 1983;24:A992.

2. Bennett A, Stamford IF, Tavares IA, et al. The biological activity of eugenol, a major constituent of nutmeg (*Myristica fragrans*): studies on prostaglandins, the intestine and other tissues. Phytother Res 1988;2(3):124–130.

3. Lis-Balchin M, Hart S. Studies on the mode of action of the essential oil of lavender (*Lavandula angustifolia* P. Miller). Phytother Res 1999;13(6):540–542.

4. al-Zuhair H, el-Sayeh B, Ameen HA, et al. Pharmacological studies of cardamom oil in animals. Pharmacol Res 1996;34(1–2):79–82.

5. Sadraei H, Ghannadi A, Malekshahi K. Relaxant effect of essential oil of *Melissa officinalis* and citral on rat ileum contractions. Fitoterapia 2003;74(5):445–452.

6. Kirov M, Vankov S. Rose oil and girosital. Med Biol Info 1988;3:3–7.

7. Rangelov A. An experimental characterization of cholagogic and cholesteric activity of a group of essential oils. Folia Med (Plovdiv) 1989;31(1):46–53.

8. Trabace L, Avato P, Mazzoccoli M, et al. Choleretic activity of some typical components of essential oils. Planta Med 1992;58(Suppl. 1):650–651.

9. The IBS Self-Help and Support Group. Available at: www.ibsgroup.org. Accessed November 25, 2004.

10. Kline RM, Kline JJ, Di Palma J, et al. Enteric-coated, pH-dependent peppermint oil capsules for the treatment of irritable bowel syndrome in children. J Paediatr 2001;138:125–128.

11. The American Gastroenterological Association. Available at: www.gastro.org. Accessed November 25, 2004.

25

Elderly Care

In developed countries, life expectancies are increasing. In 1900, life expectancy was about 49 years, and by 1960 it had gone up to 70 years. Recently the U.S. Administration on Aging estimated that a child born in 2000 could expect to live to age 76.9.[1] As a result of medical advances, better nutrition, and less strenuous physical work, people are living longer and expecting to stay healthy and active well into their seventies and eighties. In recent years, according to the Alliance for Aging Research, the proportion of older Americans who are disabled is decreasing, not increasing, and only about 5% of older people live in nursing homes.[2] This has not always been the case. Tolstoy, writing about the early nineteenth century in his book *War and Peace*, describes one older woman in this way: "The Countess was now over sixty. Her hair was quite gray and she wore a cap with ruching, which framed her whole face. Her face was wrinkled, the upper lip sunken, and her eyes were dim."[3] People in their sixties today are now often active, fit, attractive, and full of life.

Along with a longer life span, however, comes a corresponding rise in age-related illnesses and problems and an increasing interest in staving off these ill effects. Many books have been written on "anti-aging," and products promising renewed youth fill the shelves in stores. Essential oils have been investigated for their anti-aging effects, but this research is still in the experimental stages and it usually involves large doses of essential oils administered internally to animals.[4,5] However, most physicians and researchers agree that continued vitality into old age depends on a balanced lifestyle, which includes strategies to minimize discomfort and boost immunity and general functioning. Aromatherapy fits well into this kind of regime.

The Effects of Aging

As we age, various changes occur in our tissues and organs, most body systems slow down, and our body does not function as efficiently as it once did. The most immediately obvious effects are on our skin, which starts to sag and become wrinkled because of a thinning of the skin and subcutaneous tissue. This thinning has the added disadvantages of making us feel cold more easily and increasing the chance of bruising and skin injury. Other tissues below the surface also become thinner and more fragile. Bones get brittle from a decrease in various hormones, and weight-bearing joints degenerate. Vertebral discs thin, leading to spinal curvature and a loss of height, and muscle strength declines as the amount of muscle tissue decreases.

Other body systems become less elastic and less able to adapt to changing demands. Because the lungs lose their elasticity, oxygen levels in the blood decrease, and the arteries harden, leading to a risk of cardiovascular disease. The sympathetic nervous system is less efficient and vasoconstrictor fibers do not react quickly enough. Thus, many older people

may be lightheaded when they stand up quickly from a lying position, as a result of the pooling of blood in the lower extremities.

The senses tend to become less acute. For example, many older people are farsighted and are unable to read small print. Other vision problems common in old age include cataracts and glaucoma. Damage to the ears from loud noises can eventually lead to deafness. Many older adults complain that taste and smell are no longer as vivid.

The immune system is less effective in fighting pathogens because of a lowering of protective hormones and a decrease in lymphatic functioning. Together with the lowered lung functioning, this often leads to respiratory infections, which tend to last longer and be more severe. Other common infections are those of the urinary tract because kidney function decreases as we age and the urinary bladder gets smaller.

The body's metabolic rate gradually decreases, resulting in a loss of appetite and associated digestive problems as the large intestine loses muscle tone. Older people generally get less exercise, which can increase these problems, as digestion and elimination are partly dependent on skeletal muscle contraction.

Premature Aging

Some people are only in their thirties or forties but because they are overweight, smoke, and do not exercise, they look 20 years older than they should. Conversely, some older people have a healthy lifestyle, passionate interests, and a sharp mind, and they appear much younger than their years. It is fairly obvious that aging does not correspond only to chronological age: It also reflects a person's daily routine, the amount of stress one is under, and one's outlook on life. In a recent talk on healthy aging, Dr. Andrew Weil emphasized that aging is inevitable, as every living organism must change and eventually die. What is important is to age well, so that health and vitality are preserved as long as possible and old age can be enjoyed instead of dreaded.[6]

Factors that seem to lead to premature aging include:

- *Stress.* Stress activates the fight-or-flight response, flooding the body with adrenaline and exhausting the adrenal glands and, eventually, the whole body.

- *Poor diet.* Too much sugar, alcohol, caffeine, and junk food can all stress the body's detoxification and elimination organs, thereby causing damage to all body systems. Being overweight or underweight has significant health implications for the elderly.

- *Smoking.* Smoking decreases the amount of oxygen available to the body, damages various organ systems, and slows down the healing of tissues. Smoking and alcohol both can accelerate bone loss.

- *Lack of exercise.* Physical activity lowers the risk of certain chronic illnesses and helps maintain mobility and independent living. It increases cardiovascular strength, lung capacity, lymphatic flow, and elimination, and has a positive effect on all systems of the body.

How Aromatherapy Affects Older Adults

When using aromatherapy with older people (older than about age 75), aromatherapists must observe certain safety considerations.

1. Because of changes in the structure of the skin, it may be less permeable and also less prone to irritation.[7] However, this does not mean that stronger dilutions should be used. In my experience, older clients seem to be more sensitive to the effects of essential oils on the brain and in the bloodstream, and dilutions should probably be milder for clients older than 75, depending on overall health.

2. The kidneys do not function as efficiently as before and are possibly less able to handle large quantities of essential oil components. This is another reason to avoid extremely high doses or very strong dilutions of essential oils.

3. People tend to age at different rates, depending on lifestyle, stress levels, and general health. A healthy, active 80-year-old might be able to tolerate higher doses and more intense essential oils than a 65-year-old with chronic ailments and a less-than-healthy lifestyle.

Aromatherapy can be a useful support strategy for clients who may have a wide range of less serious ailments and want to use mild remedies that rarely interact with the medications that older people commonly take on a long-term basis. Although essential oils are not magic remedies, they can be used to help ease many of the symptoms associated with aging. As Marguerite Maury, the originator of holistic aromatherapy and someone who was passionately interested in the causes of aging, remarked: "When we are attacked by disease, weakness, and old age we call upon odiferous material to aid us. Nor has it ever been more faithful and more reliable than in these cases."[8]

Common Problems of Aging

All people experience different health issues or problems as they age. These problems usually develop from old injuries or illnesses that have created areas of weakness in the body or because of a genetic predisposition to certain chronic ailments. For example, someone who has injured his or her knees several times in skiing accidents is more likely to develop osteoarthritis in that area. Likewise, if a man's father and uncles have had prostate cancer, he will have a higher risk of getting this disease as he ages. Several chronic ailments commonly affect older clients no matter what their personal or family history may be. Some of these ailments

were discussed in other sections of the book, such as arthritis (see Chapter 16), high blood pressure and heart disease (see Chapter 17), Alzheimer's disease (see Chapter 19), and lowered immunity (see Chapter 20). Other health problems that may improve with aromatherapy are discussed below.

Injury and Slow Healing

For older people, injuries are likely to have more serious implications. Older people have a tendency to heal more slowly, thereby increasing the risk of bacterial infections, which a weaker immune system may not be able to counteract.

Causes. As with many other functions of the body, the mechanisms of healing tend to slow as we age. Capillaries under the skin are not as strong as before and the cushioning subcutaneous tissue is thinner, leading to increased bruising. Wounds take longer to resolve and skin is slower to heal. Some medications that are frequently prescribed for older people, such as blood thinners, contribute to this by making the blood less likely to clot. Older people also tend to undergo more medical tests and procedures, with incisions, blood pressure cuffs, and intravenous treatment causing bruising and scars.

Essential Oils. The use of essential oils as wound-healing substances may well have initiated modern aromatherapy—Gattefosse's interest was stimulated by a laboratory burn and Valnet's by his experiences with battle wounds as an army surgeon. The cicatrizant essential oils, which stimulate cell proliferation, are the ones mostly used to encourage wound healing. Because most essential oils are antibacterial, they help reduce the likelihood of bacterial infection. Lavender (*Lavandula angustifolia*),[9] German chamomile (*Matricaria recutita*),[10] frankincense (*Boswellia carteri*), myrrh (*Commiphora myrrha*), helichrysum (*Helichrysum italicum*), and neroli (*Citrus aurantium* var. *amara*) are all useful. The infused oils of St. John's wort (*Hypericum perforatum*) and calendula (*Calendula arvensis*)[11] are also cicatrizant and can be used as carriers for the essential oils.

Ron Guba, an Australian aromatherapist, conducted a study to test the effectiveness of essential oils in wound healing in six nursing homes in Melbourne from December 1995 to May 1997. The blend was used on venous ulcers, pressure ulcers, skin tears, and other superficial skin abrasions. The consensus of the nursing staff was that the essential oils definitely decreased healing times, with full healing for skin tears taking, on average, 14.5 days.[12]

For bruising, helichrysum (*Helichrysum italicum*), fennel (*Foeniculum vulgare*), hyssop (*Hyssopus officinalis*), and rosemary (*Rosmarinus officinalis*) are traditionally used in aromatherapy for their anti-inflammatory and blood-moving qualities. Donna Rona, an American aromatherapist, conducted an informal study on essential oils to treat hospital-induced trauma to the arms, mostly bruises and puncture wounds. She noted that the "normal bruising was reduced substantially and the puncture wounds healed quickly without scarring. Bruises caused by inexperienced phlebotomists healed in hours instead of days or weeks. The secondary effects of relaxation and overall anxiety reduction were noticed by all hospital personnel."[13]

Methods of Application. For wound healing, essential oils can be diluted in a carrier oil or lotion and applied as soon as the wound has closed, in a 5–25% dilution, depending on the age and health of the client and on the size of the wound. For acute bruising, essential oils can be applied under a cold compress in a 5–20% dilution, depending on the same factors. A few days later, essential oils can be applied in light massage in a 2–3% dilution to speed the complete resolution of the bruise.

Urinary Tract Infections

Infections of the bladder and the urinary tract, collectively called urinary tract infections (UTIs), are quite common and cause a significant amount of pain and discomfort. Early treatment is important because neglecting a UTI can lead to kidney damage.

Causes and Symptoms. Most UTIs are caused by *Escherichia coli*, a bacterium that is normally present in the large intestine. All the predisposing factors for UTIs are not known, and some people seem to be more prone to catching them than others. Common risk factors include some kind of obstruction of urine flow such as a kidney stone, an enlarged prostate gland, catheter use, diabetes, and immune-suppressive illnesses such as HIV/AIDS. Many of these risk factors are more commonly experienced by older people; thus, UTIs are much more common in the aging population. Symptoms include a constant urge to urinate, pain or burning sensations in the urinary tract, cloudy and/or bloody urine, and a general feeling of illness. Signs that the infection has reached the kidneys include fever, pain in the low back, nausea, and vomiting.

Essential Oils. Aromatherapy can be a useful support measure for treating UTI symptoms and avoiding further infections. However, it is important for clients who have a UTI to see their physician as soon as possible for diagnosis and treatment because serious health problems can result if the infection is left untreated for any length of time. Several essential oils are frequently used in aromatherapy to treat or help prevent infections of the urinary tract. These oils combine effective antibacterial and anti-inflammatory actions with extreme mildness on the skin and mucous membranes—ideal for treating this delicate area of the body. These oils include tea tree (*Melaleuca alternifolia*), sandalwood (*Santalum album*), lavender (*Lavandula angustifolia*), geranium (*Pelargonium graveolens*), myrrh (*Commiphora myrrha*), helichrysum (*Helichrysum angustifolia*), and juniper (*Juniperus communis*).

Methods of Application. For prevention, essential oils can be used in a low-back and lower abdominal massage in a 3–5% dilution and can be given as a take-home blend to be used in the same way. For treatment or prevention, they can be given as a take-home blend for a bath or sitz bath; 10–15 drops should be used in a regular bath and 5–8 drops in a sitz bath.

Diabetes

Type 2 diabetes, long regarded as a problem of old age, is now a major health issue in all age ranges, including children.

Causes and Symptoms. Diabetes is an illness caused by a deficiency of insulin, the hormone that enables the body to metabolize and use sugar. There are two types of diabetes. Type 1, which is genetic and most often shows up in childhood, occurs because the body does not produce enough insulin. Type 2, which is the most common form, occurs when the body either stops producing enough insulin or the cells of the body fail to use the insulin present in the bloodstream. Type 2 diabetes generally occurs in older people and has been termed adult-onset diabetes to distinguish it from type 1, which usually shows up in children or young adults. The causes of type 2 diabetes are mainly genetic predisposition, poor diet, being overweight, and lack of exercise.

Because of the lack of insulin, glucose (sugar) remains in the bloodstream, starving the body's cells of nutrition and leading to many serious health complications, such as heart disease, blindness, nerve damage, and kidney damage. Circulation to the legs may also be impaired, with the resulting risk of tissue death and gangrene.

Essential Oils. The only really effective remedies for adult-onset diabetes are insulin supplementation or a change in lifestyle, including a better diet with less sugar and saturated fats and more exercise. However, aromatherapy can help with some of the complications of diabetes and is a good support strategy for clients. The most effective use of essential oils to prevent complications in a diabetic client is to increase blood circulation to the extremities to maintain tissue health. Rosemary (*Rosmarinus officinalis*), ginger (*Zingiber officinale*), black pepper (*Piper nigrum*), juniper (*Juniperus communis*), and other rubefacient oils work well. They are warming and produce a mild irritation that draws blood to the area, improving local circulation. In Russia, the use of baths with white or yellow turpentine (usually derived from pine) was shown to improve capillary blood flow in patients with insulin-dependent diabetes.[14]

Methods of Application. Massage is extremely important for diabetic clients because it increases peripheral blood circulation and improves tissue health. Essential oils can be used in a full-body massage in a 2–3% dilution. Full baths and foot baths also can encourage better circulation; 10

drops of essential oil can be used in a bath and 4–7 drops in a foot bath. These dilutions and drop numbers should be reduced with clients who are older than 80 or who are in frail health. Both deep massage techniques and extremes of temperature in hydrotherapy are contraindicated if there is any tissue damage or loss of sensation, and massage is completely contraindicated for local damage, ulcers, gangrene, or other similar conditions.

Digestive Disorders

Problems with the digestive system are common in older adults. Being unable to eat sufficient amounts of food or digest food properly can aggravate other health problems.

Causes and Symptoms. The most common cause of digestive problems in older adults is the general slowing down of the body's metabolic processes, resulting in difficulty digesting food. Some people become overweight during this period of life from a slower "burning" of calories, and often also because of reduced levels of physical activity. Other older people frequently experience a loss of appetite because of their slower metabolic rate, and they might not consume adequate amounts of food. They become thin and frail. Constipation is common because the intestines lose their muscle tone and because of less physical exercise.

Essential Oils. Essential oils traditionally used for constipation include fennel (*Foeniculum vulgare*), rosemary (*Rosmarinus officinalis*), black pepper (*Piper nigrum*), ginger (*Zingiber officinale*), and marjoram (*Origanum majorana*). These oils help increase peristalsis. They also help increase circulation and boost metabolism slightly as a result. Other useful essential oils are those that help increase appetite, including peppermint (*Mentha piperita*), ginger (*Zingiber officinale*), cardamon (*Elletaria cardamomum*), and fennel (*Foeniculum vulgare*).

CASE STUDY 25.1

Constipation

Mr. D. is a feisty 93-year-old with chronic constipation, but otherwise he is extremely healthy. He eats fairly well and spends about 45 minutes every day walking to and from the local shops, which seems like a reasonable level of activity for his age. He refused to have massage work because he had never experienced it before and was somewhat reluctant to take off his clothes. However, he agreed to use a massage blend on his abdomen if it was made up for him to use at home. The constipation was not extreme, did not appear to be stress-based, and had been checked by his physician. Overall it seemed to be age-related.

A blend was made using the very mild essential oils of cardamon (*Elletaria cardamomum*) and marjoram (*Origanum majorana*) in a 1% dilution, because of his age. He used it for about 2 weeks but reported that there had been little change. He appeared to tolerate the oils well, so the dilution was increased to 2%. This helped the constipation considerably, and he has continued to use essential oils in this way. The blend has been varied every few weeks.

CASE STUDY 25.2

Fatigue

Ms. R., age 74, came for massage work hoping it would help relieve stress and enable her to sleep better. She reported that since menopause (about 22 years previously), she had been sleeping much more lightly and often could sleep only in 2-hour intervals during the night. She also said that she felt tired during the day. She did volunteer work for a local hospice and did not want to give that up because of her fatigue. Her stress was not related to any one thing in particular, but she said that she had always been somewhat "highly strung."

She received a 1-hour massage with essential oils of lavender (*Lavandula angustifolia*), mandarin (*Citrus reticulata*), and rose (*Rosa damascena*) in a 1% dilution, as she said that she enjoyed flower scents. She agreed to return on a twice-monthly basis for massage because her shoulders were extremely tight. The same essential oils were put into a spritzer for her to use before bedtime and at any time that she awoke during the night. A spritzer was chosen because this would be the easiest application form at any time of the night.

At her appointment 2 weeks later, she said she had slept extremely well the night after the first massage and that she had continued to sleep better than usual, waking up only once or twice during the night. She still reported feeling tired during the day, so another blend of cardamon (*Elletaria cardamomum*) and black spruce (*Picea mariana*) was made in a 4% dilution in lotion, for her to apply to her low back and/or abdomen after her shower in the mornings. At her next appointment, she looked more alert and reported that she had more energy during the day.

Methods of Application. For constipation, essential oils in a 3–5% dilution applied during an abdominal or low-back massage can be very effective. Abdominal massage can be taught to clients and the essential oils given as a take-home blend if the problem is chronic. The same oils can be used in a 1–3% dilution in full-body massage to increase metabolism. Essential oils to help improve appetite are best used as a take-home spritzer, to be used regularly throughout the day.

Fatigue

Many older people have less energy. Part of the natural process of slowing down, fatigue may also be the result of factors that can be addressed using essential oils.

Causes and Symptoms. One of the most common causes of fatigue at any age is insomnia. Many people report having difficulty sleeping as they get older, sleeping more lightly and being wakened more easily, or being unable to sleep more than 5 or 6 hours per night. They feel groggy, tired, and less mentally alert than they would otherwise. Although the causes for this lighter, shorter sleeping time are not well understood, a combination of factors is likely, including reduced levels of physical exercise.

Essential Oils. Evidence shows that using aromatherapy to counteract insomnia can work as well as, or possibly better than, conventional sedative drugs. In one study on elderly patients, diffusing lavender ensured the same amount of sleep as medications such as temazepam and clomethiazole, two commonly prescribed sedatives. Patients were also reported to be less restless when using the lavender.[15] In another study on elderly patients using lavender, nocturnal sleep increased only slightly, but daytime wakefulness and alertness improved significantly.[16]

Other essential oils commonly used to help improve sleep include Roman chamomile (*Chamaemelum nobile*), rose (*Rosa damascena*), mandarin (*Citrus reticulata*), and frankincense (*Boswellia carteri*).

Methods of Application. The most effective way to use the sedative oils is in some kind of inhalation shortly before bedtime. This might include a few drops in a bath or in a diffuser or spritzer, or simply a couple of drops placed on a tissue tucked under the pillow.

SUMMARY

- Life expectancy has increased from 49 years in 1900 to 79 years in 1997. Older people are generally fitter and healthier than before.

- Aging results in a lack of muscle tone and a thinning and hardening of tissue in most organ systems. The immune system also tends to be less effective.

- Risk factors for premature aging include stress, poor diet, smoking, and lack of exercise.

- Older skin is less sensitive to essential oils, but aromatherapy may have a stronger effect overall on elderly clients; thus, milder dilutions should probably be used for clients older than about age 75.

- Injuries can be more serious for the elderly because they take longer to heal and their risk of infection is higher. Essential oils can help resolve bruises, speed healing times for wounds and abrasions, and act as antibacterial agents.

- Essential oils can help prevent urinary tract infections because of a combination of a strong antibacterial effect and a mild action on mucous membranes.

- For diabetes, the most effective use of aromatherapy is to increase circulation to the extremities, helping avoid the risk of tissue damage. The rubefacient oils are the most useful.

- Essential oils are helpful for digestive disorders, including constipation. Oils that stimulate appetite may be useful for many older clients.

- Insomnia and the resulting fatigue can best be treated with the sedative essential oils. Research shows that using essential oils increases sleep time at night and improves alertness and energy levels the following day.

Review Questions

1. Our skin is both more sensitive and more permeable as we age. (T / F)
2. The _____ do(es) not function as efficiently as we age, with the result that essential oils would not be expelled from the body as effectively.
3. Cicatrizant essential oils are important to help wound healing. Cicatrizant means: (a) anti-inflammatory, (b) antiseptic, (c) encourages blood flow to the area, (d) encourages new cell growth.
4. What are the differences in the cause of digestive disturbances in older people and in younger people?

5. Name three oils that help to increase appetite.

6. _____ essential oils are often used to increase circulation in clients who have diabetes.

7. For urinary tract infections, essential oils are chosen for the following effects: (a) antiviral and immune boosting, (b) antibacterial and anti-inflammatory, (c) antifungal and antidepressant, (d) antianxiety and astringent.

8. What treatment methods are most effective for urinary tract infections?

9. Why do sedative essential oils help elderly people who are tired?

10. Name three sedative essential oils that are used for insomnia.

Notes

1. The U.S. Administration on Aging. Available at: www.aoa.gov /prof/statistics/profile/1.asp. Accessed April 3, 2005.

2. Alliance for Aging Research. Available at: www.agingresearch.org. Accessed April 3, 2005.

3. Tolstoy L. War and Peace, transl. by Ann Dunnigan. New York: New American Library, 1980:1392.

4. Deans SG, Noble RC, Penzes L, et al. Promotional effects of plant volatile oils on the polyunsaturated fatty acid status during ageing. Age 1993;16:71–74.

5. Deans SG, Noble RC, Hiltunen R, et al. Antimicrobial and antioxidant properties of _Syzygium aromaticum_ (L) Merr. & Perry: impact upon bacteria, fungi and fatty acid levels in ageing mice. Flavor Fragrance J 1995;10(5):323–328.

6. Weil A. Conference on Integrative Medicine, Hollyhock, BC, Canada, August 2004.

7. Buck P. Skin barrier function: effect of age, race and inflammatory disease. Int J Aromather 2004;14(2):70–76.

8. Maury M. Marguerite Maury's Guide to Aromatherapy: The Secret of Life and Youth. Essex, UK: CW Daniel, 1989:77.

9. Hartman D, Coetzee JC. Two US practitioners' experience of using essential oils for wound care. J Wound Care 2002;11(8):317–320.

10. Glowania HJ, Raulin C, Swoboda M. Effect of chamomile on wound healing—a clinical double-blind study. Z Hautkrankheiten (Berlin) 1987;62(17):1267–1271.

11. Lavagna SM, Secci D. Efficacy of hypericum and calendula oils in the epithelial reconstruction of surgical wounds in childbirth with caesarean section. Il Farmaco 2001;56:451–453.

12. Guba R. Aromatic extracts as wound healing agents (parts 1 and 2). Aromather Today 1997;3:21–25; 1997;4:5–8.

13. Rona D. The use of aromatherapy in the treatment of 'hospital induced' trauma to the arms. Int J Aromather 2003;13(4):207–209.

14. Davydova OB, Turova EA, Golovach AV. The use of white and yellow turpentine baths with diabetic patients. Vopr Kurortol Fizioter Lech Fiz Kult 1998;3:3–10.

15. Hardy M, Kirk-Smith MD, Stretch DD. Replacement of drug treatment for insomnia by ambient odor. Lancet 1995;346:701.

16. Hudson R. The value of lavender for rest and activity in the elderly patient. Complement Ther Med 1996;4:52–57.

26

End-of-Life Care

End-of-life care focuses on helping people to have as full a life as possible within the time that is left to them, while providing palliative care to reduce or eliminate pain and discomfort. The majority of people, even those diagnosed with terminal illnesses, die in their own homes. Hospice services provide specialized healthcare for people with advanced illnesses and a limited life expectancy, in a home setting or in a care facility. Hospice caregivers have experience in end-of-life care, and in addition to medical care, frequently offer other services such as counseling, companionship, dietary advice, assistance in finding other resources, help with errands, and support for bereaved families. Because of the flexibility of the service, and the support of patients remaining in their own homes if possible, hospice care is becoming increasingly common.

Aromatherapists and massage therapists can be employed by hospice services. They can also work as volunteers in either a hospice organization or a hospital, or they may have clients in their private practices who are terminally ill.

Aromatherapy in End-of-Life Care

Aromatherapy has been popular in end-of-life care for some time. Hospice programs in both the United States and Great Britain have been using essential oils in various ways to increase patient comfort and to help deal with some of the symptoms common to hospice patients. A survey in Southampton, England, of patients with cancer and their healthcare staff found that massage and aromatherapy were among the five most popular complementary health treatments.[1] This popularity exists because volunteer programs including massage and aromatherapy are common in hospice settings and because hospices seem to be more open to complementary therapies than hospitals, having the attitude that if the patient enjoys a treatment, it can only be doing some good. Hospices in the United States often offer what is called a "comfort therapy program," which provides massage, aromatherapy, music therapy, and other complementary modalities for patients.

There are many benefits to using aromatherapy in palliative and end-of-life care. It is a mild and generally pleasant therapy that can help relieve some of the physical and emotional hardships of end-of-life care. Some of these issues have already been discussed in other sections of the book, such as insomnia and pain (see Chapters 15 and 25). Other common issues are discussed below.

Pressure Sores

Pressure sores, also known as decubitus ulcers, afflict people who are paralyzed or are bedridden for long periods of time.

Causes and Symptoms. As the name suggests, they are caused by pressure or friction on tissue, often tissue covering a bony protuberance such as the ischial tuberosity or the elbow.

Pressure leads to a lack of blood flow and oxygen to the area, and eventually tissue death. The first symptoms are localized redness, heat, and hardened swelling. Later, blisters, abrasions, or ulcers can be seen. Pressure sores are a serious health hazard because they greatly increase the risk of infection, which may be difficult for a fragile immune system to fight.

Essential Oils. Essential oils can be very effective in helping relieve pressure sores. Guba had good results in Australia when he used blends to help heal various types of skin abrasions in elderly people. One example: "An 84-year-old woman had a chronic, 4 cm stage 2 pressure area on her left buttock that had remained unchanged after 6 months of conservative treatment. Wound Heal Formula was applied randomly by various nursing staff (approximately once every 2 days). The lesion healed within 3 weeks, with the patient reporting considerable pain reduction during the healing process."[2] Wound Heal Formula, a blend devised by Guba, consists of lavender (*Lavandula angustifolia*), mugwort (*Artemesia vulgaris*), sage (*Salvia officinalis*), helichrysum (*Helichrysum italicum* spp. *serotinum*), and German chamomile (*Matricaria recutita*) essential oils, with marigold (*Calendula officinalis*) CO_2 extract and calophyllum (*Calophyllum inophyllum*), borage (*Borago officinalis*), flaxseed (*Linum usitatissimum*), and Shea butter (*Butyrospermum parkii*) vegetable oils. Grapefruit (*Citrus paradisii*) seed and pulp extract and rosemary (*Rosmarinus officinalis* CT cineole) CO_2 extract are added to help preserve the blend.

The ideal essential oils for pressure sores combine a mild action on the skin with anti-inflammatory, antibacterial, and skin-healing effects. Good examples of these oils are lavender (*Lavandula angustifolia*), helichrysum (*Helichrysum italicum*), frankincense (*Boswellia carteri*), myrrh (*Commiphora myrrha*), and German chamomile (*Matricaria recutita*). Guba also suggested using essential oils high in ketones, such as mugwort (*Artemesia vulgaris*) and sage (*Salvia officinalis*), quoting the French aromatic doctors Penoël and Franchomme, who state that they have cicatrizing properties.[3]

Methods of Application. Any blend made for pressure sores should be applied, diluted, directly on the sore itself. Dilutions should be strong, as the area to be treated is small and the problem is acute. In general, dilutions of 20–40%, depending on the age and general health of the client, are appropriate. As with other strong dilutions, this application is designed for short-term treatment of an acute problem, and the period of use will probably not exceed 8 to 10 weeks, except for extremely severe and persistent sores.

Carriers for the oils should also be chosen on the basis of skin-healing properties. Aloe vera gel is an excellent carrier because of its proven anti-inflammatory and tissue-regenerating qualities.[4] Essential oils do not dissolve in the gel and might separate over time, so the mixture needs to be shaken before each use to ensure an even distribution of essential oils throughout. Some carrier oils, such as calophyllum (*Calophyllum inophyllum*) and rose hip seed (*Rosa rubiginosa*), have good reputations for skin healing, as do certain infused oils, such as calendula (*Calendula officinalis*).

Nausea and Loss of Appetite

Causes. A slight decline in appetite is common in older people because the body's metabolism slows down. However, a more extreme loss of appetite is frequently experienced by people who have advanced illnesses. This may be due to the nature of the illness itself or can be a side-effect of the treatments they are receiving.

Essential Oils. If nausea is present, peppermint (*Mentha piperita*) essential oil is the most frequently used remedy in aromatherapy, being highly effective on a short-term basis. For clients who do not have nausea but who have little appetite, essential oils such as cardamon (*Elettaria cardamomum*), lemon (*Citrus limon*), peppermint (*Mentha piperita*), bergamot (*Citrus bergamia*), fennel (*Foeniculum vulgare*), and tarragon (*Artemesia dracunculus*) can be used.

Methods of Application. A few drops of peppermint can be used in a room diffuser or on a tissue to be inhaled by the client or placed nearby, or the oil can simply be sniffed from the bottle. There seem to be no contraindications to frequent use of peppermint used in this way. Any of the essential oils listed previously can be used either as an inhalation or in a gentle abdominal massage. Dilutions are mild for massage, usually 1–3%.

Unpleasant Odors

It has been recognized for thousands of years that illnesses have their own very specific odors. Before laboratory tests were available, medical doctors would routinely diagnose diabetes, for example, by the sweet smell of the patient's skin and urine. Researchers have discovered that dogs can tell the difference in smell between a healthy cell culture and one containing cancer cells, and they can potentially be trained to give early warning of cancer growth in people.

Causes. Anyone who has worked with clients with advanced chronic illnesses knows that unpleasant odors are common in the sickroom. This might be because of the specific odor of the illness itself, because of a client's incontinence, or simply because the room may be small and rarely aired out.

Essential Oils. Essential oils are ideal for addressing this issue, which can be extremely distressing to both caregivers and the person who is ill. I frequently use citrus oils for this purpose because they are extremely volatile and easy to diffuse, even in larger spaces. Most people like citruses; they are not overly sweet and cloying and they are not likely to provoke nausea. Lemon (*Citrus limon*), lime (*Citrus aurantifolia*), and grapefruit (*Citrus x paradisii*) are excellent for clearing the air. Peppermint (*Mentha piperita*) and lemongrass (*Cymbopogon citratus*) are also useful, and the slightly crisper note of lavandin (*Lavandula x intermedia*) might be preferable to lavender for this issue.

Methods of Application. The most effective methods of application are to use a small diffuser with a candle inside, or a nebulizer of some kind. Spritzers can also be used on a regular basis. They are not as effective or thorough, but they have the advantage that they can be used by the client or the caregiver when desired.

Skin Problems

Skin problems can be an irritating addition to the discomfort experienced during chronic illness.

Causes and Symptoms. In end-of-life care, the various medications commonly used, illness itself, or old age can all cause various skin problems, the most common being dryness and itching. There might be red, dry areas on the skin, or the skin might peel or crack.

Essential Oils. Hydrosols are useful remedies for itching, particularly rose (*Rosa damascena*), lavender (*Lavandula angustifolia*), or geranium (*Pelargonium graveolens*) hydrosols,

---

CASE STUDY 26.1

Nausea

Mrs. M., age 45, had pancreatic cancer. She was experiencing nausea and vomiting and was having trouble relaxing as a result. I knew that massage would help her relax, and used cardamon (*Elettaria cardamomum*) and ginger (*Zingiber officinale*) in a massage blend for use on her feet, forearms, and abdomen. I also made a spritzer with peppermint (*Mentha piperita*) and grapefruit (*Citrus x paradisii*), which I sprayed into the air every few minutes, asking her to take a deep breath. Although her abdomen was very swollen, she enjoyed the abdominal massage most. The whole session lasted for about an hour, and she reported that she felt restful and wanted to nap. Both blends were given to her husband with instructions on how to use them.

One week later I revisited Mrs. M. She reported that she had eaten a light meal the same night as the first session, without feeling nauseous. Even though the oils used were mainly stimulating, the overall effect was relaxing, due to the easing of the nausea.

Case study provided by Aaron Glaser, an aromatherapist working for a hospice in Tacoma, Washington.

which are all relatively easy to source. Aloe vera is another useful remedy for itching, and any of the antipruritic essential oils, such as lavender (*Lavandula angustifolia*), peppermint (*Mentha piperita*), or German chamomile (*Matricaria recutita*), can be added.

Other essential oils, such as rose (*Rosa damascena*), geranium (*Pelargonium graveolens*), frankincense (*Boswellia carteri*), or mandarin (*Citrus reticulata*), can be used with infused oil of calendula (*Calendula officinalis*) to treat dry, damaged skin. Myrrh (*Commiphora myrrha*) and frankincense (*Boswellia carteri*) are helpful for cracked skin.

Methods of Application. Hydrosols provide relief when they are sprayed directly onto itchy skin or used with water to cleanse. Dilutions of essential oils in aloe vera or in a carrier oil or lotion should be mild for any skin problem—1–2% is commonly used. Peppermint should be used in no more than a 0.5% dilution because it can increase itching if more is used.

Emotional Issues

Death and dying bring up many difficult emotions, for those at the end of life as well as the people who love them. In Western culture, we often try to deny the inevitability of death, and we have few rituals to help us deal with the emotions involved. According to Michael Lerner, who works with cancer patients and has written extensively about death: "Dying is okay. That's one of the real toxicities of our culture: that it makes dying not okay. It's such a fundamental and natural act."[5] Going through a range of emotions, from anger, fear, and depression, to the eventual acceptance of death is the natural and healthy process of grieving.

Essential Oils. Because of their profound effect on the limbic system, the part of the brain involved in the recognition and processing of strong emotions and of memory, fragrances have been used for thousands of years to help people through this time of grieving and letting go. Cypress (*Cupressus sempervirens*), for example, was dedicated by both the ancient Egyptians and the Greeks to their lords of the underworld and has long been planted in cemeteries in Europe. Spikenard (*Nardus jatamansi*), frankincense (*Boswellia carteri*), sandalwood (*Santalum album*), and myrrh (*Commiphora myrrha*) have all been used in various cultures to calm the mind, enhance spiritual growth, and help manage anger, fear, and grief. Rose (*Rosa damascena*) is a traditional remedy for broken-heartedness, and neroli (*Citrus aurantium* var. *amara*) for fear and shock. The most important guideline is to use essential oils that the client likes and feels good about. Essential oils can be chosen simply because the client enjoys them or because they remind the client of happy parts of her life, such as a rose garden she loved working in.

One small study (52 patients) using essential oils in massage sessions with cancer patients found that the treatments had a "significant reducing effect on anxiety." The blend used consisted of lavender (*Lavandula angustifolia*), rosewood (*Aniba roseadora*), lemon (*Citrus limon*), rose (*Rosa damascena*), and valerian (*Valeriana officinalis*), in a 2% dilution.[6] Another study reported that using lavender (*Lavandula angustifolia*) in massage was helpful in promoting relaxation in patients with malignant brain tumors.[7]

Methods of Application. Any application that is soothing and not overwhelming can be appropriate, although the easiest are probably essential oils used in a diffuser, on a tissue, or in a mild dilution that the client's caregivers or family can use in a gentle massage on the hands or feet. Letting the client's family and friends use essential oils in some form of touching can be immensely healing to both the giver and the receiver.

CASE STUDY 26.2

Depression

Mr. G., in his seventies, had end-stage congestive heart failure. He was in a nursing home and did not have many visitors except occasionally his daughter, with whom he did not always get along. He was not getting much sleep and was not eating well. He was also in a wheelchair and told me he was not only tired but also somewhat depressed. The first time I saw him, he was lying in bed with his head covered with a cap. Not knowing how to proceed best, I made a spritzer from whole orange oil (*Citrus sinensis*) and sprayed it over his head. The sweet smell of oranges fell on his nose and he very slowly cracked a smile, removed the cap, and said hello.

I visited him once a week for several weeks, using mainly mandarin (*Citrus reticulata*) in a massage oil, and the whole orange in a spritzer. He loved the smell of the orange and said it was like a rainbow bridging his heart to his soul. After several visits, he would be sitting up in bed waiting for me. One day he was not in his room, and my heart sank. However, when I went outside I found him sitting beside his daughter. She thanked me for what I had been doing with her father, and said that since I had been seeing him they had stopped fighting and started talking about walks they used to take when she was a little girl.

Case study provided by Aaron Glaser, an aromatherapist working for a hospice in Tacoma, Washington.

SUMMARY

- Hospice services frequently provide aromatherapy and massage for patients.

- Essential oils used to treat pressure sores (decubitus ulcers) should have anti-inflammatory, antibacterial, and skin-healing properties.

- Dilutions for pressure sores are strong (20–40%) because the area treated is small and treatment normally lasts for less than 3 months.

- Good carriers for pressure sores include aloe vera, rose hip seed oil, calophyllum oil, and calendula-infused oil.

- Essential oils, such as peppermint, can be useful for the treatment of nausea and loss of appetite.

- Essential oils diffused to help with unpleasant odors should be highly volatile and not overly sweet or heavy.

- Hydrosols, or essential oils mixed with aloe vera, can be used for itchy skin.

- Calendula-infused oil, with essential oils, can be used to treat dry and damaged skin.

- Fragrances have been used for thousands of years to help people deal with the emotional issues associated with death and dying. Essential oils should be chosen for their appeal to the client, as well as their therapeutic effects.

Review Questions

1. The ideal essential oil for pressure sores are anti-_____ and anti-_____.
2. Name three oils that are useful to help heal pressure sores.
3. The best form of application for pressure sores is: (a) sitz bath, (b) direct diluted application, (c) direct undiluted application, (d) air diffusion.
4. Ideal essential oils to help with unpleasant odors will: (a) have low volatility and smell very sweet, (b) smell strong and earthy, (c) have high volatility and smell fresh.
5. Dilutions for itching should be mild; otherwise the problem could get worse. (T / F)
6. The most useful preparations for itching from medications are: (a) skin-healing carrier oils, (b) antibacterial and antifungal essential oils, (c) heavy ointments and warming essential oils, (d) hydrosols and antipruritic essential oils.
7. What methods of application are appropriate for help with emotional issues in end-of-life care?

Notes

1. Lewith GT, Broomfield J, Prescott P. Complementary cancer care in Southampton: a survey of staff and patients. Complement Ther Med 2002;10(2):100–106.
2. Guba R. Aromatic extracts as wound healing agents: part 2. Aromather Today 1997;4:5–8.
3. Guba R. Aromatic extracts as wound healing agents: part 2. Aromather Today 1997;4:5–8.
4. Avijgan M. Phytotherapy: an alternative treatment for non-healing ulcers. J Wound Care 2004;13(4):157–158.
5. Moyers B. Healing and the Mind. New York: Doubleday, 1993:339.
6. Corner J, Cawley N, Hildebrand S. An evaluation of the use of essential oils on the well-being of cancer patients. Int J Palliat Nurs 1995;1(2):67–73.
7. Hadfield N. The role of aromatherapy massage in reducing anxiety in patients with malignant brain tumors. Int J Palliat Nurs 2001; 7(6):279–285.

Answers to Review Questions

CHAPTER 1

1. F
2. (b)
3. large, small
4. F. It is more suited to acute problems.
5. T
6. They directly affect the brain; they are absorbed through the skin.
7. fats, water
8. (c)

CHAPTER 2

1. bacterial, viral, fungal
2. insects, animals, plants
3. (b)
4. wood, roots
5. labor costs
6. steam distillation
7. solvents
8. cold expression
9. T
10. solvent
11. (c)
12. F. They generally are among the least expensive oils.
13. steam distillation
14. water
15. T

CHAPTER 3

1. the perfume, food flavoring, and pharmaceutical industries
2. addition of a substance to an essential oil after distillation, generally done to make the final product greater in volume, thus increasing profits

3. Common names are unreliable, varying among different countries and even from region to region. Also, a common name may be used for several different species within one genus.
4. neroli, petitgrain, and bitter orange
5. cold expression, solvent extraction, and CO_2 extraction
6. T
7. chemical
8. extra
9. plastic
10. F. This is an oil that has been distilled again, after the initial extraction technique.
11. F. It is usually a blend of carrier oils, essential oils, and/or synthetics.
12. gas-liquid, mass
13. F. It depends on the character and volatility of the essential oil. Some oils can be kept for several years.
14. (c)

CHAPTER 4

1. because aromatic molecules are extremely small
2. olfactory bulb
3. limbic
4. T
5. endocrine
6. F. They also have a personal effect on memory and emotions.
7. F. It is used mostly to encourage relaxation.
8. F. Certain components may be found in the bloodstream 10–20 minutes after application.
9. hair follicles, sebaceous glands
10. F. Absorption is higher.
11. (c)

12. T
13. F. Broken or thin skin will make absorption faster.

CHAPTER 5

1. hydrogen, oxygen
2. T
3. T
4. F. Some essential oil components, such as alcohols, are more soluble in water.
5. (c)
6. oxygen
7. (d)
8. F. Phenols can be skin irritating.
9. (b)
10. (a)
11. burn in UV light
12. oxide

CHAPTER 7

1. T
2. F. Essential oils do not dissolve in water, and some essential oils should not be used undiluted on the face.
3. 3, 10
4. to increase absorption
5. pre-event because it is often performed through clothes
6. Undiluted essential oils can be applied directly to reflex areas on the feet or hands, or onto the appropriate acupressure points. Or a combination of essential oils can be diluted in lotion or oil and the whole foot or body massaged with this blend, after the reflexology or acupressure treatment.
7. F. The most convenient way of using compresses with aromatherapy is to apply the essential oils, either diluted or neat, to the area to be treated and cover it with the compress.
8. T
9. 3, 6
10. asthma
11. F. The skin on the face is generally more sensitive, and milder dilutions should be used.
12. F. Aroma lamps have been shown to be very effective in helping certain problems.
13. The smell can become so intense that it is difficult to remove quickly and effectively before the next client arrives.

14. shaken
15. respiratory

CHAPTER 8

1. milliliters
2. the number of drops in the bottle
3. 20–35
4. 1
5. 36
6. 100

CHAPTER 9

1. F. Light and easily absorbed carriers are more suitable for full-body massage.
2. b, d, a, c
3. oil, water
4. lipids, seeds
5. saturated, unsaturated
6. T
7. T
8. T
9. a mixture of oil and water made in such a way that they do not separate
10. calophyllum, rose hip seed oil
11. The massage therapist should regularly change the type and brand of carrier used with clients.
12. F. Commercial lotions often contain mineral oil, which blocks the absorption of essential oils.
13. oil, wax
14. to nourish the skin or to release essential oils slowly for chronic problems
15. The quality of the ingredients can be controlled by the therapist.

CHAPTER 10

1. F. Internal use is outside the scope of practice of massage therapists.
2. (a)
3. skin irritation, sensitization
4. F. Some people may experience skin irritation even with the mildest essential oils.
5. (c)
6. F. If a client has an allergic reaction to an essential oil, he or she should avoid using that oil in the future.

7. liquid soap, honey, full-fat milk, a commercial emulsifier

8. (b)

9. T

10. smells

11. (b)

12. Bergamot oil is photosensitizing, making it more likely that skin will burn in ultraviolet light.

13. F. Properties and safety indications vary between chemotypes.

14. (d)

CHAPTER 11

1. T

2. (b)

3. F. Some components of an essential oil are more volatile than others and will evaporate more quickly, changing the smell of the tester strip.

4. (d)

5. Combine base notes, essential oils that are very stable and have a long volatility, with top notes, oils that are very volatile for immediate interest, to showcase the mid notes, the medium-volatility essential oils that make up the main character of the blend.

6. a blend of two or more essential oils that together may be much more effective therapeutically than one single oil

7. F

8. T

9. (a)

10. (d)

CHAPTER 12

1. Check with your employer that they agree to your use of aromatherapy. Make sure your room is well ventilated and that smells will not drift into common use areas. Do not use diffusers or inhalers. If sharing a room, schedule clients in such a way to leave time at the end of your shift to air out the room for the next therapist.

2. for essential oils, carriers, and blending bottles or bowls

3. 1, 2

4. It is difficult to completely get rid of the smell of the original blend.

5. Small amounts of blends can be made for specific areas of the body.

6. glass, glazed ceramic, or stone

7. Standard essential oils tend to have a broader range of action, have more documented safety testing, and usually are much less expensive.

8. (a)

CHAPTER 13

1. skin sensitivity, allergies, medications, stress levels and emotional issues, scent preferences

2. wintergreen, sweet birch

3. F. There is no pollen in essential oil. However, it is probably better to avoid the essential oil from a plant to which a client has an allergy.

4. for safety reasons, to record particular blends that a client may request again, and as a reminder of how long a client has used a blend

5. the essential oils used, the dilution percentage, the method of application, and any results observed

6. The clients may have different lifestyles, constitutions, underlying issues, and scent preferences.

7. consultation, blending

8. cost of the essential oils, the extra time spent in the session

CHAPTER 14

1. making an anti-inflammatory blend for a client with an injury to help with tissue healing, making a chest rub with expectorant oils for a client with congestion, using the "learned odor response" by sending home with the client the blend used in a relaxation massage

2. insomnia, athlete's foot, fear of flying

3. (b)

4. F. Large areas, such as the back, may be difficult for clients to treat by themselves.

5. aroma lamp, tissue

6. (c)

7. Diluted blends are safer to give to clients.

8. (a)

9. how to use the blend, recommendations for dosage, recommendations for frequency of use

CHAPTER 15

1. nervous

2. F. A certain amount of stress is necessary for physical and emotional health.

3. the hypothalamus, pituitary, and adrenals

4. heat rate, blood pressure, respiratory rate, digestion

5. lavender (*Lavandula angustifolia*), mandarin (*Citrus reticulata*), Roman chamomile (*Chamaemelum nobile*), and ylang ylang (*Cananga odorata*)

6. rosemary (*Rosmarinus officinalis*), black spruce (*Picea mariana*), and ginger (*Zingiber officinale*)

7. endorphins

8. inhalation, bedtime

9. (b)

10. analgesic, parasympathetic

11. so that they can use essential oils whenever they experience a craving

CHAPTER 16

1. The cooling anti-inflammatory essential oils are ideal for acute inflammation in any form. The warming essential oils warm the tissue and increase blood flow to the area, but because they suppress hormones usually released by the body when trauma occurs, they are also classed as anti-inflammatory and work well for chronic inflammation.

2. *Cooling anti-inflammatories:* blue cypress (*Callitris intratropica*), German chamomile (*Matricaria recutita*), helichrysum (*Helichrysum italicum*), lavender (*Lavandula angustifolia*), palmarosa (*Cymbopogon martinii*), sweet birch (*Betula lenta*), turmeric (*Curcuma longa*), wintergreen (*Gaultheria procumbens*), yarrow (*Achillea millefolium*)

   Warming anti-inflammatories: black pepper (*Piper nigrum*), cardamon (*Elletaria cardamomum*), clove (*Syzygium aromaticum*), cumin (*Cuminum cyminum*), ginger (*Zingiber officinale*), nutmeg (*Myristica fragrans*).

3. (b)

4. (d)

5. Astringent essential oils can help to move lymph.

6. swelling, heat, cast

7. analgesic, antispasmodic

8. Peppermint

9. T

10. Cooling anti-inflammatory oils would be used for acute flare-ups and warming anti-inflammatory oils would be used for chronic stiffness and pain between flare-ups.

11. Inflammation is minimal with osteoarthritis.

12. warming analgesic

13. carrier oils

CHAPTER 17

1. (a) ylang ylang, (b) ginger, (c) cypress, (d) helichrysum

2. stress, control

3. full-body massage and warm bath

4. (c)

5. calming, sedative oils

6. relaxing, analgesic

7. mild, because the blend should be applied frequently

8. (a)

9. helichrysum (*Helichrysum italicum*), fennel (*Foeniculum vulgare*), hyssop (*Hyssopus officinalis*), rosemary (*Rosmarinus officinalis*), and sage (*Salvia officinalis*)

10. spleen

CHAPTER 18

1. (a) diuretic, (b) astringent, (c) hepatic

2. infection, immune, toxicity

3. grapefruit (*Citrus x paradisii*), geranium (*Pelargonium graveolens*), juniper (*Juniperus communis*), fennel (*Foeniculum vulgare*), and cypress (*Cupressus sempervirens*)

4. Peppermint, (c)

5. fat, water, toxins, connective tissue

6. (d)

7. They can cause skin irritation.

CHAPTER 19

1. (b)

2. (a) neurodepressant, (b) neurostimulant, (c) analgesic, (d) nervine

3. Local massage is contraindicated because of neuralgia and the possibility of infection. Cool baths with essential oils or self-applications of a cooling substance with essential oils are more appropriate.

4. aloe vera, hydrosols, witch hazel

5. blood, lymph

6. (c)

7. inhalation

8. lavender (*Lavandula angustifolia*) and Roman chamomile (*Chamaemelum nobile*)

9. (a)

10. stress

CHAPTER 20

1. bacterial, viral, fungal

2. They are lipophilic.

3. This is a laboratory technique designed to test various essential oils against a bacterial culture taken from a patient, to see which oil has greatest activity against that bacterial strain. Using this test, physicians can determine which essential oils are most effective for the patient.

4. (c)

5. (a)

6. inflammatory

7. Partly because treatment is often long-term, but also because the system has the potential to overreact to any substance.

8. black spruce (*Picea mariana*), pine (*Pinus sylvestris*), ginger (*Zingiber officinale*), rosemary (*Rosmarinus officinalis*), and cardamon (*Elletaria cardamomum*)

9. (a)

10. (d)

CHAPTER 21

1. (d)

2. T. Their skin is thinner and may absorb substances more quickly.

3. (a) moisturizing, (b) cicatrizant, (c) rubefacient, (d) antipruritic

4. Because it is a warming anti-inflammatory. The heat may increase skin inflammation.

5. the infused oils of calendula and St. John's wort and rose hip seed oil (*Rosa rubiginosa*) and callophyllum (*Calophyllum inophyllum*)

6. heat, healing of skin cells

7. (b)

8. yeast

9. (c)

10. soften

CHAPTER 22

1. hypothalamus

2. (d)

3. No, because they only encourage menstruation when the menstrual cycle actually occurs.

4. spasmodic, analgesic

5. T. This is because the olfactory system affects the limbic brain, including the hypothalamus.

6. geranium (*Pelargonium graveolens*), aniseed (*Pimpinella anisum*), fennel (*Foeniculum vulgare*), sage (*Salvia officinalis*), and melissa (*Melissa officinalis*)

7. (b)

8. peppermint

9. very gentle abdominal massage with essential oils such as black pepper (*Piper nigrum*), ginger (*Zingiber officinale*), rosemary (*Rosmarinus officinalis*), sweet orange (*Citrus sinensis*), or fennel (*Foeniculum vulgare*) in a 2–3% dilution

10. (c)

11. T, because it may suppress breast-milk production.

12. general balancing

13. blue cypress (*Callitris intratropica*), German chamomile (*Chamaemelum nobile*), clary sage (*Salvia sclarea*), geranium (*Pelargonium graveolens*), lavender (*Lavandula angustifolia*), palmarosa (*Cymbopogon martinii*), rose (*Rosa damascena*), and the citrus oils

14. (d)

CHAPTER 23

1. inhalation

2. (a) mucolytic, (b) antitussive, (c) decongestant, (d) expectorant

3. Peppermint, (c)

4. 10%

5. facial massage and steam inhalation

6. histamine

7. (a) inula, (b) ginger, (c) peppermint, (d) spike lavender

8. steam inhalation

9. mucolytics, expectorants

10. Chronic bronchitis. Eucalyptus (*Eucalyptus radiata*), black spruce (*Picea mariana*), and rosemary (*Rosmarinus officinalis*) will all be beneficial.

CHAPTER 24

1. internally

2. cardamon (*Elletaria cardamomum*), lemon (*Citrus limon*), peppermint (*Mentha piperita*), bergamot

(*Citrus bergamia*), fennel (*Foeniculum vulgare*), tarragon (*Artemesia dracunculus*)

3. Stress, calming
4. (b)
5. T
6. antispasmodic
7. German chamomile (*Matricaria recutita*), yarrow (*Achillea millefolium*), helichrysum (*Helichrysum italicum*), lavender (*Lavandula angustifolia*), and turmeric (*Curcuma longa*)
8. (a) sweet orange, (b) cardamon, (c) fennel, (d) rose
9. (b)

CHAPTER 25

1. F. The skin may be slightly less permeable in old age.
2. kidneys
3. (d)
4. The most common cause of digestive problems in older adults is the general slowing down of the body's metabolic processes resulting in difficulty digesting food. The most common cause of digestive problems in younger people is stress.
5. peppermint (*Mentha piperita*), ginger (*Zingiber officinale*), cardamon (*Elletaria cardamomum*), and fennel (*Foeniculum vulgare*)

6. Rubefacient
7. (b)
8. low-back and lower abdominal massage and baths or sitz baths
9. Elderly people often do not get enough sleep. Sedative oils can help to increase the length and quality of sleep.
10. lavender (*Lavandula angustifolia*), Roman chamomile (*Chamaemelum nobile*), rose (*Rosa damascena*), mandarin (*Citrus reticulata*), and frankincense (*Boswellia carteri*)

CHAPTER 26

1. inflammatory, bacterial
2. lavender (*Lavandula angustifolia*), helichrysum (*Helichrysum italicum*), frankincense (*Boswellia carteri*), myrrh (*Commiphora myrrha*), and German chamomile (*Matricaria recutita*)
3. (b)
4. (c)
5. T
6. (d)
7. essential oils used in a diffuser or on a tissue, or a mild massage lotion for the family or friends to use on the client

Appendix A: Therapeutic Guide to Ailments and Essential Oils

This guide is provided as a memory aid and quick reference check for therapists who have already read and worked with the information in the rest of the book.

addiction: citruses (*Citrus* spp.), fennel (*Foeniculum vulgare*), frankincense (*Boswellia carteri*), peppermint (*Mentha piperita*), rosemary verbenone (*Rosmarinus officinalis* CT *verbenone*)

allergy: German chamomile (*Matricaria recutita*), Roman chamomile (*Chamaemelum nobile*), Himalayan cedar (*Cedrus deodara*), lavender (*Lavandula angustifolia*), tea tree (*Melaleuca alternifolia*), turmeric (*Curcuma longa*)

Alzheimer's disease (for agitation and anxiety): Roman chamomile (*Chamaemelum nobile*), lavender (*Lavandula angustifolia*), sweet orange (*Citrus sinensis*), rose (*Rosa damascena* or *centifolia*), sandalwood (*Santalum album*), ylang ylang (*Cananga odorata*)

anger: bergamot (*Citrus x bergamia*), Roman chamomile (*Chamaemelum nobile*), frankincense (*Boswellia carteri*), lavender (*Lavandula angustifolia*), mandarin (*Citrus reticulata*)

angina: Roman chamomile (*Chamaemelum nobile*), lavender (*Lavandula angustifolia*), myrrh (*Commiphora myrrha*), sandalwood (*Santalum album*)

anxiety: basil (*Ocimum basilicum*), bergamot (*Citrus x bergamia*), cypress (*Cupressus sempervirens*), marjoram (*Origanum majorana*), neroli (*Citrus aurantium* var. *amara*), petitgrain (*Citrus aurantium* var. *amara*), ylang ylang (*Cananga odorata*)

appetite (loss of): bergamot (*Citrus x bergamia*), cardamon (*Elletaria cardamomum*), fennel (*Foeniculum vulgare*), lemon (*Citrus limon*), peppermint (*Mentha piperita*), tarragon (*Artemesia dracunculus*)

arrhythmia: lavender (*Lavandula angustifolia*), marjoram (*Origanum majorana*), neroli (*Citrus aurantium* var. *amara*), rose (*Rosa damascena* or *centifolia*), ylang ylang (*Cananga odorata*)

arthritis: See osteoarthritis; rheumatoid arthritis

asthma: German chamomile (*Matricaria recutita*), Roman chamomile (*Chamaemelum nobile*), clary sage (*Salvia sclarea*), eucalyptus (*Eucalyptus radiata*), fennel (*Foeniculum vulgare*), Himalayan cedar (*Cedrus deodara*), peppermint (*Mentha piperita*), rosemary (*Rosmarinus officinalis*), turmeric (*Curcuma longa*)

autoimmune disease (to suppress inflammatory response): cardamon (*Elletaria cardamomum*), Himalayan cedar (*Cedrus deodara*), cinnamon leaf (*Cinnamomum verum*), clove (*Syzygium aromaticum*), ginger (*Zingiber officinale*), nutmeg (*Myristica fragrans*), palmarosa (*Cymbopogon martinii*), turmeric (*Curcuma longa*)

back pain (chronic): bay laurel (*Laurus nobilis*), black pepper (*Piper nigrum*), ginger (*Zingiber officinale*)

bronchitis (chronic): clary sage (*Salvia sclarea*), frankincense (*Boswellia carteri*), marjoram (*Origanum majorana*), peppermint (*Mentha piperita*)

bronchitis (for heavy mucus): black spruce (*Picea mariana*), eucalyptus (*Eucalyptus radiata*), rosemary (*Rosmarinus officinalis*)

bruising: fennel (*Foeniculum vulgare*), helichrysum (*Helichrysum italicum*), hyssop (*Hyssopus officinalis*), rosemary (*Rosmarinus officinalis*), sage (*Salvia officinalis*)

burns: German chamomile (*Matricaria recutita*), lavender (*Lavandula angustifolia*)

bursitis: German chamomile (*Matricaria recutita*), helichrysum (*Helichrysum italicum*), lavender (*Lavandula angustifolia*), lemon eucalyptus (*Eucalyptus citriadora*), peppermint (*Mentha piperita*), sweet birch (*Betula lenta*), wintergreen (*Gaultheria procumbens*)

candidiasis: geranium (*Pelargonium graveolens*), palmarosa (*Cymbopogon martinii*), patchouli (*Pogostemon cablin*), small amounts of lemongrass (*Cymbopogon citratus*), melissa (*Melissa officinalis*)

carpal tunnel syndrome: nutmeg (*Myristica fragrans*), lavender (*Lavandula angustifolia*), eucalyptus (*Eucalyptus globulus*), marjoram (*Origanum majorana*), black pepper (*Piper nigrum*), ginger (*Zingiber officinale*)

chronic fatigue syndrome: black spruce (*Picea mariana*), cardamon (*Elletaria cardamomum*), frankincense (*Boswellia carteri*), ginger (*Zingiber officinale*), pine (*Pinus sylvestris*), rosemary (*Rosmarinus officinalis*)

chronic obstructive pulmonary disease: clary sage (*Salvia sclarea*), frankincense (*Boswellia carteri*), marjoram (*Origanum majorana*), peppermint (*Mentha piperita*)

circulation (poor): black pepper (*Piper nigrum*), eucalyptus (*Eucalyptus radiata*), ginger (*Zingiber officinale*), juniper (*Juniperus communis*), pine (*Pinus sylvestris*), rosemary (*Rosmarinus officinalis*)

colitis: See inflammatory bowel disease

concentration (difficulty with): basil (*Ocimum basilicum*), frankincense (*Boswellia carteri*), lemon (*Citrus limon*), peppermint (*Mentha piperita*), rosemary (*Rosmarinus officinalis*)

constipation: black pepper (*Piper nigrum*), fennel (*Foeniculum vulgare*), ginger (*Zingiber officinale*), marjoram (*Origanum majorana*), rosemary (*Rosmarinus officinalis*), sweet orange (*Citrus sinensis*)

cramps (menstrual): See dysmenorrhea

cramps (skeletal muscle): basil (*Ocimum basilicum*), cardamon (*Elletaria cardamomum*), clary sage (*Salvia sclarea*), Roman chamomile (*Chamaemelum nobile*), marjoram (*Origanum majorana*), tarragon (*Artemesia dracunculus*)

Crohn's disease: See inflammatory bowel disease

cystic fibrosis (for mucus): helichrysum (*Helichrysum italicum*), inula (*Inula graveolens*)

cystic fibrosis (against *Pseudomonas* bacterium): basil (*Ocimum basilicum*), clove (*Syzygium aromaticum*), cumin (*Cuminum cyminum*), lemon myrtle (*Backhousia citriadora*), oregano (*Origanum vulgare*)

cystitis: See urinary tract infection

decubitus ulcers: See pressure sores

depression: basil (*Ocimum basilicum*), citruses (*Citrus* spp.), frankincense (*Boswellia carteri*), geranium (*Pelargonium graveolens*), jasmine (*Jasminum grandiflorum*), marjoram (*Origanum majorana*), rose (*Rosa damascena* or *centifolia*)

dermatitis: calendula infused oil (*Calendula officinalis*), geranium (*Pelargonium graveolens*), mandarin (*Citrus reticulata*), palmarosa (*Cymbopogon martinii*), rose (*Rosa damascena* or *centifolia*)

dry skin: frankincense (*Boswellia carteri*), geranium (*Pelargonium graveolens*), jasmine (*Jasminum grandiflorum*), mandarin (*Citrus reticulata*), rose (*Rosa damascena* or *centifolia*)

dysmenorrhea: black pepper (*Piper nigrum*), Roman chamomile (*Chamaemelum nobile*), clary sage (*Salvia sclarea*), ginger (*Zingiber officinale*), lavender (*Lavandula angustifolia*), marjoram (*Origanum majorana*)

eczema: See dermatitis

edema: cypress (*Cupressus sempervirens*), fennel (*Foeniculum vulgare*), geranium (*Pelargonium graveolens*), grapefruit (*Citrus x paradisii*), juniper (*Juniperus communis*)

emphysema: See chronic obstructive pulmonary disease

endometriosis: black pepper (*Piper nigrum*), cypress (*Cupressus sempervirens*), ginger (*Zingiber officinale*), lavender (*Lavandula angustifolia*), peppermint (*Mentha piperita*)

epilepsy: bergamot (*Citrus x bergamia*), Roman chamomile (*Chamaemelum nobile*), lavender (*Lavandula angustifolia*), marjoram (*Origanum majorana*), ylang ylang (*Cananga odorata*)

fatigue: black spruce (*Picea mariana*), pine (*Pinus sylvestris*), rosemary (*Rosmarinus officinalis*), cardamon (*Elletaria cardamomum*), ginger (*Zingiber officinale*)

fibromyalgia: bay laurel (*Laurus nobilis*), black pepper (*Piper nigrum*), eucalyptus (*Eucalyptus globulus*), ginger (*Zingiber officinale*)

gout: carrot (*Daucus carota*), grapefruit (*Citrus x paradisii*), helichrysum (*Helichrysum italicum*), juniper (*Juniperus communis*), lavender (*Lavandula angustifolia*), peppermint (*Mentha piperita*)

hay fever: See respiratory allergies

headache (tension): basil (*Ocimum basilicum*), peppermint (*Mentha piperita*), lavender (*Lavandula angustifolia*), Roman chamomile (*Chamaemelum nobile*), rosemary (*Rosmarinus officinalis*)

healing (slow): frankincense (*Boswellia carteri*), helichrysum (*Helichrysum italicum*), myrrh (*Commiphora myrrha*), neroli (*Citrus aurantium* var. *amara*), infused oils of calendula (*Calendula officinalis*), St. John's wort (*Hypericum perforatum*)

hot flashes: blue cypress (*Callitris intratropica*), clary sage (*Salvia sclarea*), geranium (*Pelargonium graveolens*), German chamomile (*Matricaria recutita*), lavender (*Lavandula angustifolia*), lemon (*Citrus limon*), palmarosa (*Cymbopogon martinii*), rose (*Rosa damascena* or *centifolia*)

hypertension: basil (*Ocimum basilicum*), cedar (*Cedrus atlantica* or *deodara*), celery seed (*Apium graveolens*), geranium (*Pelargonium graveolens*), marjoram (*Origanum majorana*), neroli (*Citrus aurantium* var. *amara*), spikenard (*Nardus jatamansi*), ylang ylang (*Cananga odorata*)

immunity (depressed): bay laurel (*Laurus nobilis*), frankincense (*Boswellia carteri*), geranium (*Pelargonium graveolens*), lemon (*Citrus limon*), marjoram (*Origanum majorana*), myrrh (*Commiphora myrrha*), palmarosa (*Cymbopogon martinii*), petitgrain (*Citrus aurantium* var. *amara*), thyme (*Thymus vulgaris* CT linalool)

inflammation (skin): German chamomile (*Matricaria recutita*), Roman chamomile (*Chamaemelum nobile*), lavender (*Lavandula angustifolia*), rose (*Rosa damascena* or *centifolia*), yarrow (*Achillea millefolium*)

inflammatory bowel disease: German chamomile (*Matricaria recutita*), helichrysum (*Helichrysum italicum*), lavender (*Lavandula angustifolia*), turmeric (*Curcuma longa*), yarrow (*Achillea millefolium*)

injury (acute): blue cypress (*Callitris intratropica*), cypress (*Cupressus sempervirens*), German chamomile (*Matricaria recutita*), lavender (*Lavandula angustifolia*), sweet birch (*Betula lenta*), turmeric (*Curcuma longa*), wintergreen (*Gaultheria procumbens*)

insomnia (with anxiety): mandarin (*Citrus reticulata*), neroli (*Citrus aurantium* var. *amara*)

insomnia (with emotional upset): rose (*Rosa damascena* or *centifolia*)

insomnia (general): lavender (*Lavandula angustifolia*), bitter orange (*Citrus aurantium* var. *amara*)

insomnia (with mental agitation): frankincense (*Boswellia carteri*)

insomnia (with nervous exhaustion): marjoram (*Origanum majorana*)

irritable bowel syndrome: basil (*Ocimum basilicum*), peppermint (*Mentha piperita*), Roman chamomile (*Chamaemelum nobile*), tarragon (*Artemesia dracunculus*)

itching: German chamomile (*Matricaria recutita*), lavender (*Lavandula angustifolia*), peppermint (*Mentha piperita*)

lymphedema: See edema

memory (poor): basil (*Ocimum basilicum*), frankincense (*Boswellia carteri*), rosemary (*Rosmarinus officinalis*)

menopause (general balancing): aniseed (*Pimpinella anisum*), fennel (*Foeniculum vulgare*), geranium (*Pelargonium graveolens*), melissa (*Melissa officinalis*), sage (*Salvia officinalis*), vitex (*Vitex agnus castus*)

migraine headache: basil (*Ocimum basilicum*), lavender (*Lavandula angustifolia*), lemon (*Citrus limon*), peppermint (*Mentha piperita*)

mood swings: bergamot (*Citrus x bergamia*), cardamon (*Elletaria cardamomum*), clary sage (*Salvia sclarea*), jasmine (*Jasminum grandiflorum*), rose (*Rosa damascena* or *centifolia*), ylang ylang (*Cananga odorata*)

morning sickness: peppermint (*Mentha piperita*)

muscle (spasm): basil (*Ocimum basilicum*), cardamon (*Elletaria cardamomum*), clary sage (*Salvia sclarea*), marjoram (*Origanum majorana*), black pepper (*Piper nigrum*), petitgrain (*Citrus aurantium* var. *amara*), tarragon (*Artemesia dracunculus*)

muscle (overworked): ginger (*Zingiber officinale*), nutmeg (*Myristica fragrans*), black pepper (*Piper nigrum*)

nausea: peppermint (*Mentha piperita*)

nerve pain: See neuralgia

neuralgia: black pepper (*Piper nigrum*), eucalyptus (*Eucalyptus radiata*), ginger (*Zingiber officinale*), lavender (*Lavandula angustifolia*), nutmeg (*Myristica fragrans*), marjoram (*Origanum majorana*)

odors (unpleasant): grapefruit (*Citrus x paradisii*), lavandin (*Lavandula x intermedia*), lemon (*Citrus limon*), lemongrass (*Cymbopogon citratus*), lime (*Citrus aurantiifolia*), peppermint (*Mentha piperita*), spearmint (*Mentha spicata*)

osteoarthritis: bay laurel (*Laurus nobilis*), black pepper (*Piper nigrum*), ginger (*Zingiber officinale*), nutmeg (*Myristica fragrans*), rosemary (*Rosmarinus officinalis*)

pain (chronic): clove bud (*Syzygium aromaticum*), lavender (*Lavandula angustifolia*), nutmeg (*Myristica fragrans*), myrrh (*Commiphora myrrha*), spike lavender (*Lavandula latifolia*), sweet birch (*Betula lenta*), wintergreen (*Gaultheria procumbens*)

paralysis (maintaining tissue health): bay laurel (*Laurus nobilis*), black pepper (*Piper nigrum*), cypress (*Cupressus sempervirens*), eucalyptus (*Eucalyptus radiata*), geranium (*Pelargonium graveolens*), grapefruit (*Citrus x paradisii*), rosemary (*Rosmarinus officinalis*)

perspiration (excessive): cypress (*Cupressus sempervirens*), grapefruit (*Citrus x paradisii*), juniper (*Juniperus communis*), lemon (*Citrus limon*)

plantar fasciitis: German chamomile (*Matricaria recutita*), helichrysum (*Helichrysum italicum*), lavender (*Lavandula angustifolia*), peppermint (*Mentha piperita*), sweet birch (*Betula lenta*), wintergreen (*Gaultheria procumbens*)

postnatal depression: fennel (*Foeniculum vulgare*), geranium (*Pelargonium graveolens*), grapefruit (*Citrus x paradisii*), marjoram (*Origanum majorana*), rose (*Rosa damascena* or *centifolia*), ylang ylang (*Cananga odorata*)

premenstrual syndrome: aniseed (*Pimpinella anisum*), fennel (*Foeniculum vulgare*), geranium (*Pelargonium graveolens*), melissa (*Melissa officinalis*), sage (*Salvia officinalis*)

pressure sores: frankincense (*Boswellia carteri*), German chamomile (*Matricaria recutita*), helichrysum (*Helichrysum italicum*), lavender (*Lavandula angustifolia*), myrrh (*Commiphora myrrha*)

respiratory allergies: German chamomile (*Matricaria recutita*), himalayan cedar (*Cedrus deodara*), lavender (*Lavandula angustifolia*), Roman chamomile (*Chamaemelum nobile*), tea tree (*Melaleuca alternifolia*), turmeric (*Curcuma longa*)

rheumatoid arthritis (flare-up): German chamomile (*Matricaria recutita*), lemon eucalyptus (*Eucalyptus citriadora*), peppermint (*Mentha piperita*), spike lavender (*Lavandula latifolia*), sweet birch (*Betula lenta*), turmeric (*Curcuma longa*), wintergreen (*Gaultheria procumbens*)

scars: frankincense (*Boswellia carteri*), helichrysum (*Helichrysum italicum*), lavender (*Lavandula angustifolia*), lavandin (*Lavandula x intermedia*), myrrh (*Commiphora myrrha*), rose (*Rosa damascena* or *centifolia*); infused oils of calendula (*Calendula officinalis*) and St. John's wort (*Hypericum perforatum*); carrier oils calophyllum (*Calophyllum inophyllum*) and rose hip seed (*Rosa rubiginosa*)

scar tissue: helichrysum (*Helichrysum italicum*), juniper (*Juniperus communis*), lavender (*Lavandula angustifolia*), rosemary (*Rosmarinus officinalis*)

sciatica: black pepper (*Piper nigrum*), eucalyptus (*Eucalyptus radiata*), ginger (*Zingiber officinale*), lavender (*Lavandula angustifolia*), marjoram (*Origanum majorana*), nutmeg (*Myristica fragrans*)

scleroderma: geranium (*Pelargonium graveolens*), palmarosa (*Cymbopogon martinii*), rock rose (*Cistus ladaniferus*), rose (*Rosa damascena* or *centifolia*), sandalwood (*Santalum album*); carrier oils calophyllum (*Calophyllum inophyllum*) and rose hip seed (*Rosa rubiginosa*); infused oil calendula (*Calendula officinalis*)

shin splints: German chamomile (*Matricaria recutita*), helichrysum (*Helichrysum italicum*), lavender (*Lavandula angustifolia*), peppermint (*Mentha piperita*), sweet birch (*Betula lenta*), wintergreen (*Gaultheria procumbens*)

shingles (associated nerve pain): See neuralgia

shingles (rash): German chamomile (*Matricaria recutita*), helichrysum (*Helichrysum italicum*), lavender (*Lavandula angustifolia*), small amounts of peppermint (*Mentha piperita*)

sinusitis: eucalyptus (*Eucalyptus radiata*), peppermint (*Mentha piperita*), rosemary (*Rosmarinus officinalis*), spike lavender (*Lavandula latifolia*)

sinusitis (for thick mucus): helichrysum (*Helichrysum italicum*), inula (*Inula graveolens*)

sprains: See injury

strains: See injury

stress (relaxation for short-term stress): frankincense (*Boswellia carteri*), lavender (*Lavandula angustifolia*), mandarin (*Citrus reticulata*), neroli (*Citrus aurantium* var. *amara*), Roman chamomile (*Chamaemelum nobile*), ylang ylang (*Cananga odorata*)

stress (strengthening for long-term stress): basil (*Ocimum basilicum*), black spruce (*Picea mariana*), clary sage (*Salvia sclarea*), pine (*Pinus sylvestris*), rosemary (*Rosmarinus officinalis*)

stretch marks (prevention): helichrysum (*Helichrysum italicum*), lavender (*Lavandula angustifolia*), mandarin (*Citrus reticulata*), neroli (*Citrus aurantium* var. *amara*)

temporomandibular joint dysfunction: basil (*Ocimum basilicum*), German chamomile (*Matricaria recutita*), marjoram (*Origanum majorana*), black pepper (*Piper nigrum*), sweet birch (*Betula lenta*), wintergreen (*Gaultheria procumbens*)

tendonitis: German chamomile (*Matricaria recutita*), helichrysum (*Helichrysum italicum*), lavender (*Lavandula angustifolia*), peppermint (*Mentha piperita*), sweet birch (*Betula lenta*), wintergreen (*Gaultheria procumbens*)

thoracic outlet syndrome: black pepper (*Piper nigrum*), eucalyptus (*Eucalyptus radiata*), ginger (*Zingiber officinale*), lavender (*Lavandula angustifolia*), marjoram (*Origanum majorana*), nutmeg (*Myristica fragrans*)

tiredness: See fatigue

urethritis: See urinary tract infection

urinary tract infection: geranium (*Pelargonium graveolens*), helichrysum (*Helichrysum italicum*), juniper (*Juniperus communis*), lavender (*Lavandula angustifolia*), myrrh (*Commiphora myrrha*), sandalwood (*Santalum album*), tea tree (*Melaleuca alternifolia*)

varicose veins: cypress (*Cupressus sempervirens*), helichrysum (*Helichrysum italicum*), juniper (*Juniperus communis*), lemon (*Citrus limon*), mastic (*Pistacia lentiscus*), peppermint (*Mentha piperita*)

viral infection: cardamon (*Elletaria cardamomum*), eucalyptus (*Eucalyptus radiata*), ginger (*Zingiber officinale*), marjoram (*Origanum majorana*), tea tree (*Melaleuca alternifolia*)

Appendix B: Suppliers

There are many good retailers of essential oils and other supplies. I have included only those with whom I have had first-hand experience.

ESSENTIAL OIL SUPPLIERS

Florial
Florihana distillerie
Les Grands Prés
06460 Caussols, France
Phone: +33 (0) 493 09 0609
Fax: +33 (0) 493 09 8685
E-mail: info@florial.com
Website: www.florihana.com

Fragrant Earth
Orchard Court
Magdalene Street
Glastonbury, England BA6 9EW
Phone: +44 (0) 1458 831216
Fax: +44 (0) 1458 831361
E-mail: all-enquiries@fragrant-earth.com
Website: www.fragrant-earth.com
(U.S. suppliers: www.essentialspirit.net)

John Steele
3949 Longridge Ave.
Sherman Oaks, CA 91423
Phone: (818) 986-0594

Northwest Essence, Inc.
PO Box 550
Lakebay, WA 98349
Phone: (253) 884-5600
Fax: (253) 884-5610
E-mail: northwestessence@earthlink.net
Website: www.northwestessence.com

Primafleur
1525 E. Francisco Blvd., Suite 16
San Rafael, CA 94901
Phone: (415) 455-0957
Fax: (415) 455-0956
E-mail: sales@primafleur.com
Website: www.primafleur.com

Primavera
Website: www.primavera-life.de
There are many U.S. suppliers of this German company. Do a Web search for those in your area.

Solen Aromatics
6403 15th Ave NW #300
Seattle, WA 98107
Phone: (206) 465-4868
E-mail: ingrid@solenaromatics.com
Website: www.solenaromatics.com

HYDROSOL SUPPLIERS

Acqua Vita
85 Arundel Ave
Toronto, ON M4K 3A3
Phone: (416) 405-8855
Fax: (416) 405-8185
E-mail: info@acqua-vita.com
Website: www.hydrosols.com

Nature's Gift
Website: www.naturesgift.com

CARRIER AND VEGETABLE OIL SUPPLIERS

Essential Wholesale
8850 SE Herbert Court
Clackamas, OR 97015
Phone: (503) 722-7557
Fax: (503) 296-5631
E-mail: info@essentialwholesale.com
Website: www.essentialwholesale.com

BOTTLE AND CONTAINER SUPPLIERS

Lavender Lane Forever
PO Box 600
Merlin, OR 97532
Phone: (888) 593-4400
Fax: (541) 474-3551
Website: www.lavenderlane.com

SKS Bottle
3 Knaber Road
Mechanicville, NY 12118
Phone: (518) 899-7488 Ext 1
Fax: (800) 810-0440
Website: www.sks-bottle.com

Specialty Bottle LLC
5215 5th Ave. S
Seattle, WA 98108
Phone: (206) 340-0459
Fax: (206) 903-0785
E-mail: service@specialtybottle.com
Website: www.specialtybottle.com

Appendix C: Training Courses in Aromatherapy

Because there are no licensing standards for aromatherapy in most countries, including the United States and Britain, courses vary greatly, in both content and length. Some of the teachers or schools below concentrate on courses for students starting off in aromatherapy, while others are more advanced and require some previous training and/or experience.

UNITED STATES

R. J. Buckle Associates
E-mail: info@rjbuckle.com
Website: www.rjbuckle.com

Institute of Traditional Herbal Medicine and Aromatherapy
180 Allen Road Suite 103 North
Atlanta, GA 30328
Phone: (866) 420-8484
E-mail: info@aromatherapy-studies.com
Website: www.aromatherapy-studies.com

Ingrid Martin (Solen Aromatics)
6403 15th Ave. NW #300
Seattle, WA 98107
Phone: (206) 465 4868
E-mail: ingrid@solenaromatics.com
Website: www.solenaromatics.com

Cheryl Young
PO Box 550
Lakebay, WA 98349
Phone: (253) 884-5600
Fax: (253) 884-5610
E-mail: northwestessence@earthlink.net
Website: www.northwestessence.com

GREAT BRITAIN

Institute of Traditional Herbal Medicine and Aromatherapy
Oaklands,
Postmans Lane
Little Baddow
Chelmsford, England CM3 4SF
Phone: 144 (0)1245 223871
E-mail: info@aromatherapy-studies.com
Website: www.aromatherapy-studies.com

Shirley Price International College of Aromatherapy
Essentia House
Upper Bond Street
Hinckley
Leicestershire, England LE10 1RS
Phone: +44 (0)1455 633231

FRANCE

Essential Oil Resource Consultants
Au Village
83840 La Martre
France
Phone/Fax: +33 494 84 2993
E-mail: essentialorc@aol.com
Website: www.essentialorc.com

Appendix D: Research Resources

WEBSITES

Aromatherapy Database
Au Village
83840 La Martre
France
Phone/Fax: +33 494 84 2993
E-mail: essentialorc@aol.com
Website: www.aromatherapydatabase.com

Essential Oil Crop Calendar
Website: www.manheimer.com/html/cropchar.htm

Herb Research Foundation
Website: www.herbs.org

International Fragrance Association
Website: www.ifra.org

Monell Chemical Sense Center
Website: www.monell.org

Phytochemical and Ethnobotanical Databases
Website: www.ars-grin.gov/duk/index.html

PubMed
Website: www.ncbi.nim.nih.gov/PubMed

Review of Aromatic and Medicinal Plants Journal
Website: www.cabi-publishing.org

ORGANIZATIONS

International Federation of Professional Aromatherapists (IFPA)
82 Ashby Road
Hinckley
Leicestershire, England LE10 1SN
Phone/Fax: +44 20 8653 9152
E-mail: aromatherapyUK@aol.com
Website: www.aromatherapyuk.net
The IFPA also produces its own journal: *In Essence*

The National Association of Holistic Aromatherapists (NAHA)
4509 Interlake Ave. N, #233
Seattle, WA 98103-6773
Phone: (206) 256-0741
E-mail: info@naha.org
Website: www.naha.org
NAHA also produces its own journal: *Aromatherapy Journal*

JOURNALS

Aromatherapy Today
PO Box 211
Kellyville NSW
Australia 2155
Phone +61 2 9894 9933
Fax: +61 2 9894 0199
Website: www.aromatherapytoday.com

The International Journal of Aromatherapy
Journals Marketing Department
Elsevier Science
PO Box 945
New York, NY 10159-0945
Phone: (888) 437-4636
Fax: (212) 633-3680
E-mail: usinfo-f@elsevier.com

GLOSSARY

abortifacient Referring to a substance that can induce a miscarriage.

absolute An extract produced by solvent extraction of aromatic plant material.

acquired immunity Immunity produced by exposure to a harmful organism.

adaptogenic Referring to a substance that helps the body return to homeostasis and manage stress.

adrenal burnout Extreme fatigue caused by chronic stress.

adrenaline A hormone secreted by the adrenal medulla, especially during stress.

adulteration The addition of a substance to an essential oil after distillation, generally done to make the final product greater in volume, thus increasing profits.

alcohol A molecule with a hydroxyl functional group and based on a carbon chain.

aldehyde A molecule with a carbonyl functional group attached.

aliphatic compound *See* terpenoid.

allopathic medication Standard Western medical drugs.

amygdala A structure in the limbic system of the brain, specialized in recognizing the emotional significance of events.

analgesic Pain relieving.

anesthetic Numbing.

anticoagulant Referring to a substance that hinders blood clotting.

antigalactagogue Referring to a substance that stops or reduces the flow of breast milk.

antihematomic Referring to a substance that stops or reduces bleeding.

antipruritic Referring to a substance that prevents or stops itching.

antitussive Referring to a substance that reduces coughing, by calming the cough reflex.

anxiolytic Referring to a substance that reduces anxiety.

aroma lamp A device for diffusing essential oils, usually made of pottery or glass, with a small candle to provide heat. Also called oil burner.

aromatherapy The use of essential oils for healing purposes.

aromatherapy oil A blend of carrier oil, essential oils, and/or synthetics.

aromatic phenol A phenol formed along the mevalonate pathway.

aromatic plant A plant that produces essential oils and has a distinct and unique smell.

aromatogram A laboratory technique used in France to test the effectiveness of certain essential oils against specific strains of bacteria.

arrhythmia An irregular heart beat.

arteriosclerosis The end stage of a disease that starts as atherosclerosis.

astringent Referring to a substance that contracts tissue.

atherosclerosis A narrowing of the arteries caused by a thickening of the artery walls.

base note An essential oil with a deep, very long-lasting scent; used in perfumery work.

base oil A vegetable oil. Also called carrier oil, fixed oil.

bleaching A stage in the processing of commercially produced vegetable oils.

botanical name The internationally recognized Latin name of a plant.

carbon dioxide extract An aromatic extract, using liquid CO_2 as a solvent.

carbonyl group A functional group with a carbon and an oxygen atom double bonded together.

carcinogenic A substance that can cause cancer.

carminative Referring to a substance that relieves flatulence and digestive pain or discomfort.

carrier A substance used to dilute essential oils.

carrier oil A vegetable oil used to dilute essential oils, often for massage. Also called base oil, fixed oil.

cephalic Stimulating or clearing to the head or brain.

chakras Energy centers of the body.

character A description of the aroma of an essential oil.

chemotype One of two of the same species of plant having consistently different chemistry when distilled.

cholagogue Referring to a substance that stimulates the flow of bile from the gallbladder to the small intestine.

cicatrizant Referring to a substance that encourages the formation of scar tissue, and therefore rapid healing.

clinical aromatherapy Aromatherapy used externally or in inhalation as a support therapy for serious illnesses, or in hospitals; often practiced by nurses and other health professionals.

CO_2 extract *See* carbon dioxide extract.

cold expression Referring to the extraction of essential oils by means of pressure; only used for citrus rinds.

cold-pressed Referring to the extraction of vegetable oil by pressure without added heat.

complete In reference to ylang ylang, a mixture of several grades, usually extra, first grade, and second grade.

concrete A transitional stage in the preparation of an absolute, before the plant waxes have been removed.

cortisol A hormone produced by the adrenal cortex in response to stress.

cramp A painful muscle spasm.

cream A semi-solid emulsion of oil and water.

cytophylactic Referring to a substance that encourages the growth of cells.

cytotoxicity Damage to cells.

decongestant Referring to a substance that clears congestion in the respiratory system.

degumming One of the stages in the commercial refining process of vegetable oil.

dermis A layer of connective tissue below the epidermis.

diffuser A device for evaporating essential oils into the air.

dislocation A dissociation of the articulating surfaces of a joint.

distillation The extraction of essential oils by the use of heat and water or steam.

diterpene A hydrocarbon with 20 carbon atoms; very rare in essential oil chemistry.

diterpene alcohol An alcohol based on a 20-carbon atom chain.

diuretic A substance that increases the flow of urine.

dysmenorrhea Painful menstruation.

edema An accumulation of protein and fluid in the interstitial spaces.

emmenagogue A substance that increases menstrual flow.

endometriosis A disease in which the lining of the uterus (endometrium) migrates to other areas of the pelvis.

endorphin An opioid produced by the body, with painkilling and euphoric effects.

enfleurage A method of extraction by placing plant material on trays covered with fat, which absorbs the essential oils.

essence *See* expressed oil.

essential fatty acid (EFA) A fatty acid that the body must have but cannot manufacture; linoleic acid and alpha-linoleic acid are examples.

essential oil An aromatic extract obtained by some form of distillation.

ester A molecule produced by the reaction of an alcohol (or phenol) and a carboxylic acid.

estrogenic Referring to a substance that produces similar effects to the hormone estrogen.

ether A molecule with an oxygen atom linking two carbon atoms.

expectorant A substance that loosens phlegm in the lungs, making it easier to expel.

expeller-pressed *See* cold-pressed.

expressed oil An essential oil extracted by means of pressure.

extended oil An essential oil with natural or synthetic ingredients added to it. Also called reconstituted oil.

extra The highest, most expensive grade of ylang ylang.

fan diffuser A device with a fan for evaporating essential oils into the air.

family A large group of closely related plants.

fatty acid The main component of all the fats in the body.

fetotoxic Dangerous or damaging to the fetus.

fight-or-flight response The response of the sympathetic nervous system to a threat.

fixed oil A vegetable oil. Also called carrier oil, base oil.

folded oil An essential oil (usually a citrus) that is redistilled several times to increase concentration; usually used in the food industry.

fractional distillation A distillation method that is interrupted every few hours; the different grades produced are sold separately; most commonly used with ylang ylang.

functional group An atom or group of atoms added to a hydrocarbon; usually makes the molecule more reactive.

gas-liquid chromatography (GC) A laboratory technique used to separate the different components of a substance and identify them.

gel A nongreasy liquid emulsion of oil and water.

general adaptation syndrome A theory of how the body responds to stress; developed in the 1930s by Hans Selye.

genus A small group of very closely related plants.

glucose A simple sugar produced by plants.

hepatic Referring or relating to the liver.

hepatotoxicity Damage to the liver.

herbalism The use of medicinal plants for healing purposes.

holistic aromatherapy The use of essential oils to heal body, mind, and spirit; generally used in mild dilutions, externally or in inhalation.

hydrocarbon A molecule formed of carbon and hydrogen only, that is common in essential oils.

hydrodiffusion A distillation method in which steam is forced through the plant material from above.

hydrolat *See* hydrosol.

hydrophilic Having an attraction for water; soluble in water.

hydrosol A dilute aromatic substance, soluble in water; a by-product of distillation. Also called hydrolat.

hydroxyl group A functional group made up of a hydrogen atom and an oxygen atom.

hypertension High blood pressure.

hypertensive Referring to a substance that raises blood pressure.

hypertonicity The state in which muscles are abnormally tight and often painful.

hypotensive Referring to a substance that helps lower high blood pressure.

hypothalamus A structure in the limbic system of the brain; regulator of the nervous and endocrine systems.

hypoxemia A lack of oxygen in the tissues of the body.

immunosuppressive A substance that suppresses or reduces the immune system's allergic reaction.

infusion A method of producing a scented oil by soaking aromatic plant material in vegetable oil.

innate immunity A type of immunity that is genetically determined and prevents organisms that infect animals from affecting humans.

intensity The strength of the aroma of an essential oil.

isoprene unit The basic building block for terpenes; made up only of carbon and hydrogen atoms.

ketone A molecule with a carbonyl functional group attached.

lactone An ester with a functional group incorporated into a carbon ring.

learned odor response A conditioned physical or emotional response to an odor.

limbic system A part of the brain that regulates emotion, appetite, and survival responses.

lipid A fat or oil.

lipophilic Having an attraction for fats; soluble in fats.

lotion A liquid emulsion of oil and water.

macerated oil An oil produced by soaking aromatic material in vegetable oil.

maceration The process of soaking aromatic plant material in vegetable oil.

masking fragrance A fragrance used to cover up undesirable odors; usually found in commercial cosmetic preparations.

mass spectroscopy (MS) A lab technique used to identify components in a substance by determining their atomic or molecular masses.

medical aromatherapy Aromatherapy used in larger doses, often internally; generally used by medical doctors in France.

mevalonate pathway One of the two most common chemical sequences within a plant that produces essential oils. *See also* shikimate pathway.

mid note An essential oil with a warm scent and medium volatility; used in perfumery work.

monoterpene The smallest and most common type of molecule found in essential oils; has 10 carbon atoms.

monoterpene alcohol An alcohol based on a 10-carbon chain.

morphological blending In aromatherapy, a technique in which essential oils from different plants but the same plant part are blended for therapeutic reasons.

mucolytic Referring to a substance that breaks down and dissolves mucus.

natural oil A designation often found on scented oils; has no legal meaning.

nature identical oil A compound of naturally extracted and/or synthetic aromatic oils.

neat Undiluted.

nebulizer A device for diffusing essential oils, without heat, usually by forcing air through them.

nervine Strengthening or stimulating to the nervous system.

neurodepressant A substance that calms the nervous system.

neurostimulant A substance that stimulates the nervous system.

neurotoxicity Damage to the nervous system.

nonspecific immunity A generalized immune response to any pathogen.

nut *See* seed.

occlude To cover; in aromatherapy, to prevent the escape of essential oils and increase absorption.

oil burner *See* aroma lamp.

ointment A substance that is heavier than a lotion or a cream; usually made of a mixture of oil and wax.

olfaction The sense of smell.

olfactory bulb The primary organ of smell.

olfactory cortex The part of the cerebral cortex of the brain that deals with olfaction.

olfactory tract A bundle of nerve fibers that transport impulses from the olfactory bulb to the brain.

organic chemistry The chemistry of substances containing carbon (includes all plant chemistry).

oxide A molecule with an atom within a carbon ring structure; evolved from an alcohol.

oxidize To react with oxygen, usually causing faster degradation.

patch testing The application of a strong dilution of essential oil to the skin to test for an allergic reaction.

percent dilution The percentage of essential oil to carrier.

phenol A molecule with a hydroxyl functional group and based on a phenyl ring.

phenyl ring A ring of six carbon atoms with stable bonds between each atom.

phenylpropanoid A compound formed along the shikimate pathway.

phenylpropanoid aldehyde An aldehyde formed along the shikimate pathway.

phenylpropanoid phenol A phenol formed along the shikimate pathway.

photosensitizing Referring to a substance that increases the sensitivity of the skin to UV light. Also called phototoxic.

photosynthesis The process by which a plant uses sunlight as energy to make glucose from carbon dioxide and water.

phototoxic *See* photosensitizing.

phytoestrogen A plant hormone similar in form and action to the human hormone estrogen.

primary alcohol An alcohol with a hydroxyl group bonded to a carbon at the end of the carbon chain.

primary metabolite A substance a plant produces for its own survival, such as sugar (glucose).

prostaglandin A hormone-like substance, involved in the inflammatory response.

pruritus Itching.

psychoneuroimmunology The study of the interconnections of the mind, the nervous system, and the immune system.

pure oil A designation often found on scented oils; has no legal meaning.

reconstituted oil *See* extended oil.

rectified oil An essential oil that has been distilled more than once to remove undesired components. Also called redistilled oil.

redistilled oil *See* rectified oil.

refined oil A vegetable oil from which the constituents most likely to degrade have been extracted.

refining A stage in the commercial processing of a vegetable oil.

rose otto The steam distilled essential oil of rose.

rubefacient Referring to a substance that stimulates blood flow to the skin, causing the area to become red.

saturated fatty acid Part of a fat molecule that is made of long straight carbon chains; solid at room temperature and very stable.

secondary metabolite A secondary substance that a plant produces, such as an essential oil.

seed The reproductive part of a plant. Also called nut.

sesquiterpene A hydrocarbon molecule with 15 carbon atoms.

sesquiterpene alcohol An alcohol based on a 15-carbon chain.

shikimate pathway One of the two most common chemical sequences within a plant that produces essential oils. *See also* mevalonate pathway.

skin irritation Redness, rash, and occasional damage to skin or mucous membrane.

skin sensitization An allergic reaction to a substance involving skin irritation.

solvent extraction A method of extracting essential oils using solvents such as hexane and butane; the products are called absolutes.

soporific Referring to a substance that causes drowsiness or sleep.

spasm A persistent muscle contraction that cannot be released at will.

species A particular plant within a genus group.

specific immunity An immune response to a specific pathogen.

sprain An injury caused by overstretching a ligament.

spritzer A blend of essential oils mixed with water in a spray bottle.

steam distillation A method of essential oil extraction using steam.

steam inhalation The inhalation of volatile essential oils placed in hot water.

still note An unpleasant odor connected with a freshly distilled essential oil.

strain An injury caused by overstretching a muscle-tendon unit.

stratum corneum The most superficial outer layer of the epidermis, consisting mostly of dead cells and keratin.

stress A reaction to circumstances that affects homeostasis of the body.

synergy A blend of essential oils that has a greater therapeutic effect than any one of the oils used separately.

systemic toxin A substance that is harmful to the entire body.

tachycardia An unusually rapid heartbeat.

terpenoid A compound formed along the mevalonate pathway.

terpenoid aldehyde An aldehyde formed along the mevalonate pathway.

terrain support An essential oil appropriate for long-term use to support overall immune functioning.

therapeutic-grade essential oil An unadulterated essential oil knowledgeably and carefully extracted from a single, high-quality botanical source.

top-mid-base note blending A method of perfume blending.

top note An essential oil with a high scent and very high volatility; used in perfumery work.

toxicity Poisoning.

triethanolamine (TEA) A common constituent of commercially produced creams and lotions.

unsaturated fatty acid Part of a fat molecule that is made of bent carbon chains; liquid at room temperature and less stable than saturated fatty acids.

vegetable oil A fatty oil extracted from a plant (e.g., olive oil).

vermifuge A substance that destroys intestinal worms.

volatile Referring to a substance that evaporates at room temperature.

volatility The rate at which an essential oil evaporates at room temperature.

vulnerary Substance that helps in tissue healing.

water distillation A gentle form of distillation, in which the plant material is placed in water, which is then heated; the method is used less today.

winterizing A stage in the commercial refining process of vegetable oils.

yield The amount of essential oil extracted from a plant.

Index

Note: Page numbers in *italics* denote figures; those followed by t denote tables.